W9-AZQ-408

MICROBIAL THREATS TO HEALTH

EMERGENCE, DETECTION, AND RESPONSE

Mark S. Smolinski, Margaret A. Hamburg,
and Joshua Lederberg, *Editors*

Committee on Emerging Microbial Threats to Health
in the 21st Century

Board on Global Health

INSTITUTE OF MEDICINE
OF THE NATIONAL ACADEMIES

THE NATIONAL ACADEMIES PRESS
Washington, D.C.
www.nap.edu

THE NATIONAL ACADEMIES PRESS 500 Fifth Street, N.W.   Washington, DC 20001

NOTICE: The project that is the subject of this report was approved by the Governing Board of the National Research Council, whose members are drawn from the councils of the National Academy of Sciences, the National Academy of Engineering, and the Institute of Medicine. The members of the committee responsible for the report were chosen for their special competences and with regard for appropriate balance.

Support for this project was provided by the Centers for Disease Control and Prevention's National Center for Infectious Diseases (Contract No. H75/CCH311468, TO#8), the U.S. Department of Defense (Contract No. DAMD17-01-2-0040), the U.S. Agency for International Development (Contract No. HRN-A-00-00-00012-00), the U.S. Department of Agriculture's Food Safety and Inspection Service (Contract No. 590-0790-1-188), the National Institutes of Health's National Institute of Allergy and Infectious Diseases, the National Institutes of Health's Fogarty International Center, the Ellison Medical Foundation, the U.S. Food and Drug Administration, and the U.S. Joint Institute for Food Safety Research. The views presented in this report are those of the Institute of Medicine Committee on Emerging Microbial Threats to Health in the 21st Century and are not necessarily those of the funding agencies.

Library of Congress Cataloging-in-Publication Data

Microbial threats to health : emergence, detection, and response / Mark S. Smolinski, Margaret A. Hamburg, and Joshua Lederberg, editor(s) ; Committee on Emerging Microbial Threats to Health in the 21st Century, Board on Global Health.
      p. ; cm.
Includes bibliographical references.
  ISBN 0-309-08864-X (hardcover) — ISBN 0-309-50730-8 (PDF)
  1. Communicable diseases—United States. 2. Public health—United States.
  [DNLM: 1. Communicable Diseases, Emerging—epidemiology. 2. Communicable Diseases, Emerging—prevention & control. 3. Communicable Disease Control. WA 110 M626 2003] I. Smolinski, Mark S. II. Hamburg, Margaret A. III. Lederberg, Joshua. IV. Institute of Medicine (U.S.). Committe on Emerging Microbial Threats to Health in the 21st Century.
  RA643.5.M53 2003
  614.5'7—dc21

                        2003008754

Additional copies of this report are available from the National Academies Press, 500 Fifth Street, N.W., Lockbox 285, Washington, DC 20055; (800) 624-6242 or (202) 334-3313 (in the Washington metropolitan area); Internet, http://www.nap.edu.

For more information about the Institute of Medicine, visit the IOM home page at: www.iom.edu.

Copyright 2003 by the National Academy of Sciences. All rights reserved.

Printed in the United States of America.

The serpent has been a symbol of long life, healing, and knowledge among almost all cultures and religions since the beginning of recorded history. The serpent adopted as a logotype by the Institute of Medicine is a relief carving from ancient Greece, now held by the Staatliche Museen in Berlin.

"Knowing is not enough; we must apply.
Willing is not enough; we must do."
—Goethe

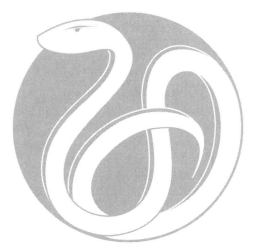

INSTITUTE OF MEDICINE
OF THE NATIONAL ACADEMIES

Shaping the Future for Health

THE NATIONAL ACADEMIES
Advisers to the Nation on Science, Engineering, and Medicine

The **National Academy of Sciences** is a private, nonprofit, self-perpetuating society of distinguished scholars engaged in scientific and engineering research, dedicated to the furtherance of science and technology and to their use for the general welfare. Upon the authority of the charter granted to it by the Congress in 1863, the Academy has a mandate that requires it to advise the federal government on scientific and technical matters. Dr. Bruce M. Alberts is president of the National Academy of Sciences.

The **National Academy of Engineering** was established in 1964, under the charter of the National Academy of Sciences, as a parallel organization of outstanding engineers. It is autonomous in its administration and in the selection of its members, sharing with the National Academy of Sciences the responsibility for advising the federal government. The National Academy of Engineering also sponsors engineering programs aimed at meeting national needs, encourages education and research, and recognizes the superior achievements of engineers. Dr. Wm. A. Wulf is president of the National Academy of Engineering.

The **Institute of Medicine** was established in 1970 by the National Academy of Sciences to secure the services of eminent members of appropriate professions in the examination of policy matters pertaining to the health of the public. The Institute acts under the responsibility given to the National Academy of Sciences by its congressional charter to be an adviser to the federal government and, upon its own initiative, to identify issues of medical care, research, and education. Dr. Harvey V. Fineberg is president of the Institute of Medicine.

The **National Research Council** was organized by the National Academy of Sciences in 1916 to associate the broad community of science and technology with the Academy's purposes of furthering knowledge and advising the federal government. Functioning in accordance with general policies determined by the Academy, the Council has become the principal operating agency of both the National Academy of Sciences and the National Academy of Engineering in providing services to the government, the public, and the scientific and engineering communities. The Council is administered jointly by both Academies and the Institute of Medicine. Dr. Bruce M. Alberts and Dr. Wm. A. Wulf are chair and vice chair, respectively, of the National Research Council.

www.national-academies.org

COMMITTEE ON MICROBIAL THREATS TO HEALTH IN THE 21ST CENTURY

MARGARET A. HAMBURG (*Co-chair*), Vice President for Biological Programs, Nuclear Threat Initiative

JOSHUA LEDERBERG (*Co-chair*), Professor Emeritus and Sackler Foundation Scholar, The Rockefeller University

BARRY BEATY, Professor of Microbiology, Colorado State University

RUTH BERKELMAN, Professor, Department of Epidemiology, Rollins School of Public Health, Emory University

DONALD BURKE, Professor, Departments of International Health and Epidemiology, Bloomberg School of Public Health, Johns Hopkins University

GAIL CASSELL, Vice President of Scientific Affairs and Distinguished Research Scholar in Infectious Diseases, Eli Lilly and Company

JIM YONG KIM, Co-director of program in Infectious Disease and Social Change, Department of Medicine, Harvard University

KEITH KLUGMAN, Professor of International Health, Department of International Health, Rollins School of Public Health; Professor of Medicine, Division of Infectious Diseases, School of Medicine, Emory University

ADEL MAHMOUD, President, Merck Vaccines, Merck and Co, Inc.

LINDA MEARNS, Scientist and Deputy Director, Environmental and Societal Impacts Group, National Center for Atmospheric Research

FREDERICK MURPHY, Professor, Schools of Veterinary Medicine and Medicine, University of California, Davis

MICHAEL OSTERHOLM, Director, Center for Infectious Disease Research and Public Policy, Professor, School of Public Health, University of Minnesota

CLARENCE PETERS, Professor, Departments of Microbiology and Immunology and Pathology, University of Texas Medical Branch

PATRICIA QUINLISK, Iowa State Epidemiologist, Iowa Department of Public Health

FREDERICK SPARLING, Professor of Medicine and Microbiology and Immunology, University of North Carolina, Chapel Hill

ROBERT WEBSTER, Professor, Virology Division, Department of Infectious Diseases, Rose Marie Thomas Chair, St. Jude Children's Research Hospital

MARK WILSON, Director, Global Health Program, Associate Professor of Epidemiology, University of Michigan

MARY WILSON, Associate Professor of Medicine, Harvard Medical School, Associate Professor of Population and International Health, Harvard School of Public Health

Staff

MARK S. SMOLINSKI, Study Director
PATRICIA A. CUFF, Research Associate
KATHERINE A. OBERHOLTZER, Project Assistant
RICHARD MILLER, Director, Medical Follow-up Agency

Reviewers

This report has been reviewed in draft form by individuals chosen for their diverse perspectives and technical expertise, in accordance with procedures approved by the NRC's Report Review Committee. The purpose of this independent review is to provide candid and critical comments that will assist the institution in making its published report as sound as possible and to ensure that the report meets institutional standards for objectivity, evidence, and responsiveness to the study charge. The review comments and draft manuscript remain confidential to protect the integrity of the deliberative process. We wish to thank the following individuals for their review of this report:

John G. Bartlett, The Johns Hopkins University, Baltimore, Maryland
Michael G. Groves, Louisiana State University, Baton Rouge, Louisiana
Marcelle C. Layton, New York City Department of Health, New York, New York
Lord Robert May, University of Oxford, Oxford, United Kingdom
Mark Nichter, University of Arizona, Tucson, Arizona
Jonathan Patz, The Johns Hopkins University, Baltimore, Maryland
Regina Rabinovich, Malaria Vaccine Initiative, Rockville, Maryland
Bill Roper, University of North Carolina, Chapel Hill, North Carolina
Robert Shope, University of Texas, Galveston, Texas
Andrew Spielman, Harvard University, Boston, Massachusetts
Robert A. Weinstein, Cook County Hospital, Chicago, Illinois

Although the reviewers listed above have provided many constructive comments and suggestions, they were not asked to endorse the conclusions or recommendations nor did they see the final draft of the report before its release. The review of this report was overseen by **Ronald W. Estabrook, the University of Texas Southwestern, Dallas, Texas, and Samuel L. Katz, Duke University, Durham, North Carolina.** Appointed by the National Research Council and Institute of Medicine, they were responsible for making certain that an independent examination of this report was carried out in accordance with institutional procedures and that all review comments were carefully considered. Responsibility for the final content of this report rests entirely with the authoring committee and the institution.

Cover Artwork

INFLUENZA*

The global nature of influenza and the aqueous environment needed for virus spread are depicted by the world viewed from space and its aqueous environs (blue globe). Gulls and wild ducks are the natural host of all known influenza A viruses. During evolution these viruses adapted to migratory birds that travel long distances and spread virus by transmission to mammals (lines of migration and interspecies spread). Pigs act as intermediate hosts with receptors for avian and mammalian influenza viruses and occasionally transmit the viruses to humans.

There are 15 different subtypes of influenza A viruses (different shades of virus particles) that vary in shape and size. After transmission to mammalian hosts influenza viruses evolve rapidly. The segmented RNA genomes (8 segments per virion) permit related viruses to reassort (virus particle with 14 genes—should be 16—artistic license). In mammalian hosts

*A stained glass window 21 × 56" depicting the natural history of influenza viruses and zoonotic exchange in the emergence of new strains is shown in reduced size on the back cover of this report. A detailed section of the image was used to design the front cover. Based on the work done at St. Jude Children's Research Hospital supported by American Lebanese Syrian Associated Charities (ALSAC) and the National Institute of Allergy and Infectious Diseases (NIAID).

Artist: Jenny Hammond, Highgreenleycleugh, Northumberland, England
Commissioned by Rob and Marjorie Webster.

the ever-changing spike glycoproteins (spike-like fringe on particles) permit the virus to evade the immune response resulting in annual disease outbreaks. At irregular intervals the reassortment of viruses gives rise to pandemic strains with the potential of devastating disease. The yearly outbreaks of influenza and occasional pandemics cause high fever (red) and excess mortality.

Preface

As we enter the twenty-first century, infectious diseases continue to burden populations around the world. Both naturally occurring and intentionally introduced biological threats hold increasing potential to cause disease, disability, and death. And beyond disease itself, the ability of infectious agents to destabilize populations, economies, and governments is fast becoming a sad fact of life. The prevention and control of infectious diseases are fundamental to individual, national, and global health and security; failure to recognize—and act on—this essential truth will surely lead to disaster. Over the past decade, the United States has taken important steps to strengthen its capacity to address the threats posed by these diseases. However, we must do more to improve our ability to detect, prevent, and control emerging and resurging diseases if we are to be better prepared for future microbial threats to health.

In 1992, the Institute of Medicine published a landmark report, *Emerging Infections: Microbial Threats to Health in the United States*, which pointed to major challenges for the public health and medical care communities in detecting and managing infectious disease outbreaks and monitoring the prevalence of endemic diseases. Completed just about a decade ago, it reflected the consensus of a wide-ranging group of specialists that America needed a wake-up call, that infectious diseases remained a tangible threat to our security, and that the comfort and complacency that overtook us in the 1960s with the advent of wonder drugs and vaccines might be short-lived. That report was a stimulus for numerous other studies and policy actions, many in response to the harsh realities of the spread of HIV/AIDS, the emergence of new or previously unrecognized diseases, the resurgence of old diseases, and the looming failure of technological innovation in antimicrobial drugs to keep up with the constant evolution of microbial resistance.

The 1990s also saw a revolution in globalization in all spheres: political, economic, cultural, technological, and informational. This revolution included the breakdown of cold war politics and the ever broader engagement of the United States in every geographic region; the progressive breakdown of national barriers to trade and migration and the emergence of a global economy; and the wonders of information technology, especially Internet access to ideas and information. These developments offered new opportunities and exigent challenges as infectious agents piggybacked on the internationalization of people and goods. More recently, the new global environment has brought home our vulnerability to malicious attacks on our homeland, including events that have led the words "anthrax" and "smallpox" to appear in banner headlines. All this has occurred in an era that has seen us identify the complete genomic codes not merely for mice and humans, but also for a host of their parasites.

As we conclude our work for the current study, we must continue to trumpet the message of urgency and concern, but our more demanding task is to take stock of existing preventive and remedial measures, and to consider what further investments of fiscal and political capital are needed if we are to keep pace with our microbial competitors. We need no longer limit our concern to the United States as the venue for microbial threats to health, as it is now widely understood that our borders offer trivial impediment to such threats. Nor need we have an exclusive focus on emerging diseases when we have so far to go in dealing globally with tuberculosis, malaria, and HIV/AIDS, which emerge and reemerge with violent fluctuations of intensity in different parts of the world.

This report is entitled *Microbial Threats to Health* with the tacit understanding that the phrase embraces all of the above. Information resources such as the Internet, with content provided by a multitude of governmental and academic sources (most notably Medline and PromedMail), obviate the need to catalogue the details of the thousand or so microbial agents of most urgent concern, especially with information on new threats appearing monthly. Yet we have included important narratives to illustrate the complexity of disease and the intertwining of the biological, environmental, ecological, social, and political factors that must all be taken into account to understand the threats that confront us, and to define meaningful and sustainable solutions.

We must also note that soon after the work of this committee began, the world was rocked by the attacks of September 11, 2001, and the subsequent dissemination of anthrax as a biological weapon through the mail. In the wake of these tragic events, a new imperative animated our discussions and reinvigorated our work. Suddenly a spotlight was cast on the serious and frightening reality of the intentional use of a microbial agent. With this heightened awareness came increased conviction that the best defense against any disease outbreak is a robust public health science and practice, underscoring the need to devote markedly greater attention and resources to meeting this critical need.

Of course, it is often easier to delineate problems than to design and execute remedies, though the former is obviously an obligatory first step. In the triad of *Emergence, Detection, and Response*, the last decade has seen important improvements—perhaps most dramatically in technologies that enable us to detect previously unknown pathogens. The most problematic need is perhaps for incentives for the necessary investments in preventive and therapeutic technologies (i.e., vaccines and antimicrobials) to bring them from the laboratory to public use. While there was consensus among the committee members that the nation is well into a crisis with regard to microbial threats to health, our most contentious discussions concerned the precise details of how the enormous power (and political sensitivity) of government can be applied in partnership with the private sector to meet public needs.

The next decade will surely see a broader range of further scientific advances in our fundamental understanding of pathogenesis, host–parasite co-evolution, and intertwined genomics and physiology. Comparable leaps of political will and public understanding will be required to enable these fruits of scientific endeavor to benefit a humankind that still suffers many burdens whose alleviation is scandalously within our technical grasp.

Margaret A. Hamburg
Joshua Lederberg
Co-chairs

Acknowledgments

The committee is indebted to the researchers, administrators, and public health professionals who presented informative talks to the committee and participated in lively discussions at the open meetings, including James Hughes, Carol Heilman, Gerald Keusch, Richard Sprott, Stephanie James, Murray Trostle, Patrick Kelley, Michael Zeilinger, Kaye Wachsmuth, Walter Hill, Jerry Gillespie, Jessie Goodman, Byron Wood, Alexandra Levitt, Ray Arthur, Mary Gilchrist, Julie Gerberding, Douglas Hamilton, Joel Breman, Claude Earl Fox, Richard Wansley, and Bob England (see Appendix A for affiliations and discussion topics). The committee is also grateful to Jo Ivey Boufford, John Edman, Bruce Eldridge, and Stanley Oaks who graciously made themselves available for consultation and technical reviews.

Of particular note, the following individuals directly contributed to the report by drafting commissioned papers in their areas of expertise. Aaron Shakow, Paul Farmer, and William Rodriguez contributed to a review of the social and economic determinants of infectious disease that made a substantial contribution to the report. A paper by Kelly Henning provided important background on syndromic surveillance (see Appendix B), and another by David Relman provided insight to modern methods of pathogen discovery, detection, and diagnostics (see Appendix C). Thanks also to Lawrence Gostin for his contributions on public health law, which were replicated in that section of the report.

The committee would like to thank the staff and members of the Institute of Medicine's Forum on Emerging Infections for their support in conducting three workshops over the course of the study that served to inform

xv

the committee's deliberations on assessing the science and response capabilities regarding the intentional use of biological agents, the growing threat of antimicrobial resistance, and the impact of globalization on emerging infectious diseases (see Appendix D for Forum membership and list of publications).

The committee wishes to express its sincere appreciation to the devoted project staff. As study director, Mark Smolinski ensured the success of this project through his dedication, diligence, creativity, and leadership. This study would not have been possible without Dr. Smolinski's oversight and coordination of the work of the committee and his insightful and careful drafting of the report. Additional praise goes to Patricia Cuff for her analytic proficiency and perseverance in completing the daunting task of reviewing the literature, verifying references, and drafting text. Pat's contributions were instrumental to the evidence-based rigor of the report. Katherine Oberholtzer was outstanding in her meticulous attention to detail, great finesse in the organizational work of the committee, and numerous contributions to supporting the research and editing of the report.

Many other individuals within the Institute of Medicine and the National Academies were instrumental in seeing the project to completion. A special note of appreciation goes to Judith Bale for her continuous encouragement, Dick Miller for his leadership and guidance, and Stacey Knobler for her invaluable assistance through her work with the Forum on Emerging Infections. Thanks also to Clyde Behney, Andrea Cohen, Bronwyn Schrecker, Jennifer Otten, Jennifer Bitticks, Carlos Orr, Marjan Najafi, Lois Joellenbeck, Janice Mehler, and the NAP production staff. Thanks are also due to writing and editorial consultants Leslie Pray, Beth Gyorgy, and especially Rona Briere who helped polish brass into gold.

The committee would like to thank the following agencies and organizations who generously provided funding for this study: the Centers for Disease Control and Prevention's National Center for Infectious Diseases, the National Institutes of Health's National Institute of Allergy and Infectious Diseases, the National Institutes of Health's Fogarty International Center, the Ellison Medical Foundation, the U.S. Agency for International Development, the U.S. Department of Defense, the U.S. Department of Agriculture's Food Safety and Inspection Service, the U.S. Food and Drug Administration, and the U.S. Joint Institute for Food Safety Research. Finally, the committee would like to acknowledge the support of the Board on Global Health (see Appendix D) as part of its continuing pursuit to improve the health of the global community.

Synopsis

Infectious diseases continue to be a serious burden around the world, in developing and industrialized countries alike. Whether naturally occurring or intentionally inflicted, microbial agents can cause illness, disability, and death in individuals while disrupting entire populations, economies, and governments. In the highly interconnected and readily traversed "global village" of our time, one nation's problem soon becomes every nation's problem as geographical and political boundaries offer trivial impediments to such threats. The United States has shown leadership in the past by strengthening its own and others' capacities to deal with infectious diseases, but the present reality is that the public health, veterinary, and medical-care communities are inadequately prepared. We must do more to improve our ability to prevent, detect, and control microbial threats to health.

We must understand that pathogens are endlessly resourceful in adapting to and breaching our defenses. We must also recognize that factors relating to society, the environment, and our increasing global interconnectedness actually enhance the likelihood of disease emergence and spread. Moreover, it is a sad reality that today we must also grapple with the intentional use of biological agents to do harm, human against human. In fact, thirteen individual factors—some reflecting the ways of nature, most of them reflecting our ways of life—account for the emergence of infectious disease. Any of these factors alone can trigger problems, but their convergence creates especially high-risk environments where infectious diseases may readily emerge, or re-emerge.

Dramatic advances in science, technology, and medicine have enabled us to make great strides forward in our struggle to prevent and control infectious diseases, yet we cannot fall prey to an illusory complacency. The magnitude of the problem requires renewed commitment. As we look at our prospects, it is clear that a robust public health system—in its science, capacity, practice, and through its collaborations with clinical and veterinary medicine, academia, industry, and other public and private partners—is the best defense against any microbial threat.

Contents

List of
Figures, Tables, and Boxes

FIGURES

TABLES

BOXES

Acronyms

ABCs:	Active Bacterial Core Surveillance
AFO:	animal feeding operation
AIDS:	acquired immunodeficiency syndrome
APHIS:	Animal and Plant Health Inspection Service
APUA:	Alliance for the Prudent Use of Antibiotics
ARS:	Agricultural Research Service
BSE:	bovine spongiform encephalopathy
BSI:	blood stream infection
CAFO:	concentrated animal feeding operation
CAREC:	Caribbean Epidemiology Center
CDC:	Centers for Disease Control and Prevention
CIN:	cervical intraepithelial neoplasia
CJD:	Creutzfeldt-Jakob disease
CLIA:	Clinical Laboratory Improvement Amendments
CMV:	cytomegalovirus
CSTE:	Council of State and Territorial Epidemiologists
CWD:	chronic wasting disease
DARPA:	Defense Advanced Research Projects Agency
DHF-SS:	dengue hemorrhagic fever and shock syndrome
DNA:	deoxyribonucleic acid
DOD:	Department of Defense

DOT:	directly observed therapy
DOTS:	directly observed therapy, short course
DTP:	diptheria, tetanus, and pertussis vaccine
EBV:	Epstein-Barr virus
EIP:	Emerging Infections Program
EIS:	Epidemic Intelligence Service
EMS:	Emergency Medical System
Epi-X:	Epidemic Information Exchange
ESSENCE:	Electronic Surveillance System for Early Notification of Community-Based Epidemics
EU:	European Union
EWORS:	Early Warning Outbreak Recognition System
FADDL:	Foreign Animal Disease Diagnostic Laboratory
FAO:	Food and Agriculture Organization
FDA:	Food and Drug Administration
FETP:	Field Epidemiology Training Programs
FIC:	National Institutes of Health Fogarty International Center for Advanced Study in the Health Sciences
FoodNet:	Foodborne Disease Active Surveillance Network
GAO:	General Accounting Office
GDP:	gross domestic product
GEIS:	Global Emerging Infections Surveillance
GIS:	geographic information system
GISP:	Gonococcal Isolate Surveillance Project
GOCO:	government owned, contractor operated
GPHIN:	Global Public Health Intelligence Network
HA:	hemagglutinin
HERV:	human endogenous retrovirus
HFRS:	hemorrhagic fever with renal syndrome
HHV-8:	human herpesvirus-8
HIV:	human immunodeficiency virus
HLA:	human leukocyte antigen
HMO:	health maintenance organization
HPS:	hantavirus pulmonary syndrome
HPV:	human papilloma virus
HRSA:	Health Resources and Services Administration
HSV:	herpes simplex virus
HTLV:	human T-cell lymphotropic viruses
HUS:	hemolytic uremic syndrome

ICC: immunocytochemical
ICD-9:   International Classification of Diseases, 9th Revision
ICIDR: International Collaborations in Infectious Disease Research
ICU: intensive-care unit
IOM: Institute of Medicine

KSHV: kaposi's sarcoma-associated herpesvirus

MDR: multidrug-resistant
MDR-TB: multidrug-resistant tuberculosis
MRSA: methicillin-resistant *Staphylococcus aureus*

NA: neuraminidase
NCHS: National Center for Health Statistics
NEDSS: National Electronic Disease Surveillance System
NETSS: National Electronic Telecommunications System for
            Surveillance
NIAID: National Institute of Allergy and Infectious Diseases
NIH: National Institutes of Health
NNDSS: National Notifiable Diseases Surveillance System
NNIS: National Nosocomial Infections Surveillance System
NRC: National Research Council
NSF: National Science Foundation

OIE: Office International des Epizooties

PAHO: Pan American Health Organization
PCR: polymerase chain reaction

QRNG: fluoroquinolone-resistant *Neisseria gonorrhoeae*

rDNA: ribosomal DNA
RNA: ribonucleic acid
RSVP: Rapid Syndrome Validation Program
RVF: Rift Valley fever

SIV: simian immunodeficiency viruses
SNV: Sin Nombre virus
STD: sexually transmitted disease
STI: strategic treatment interruption
SV: Simian virus

TB: tuberculosis
TLR: TOLL-like receptors
TSE: transmissible spongiform encephalopathy
TTV: TT virus

UNAIDS: Joint United Nations Programme on HIV/AIDS
UNICEF: United Nations Children's Fund
USAID: U.S. Agency for International Development
USDA: U.S. Department of Agriculture
UTI: urinary tract infection

VA: Department of Veterans Affairs
vCJD: variant Creutzfeldt-Jakob disease

WHO: World Health Organization
WTO: World Tourism Organization

YF: yellow fever

MICROBIAL THREATS TO HEALTH

EMERGENCE, DETECTION, AND RESPONSE

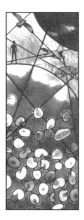

Executive Summary

Microbes live in every conceivable ecological niche on the planet and have inhabited the earth for many hundreds of millions of years. Indeed, microbes may be the most abundant life form by mass, and they are highly adaptable to external forces. The vast majority of microbes are essential to human, animal, and plant life. Occasionally, however, a microbe is identified as a pathogen because it causes an acute infectious disease or triggers a pathway to chronic diseases, including some cancers. Certainly, humankind remains ignorant of the full scope of diseases caused by microbial threats, as only a small portion of all microbes have been identified by currently available technologies.

Microbial threats continue to emerge, reemerge, and persist. Some microbes cause newly recognized diseases in humans; others are previously known pathogens that are infecting new or larger population groups or spreading into new geographic areas. Within the last 10 years, newly discovered infectious diseases have emerged in the United States (e.g., hantavirus pulmonary syndrome from Sin Nombre virus) and abroad (e.g., viral encephalitis from Nipah virus). During the same time, the worldwide resurgence of long-recognized infectious diseases (e.g., tuberculosis, malaria, cholera, and dengue) has gained in force. The United States has seen the importation of infectious diseases, such as West Nile encephalitis, measles, multidrug-resistant tuberculosis, malaria, and cyclosporiasis, from immigrants, U.S. residents returning from foreign destinations, and products of international commerce.

The realization of just how quickly newly discovered infectious diseases

FACTORS IN EMERGENCE

The convergence of any number of factors can create an environment in which infectious diseases can emerge and become rooted in society. A model was developed to illustrate how the convergence of factors in four domains impacts on the human–microbe interaction and results in infectious disease (see Figure ES-1). Ultimately, the emergence of a microbial threat derives from the convergence of (1) genetic and biological factors; (2) physical environmental factors; (3) ecological factors; and (4) social, political, and economic factors. As individual factors are examined, each can be envisioned as belonging to one or more of these four domains. The following individual factors in emergence are examined in this report:

Microbial adaptation and change. Microbes are continually undergoing adaptive evolution under selective pressures for perpetuation. Through structural and functional genetic changes, they can bypass the human immune system and infect human cells. The tremendous evolutionary potential of microbes makes them adept at developing resistance to even the most potent drug therapies and complicates attempts at creating effective vaccines.

Human susceptibility to infection. The human body has evolved with an abundance of physical, cellular, and molecular barriers that protect it from microbial infection. Susceptibility to infection can result when normal defense mechanisms are altered or when host immunity is otherwise impaired by such factors as genetically inherited traits and malnutrition.

Climate and weather. Many infectious diseases either are strongly influenced by short-term weather conditions or display a seasonality indicating the possible influence of longer-term climatic changes. Climate can directly impact disease transmission through its effects on the replication and movement (perhaps evolution) of pathogens and vectors; climate can also operate indirectly through its impacts on ecology and/or human behavior.

Changing ecosystems. In general, changes in the environment tend to have the greatest influence on the transmission of microbial agents that are waterborne, airborne, foodborne, or vector-borne, or that have an animal reservoir. Given today's rapid pace of ecological change, understanding how environmental factors are affecting the emergence of infectious diseases has assumed an added urgency.

Economic development and land use. Economic development activities can have intended or unintended impacts on the environment, resulting in eco-

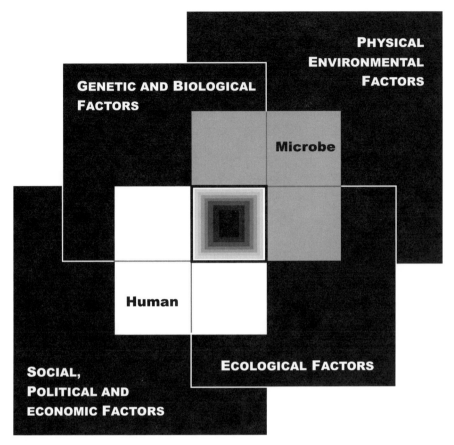

FIGURE ES-1 The Convergence Model. At the center of the model is a box representing the convergence of factors leading to the emergence of an infectious disease. The interior of the box is a gradient flowing from white to black; the white outer edges represent what is known about the factors in emergence, and the black center represents the unknown (similar to the theoretical construct of the "black box" with its unknown constituents and means of operation). Interlocking with the center box are the two focal players in a microbial threat to health—the human and the microbe. The microbe–host interaction is influenced by the interlocking domains of the determinants of the emergence of infection: genetic and biological factors; physical environmental factors; ecological factors; and social, political, and economic factors.

logical changes that can alter the replication and transmission patterns of pathogens. A growing number of emerging infectious diseases arise from increased human contact with animal reservoirs as a result of changing land use patterns.

Human demographics and behavior. An infectious disease can result from a behavior that increases an individual's risk of exposure to a pathogen, or from the increased probability of exchange of a communicable infectious disease between humans as the world's population increases in absolute number. Additional factors include demographic changes such as urbanization and the growth of megacities; the aging of the world's population and the associated increased risk of infection; and the growing number of individuals immunocompromised by cancer chemotherapy, chronic diseases, or infection with HIV.

Technology and industry. Infectious diseases have emerged as a direct result of changes in technology and industry. Advances in medical technologies, such as blood transfusions, human organ and tissue transplants, and xenotransplantation (using an animal source), have created new pathways for the spread of certain infections. Even the manner in which animals are raised as food products, such as the use of antimicrobials for growth production, has abetted the rise in infectious diseases by contributing to antimicrobial resistance.

International travel and commerce. The rapid transport of humans, animals, foods, and other goods through international travel and commerce can lead to the broad dissemination of pathogens and their vectors throughout the world. Microbes that can colonize without causing symptoms (e.g., *Neisseria meningitidis*) or can infect and be transmissible at a time when infection is asymptomatic (e.g., HIV, hepatitis B, and hepatitis C) can spread easily in the absence of recognition in traveling or migrant hosts. Pathogens in meat and poultry, such as the agents of "mad cow disease," can also be delivered unintentionally across borders, while the vectors of tropical diseases can be transported in cargo holds or in the wheel wells of international aircraft.

Breakdown of public health measures. A breakdown or absence of public health measures—especially a lack of potable water, unsanitary conditions, and poor hygiene—has had a dramatic effect on the emergence and persistence of infectious diseases throughout the world. The breakdown of public health measures in the United States has resulted in an increase in nosocomial infections, difficulties in maintaining adequate supplies of vaccines in recent years, immunization rates that are far below national targets for many population groups (e.g., influenza and pneumococcal immunizations in adults), and a paucity of needed expertise in vector control for diseases such as West Nile encephalitis.

Poverty and social inequality. At the same time that infectious diseases have significant and far-reaching economic implications, social inequality, driven in large part by poverty, is a major factor in emergence. Mortality from infectious diseases is closely correlated with transnational inequalities in income. Global economic trends affect not only the personal circumstances of those at risk for infection, but also the structure and availability of public health institutions necessary to reduce risks.

War and famine. War and famine are closely linked to each other and to the spread of infectious diseases. Displacement due to war and the fairly consistent sequelae of malnutrition due to famine can contribute significantly to the emergence and spread of infectious diseases such as malaria, cholera, and tuberculosis.

Lack of political will. If progress is to be made toward the control of infectious diseases, the political will to do so must encompass not only governments in the regions of highest disease prevalence, but also corporations, officials, health professionals, and citizens of affluent regions who ultimately share the same global microbial landscape. The complacency toward the threat of infectious diseases that has become somewhat entrenched in developed countries must reverse in direction if we are to avoid losing windows of opportunity to reduce the global burden of infection.

Intent to harm. The world today is vulnerable to the threat of intentional biological attacks, and the likelihood of such an event is high. The U.S. public health system and health care providers should be prepared to address various biological agents that pose a risk to national security because of their potential to cause large numbers of deaths and widespread social disruption.

Recognizing and addressing the ways in which the factors in emergence converge to change vulnerability to infectious diseases is essential to the development and implementation of effective prevention and control strategies. Detecting and responding to global infectious disease threats is in the economic, humanitarian, and national security interests of the United States and essential to the health of its people.

ADDRESSING THE THREATS:
CONCLUSIONS AND RECOMMENDATIONS

The response to a microbial threat—from detection to prevention and control—is a multidisciplinary effort involving all sectors of the public health, clinical medicine, and veterinary medicine communities. The committee's recommendations emerged from focused deliberations and application of the criteria of urgency, priority, and amenability to immediate action. Given that infectious diseases are a significant threat to the health of the world's population, several of the committee's recommendations could be justified solely on the basis of humanitarian need; *all* are justified as being in the best interest of the United States to protect the health of its own citizens.

Enhancing Global Response Capacity

Infectious diseases are a global threat and therefore require a global response. Nations not only must be concerned about the endemic diseases that plague their own citizens, but also must expand their concerns to include the global burden of disease that ultimately encompasses the gamut of potential threats—even if these threats are not currently found within their borders. While the true burden of infectious diseases in many areas of the world is unknown, the greatest burden occurs within developing countries, where an estimated one in every two persons dies from such a disease. The United States' capacity to respond to microbial threats must therefore include a significant investment in the capacity of developing countries to monitor and address microbial threats as they arise.

The United States should seek to enhance the global capacity for response to infectious disease threats, focusing in particular on threats in the developing world. Efforts to improve the global capacity to address microbial threats should be coordinated with key international agencies such as the World Health Organization (WHO) and based in the appropriate U.S. federal agencies (e.g., the Centers for Disease Control and Prevention [CDC], the Department of Defense [DOD], the National Institutes of Health [NIH], the Agency for International Development [USAID], the Department of Agriculture [USDA]), with active communication and coordination among these agencies and in collaboration with private organizations and foundations. Investments should take the form of financial and technical assistance, operational research, enhanced surveillance, and efforts to share both knowledge and best public health practices across national boundaries.

Improving Global Infectious Disease Surveillance

Global surveillance, especially for newly recognized infectious diseases, is crucial to responding to and containing microbial threats before isolated outbreaks develop into regional or worldwide pandemics.

The United States should take a leadership role in promoting the implementation of a comprehensive system of surveillance for global infec-

tious diseases that builds on the current global capacity of infectious disease monitoring. This effort, of necessity, will be multinational and will require regional and global coordination, advice, and resources from participating nations. A comprehensive system is needed to accurately assess the burden of infectious diseases in developing countries, detect the emergence of new microbial threats, and direct prevention and control efforts. To this end, CDC should enhance its regional infectious disease surveillance; DOD should expand and increase in number its Global Emerging Infections Surveillance (GEIS) overseas program sites; and NIH should increase its global surveillance research. In addition, CDC, DOD, and NIH should increase efforts to develop and arrange for the distribution of laboratory diagnostic reagents needed for global surveillance, transferring technology to other nations where feasible to ensure self-sufficiency and sustainable surveillance capacity. The overseas disease surveillance activities of the relevant U.S. agencies (e.g., CDC, DOD, NIH, USAID, USDA) should be coordinated by a single federal agency, such as CDC. Sustainable progress and ultimate success in these efforts will require health agencies to broaden partnerships to include nonhealth agencies and institutions, such as the World Bank.

Rebuilding Domestic Public Health Capacity

Strong and well-functioning local, state, and federal public health agencies working together represent the backbone of an effective response to infectious diseases. The U.S. capacity to respond to microbial threats is contingent upon a public health infrastructure that has suffered years of neglect. Upgrading current public health capacities will require considerably increased, sustained investments.

U.S. federal, state, and local governments should direct the appropriate resources to rebuild and sustain the public health capacity necessary to respond to microbial threats to health, both naturally occurring and intentional. The public health capacity in the United States must be sufficient to respond quickly to emerging microbial threats and monitor infectious disease trends. Prevention and control measures in response to microbial threats must be expanded at the local, state, and national levels and be executed by an adequately trained and competent workforce. Examples of such measures include surveillance (medical, veterinary, and entomological); laboratory facilities and capacity; epidemiological, statistical, and communication skills; and systems to ensure the rapid utility and sharing of information.

Improving Domestic Surveillance Through Better Disease Reporting

Open lines of communication and good working relationships among health care providers, clinical laboratories, and public health authorities are essential to robust systems of surveillance and effective implementation of disease investigation and response activities. The reporting of infectious diseases by health care providers and laboratories, however, remains inadequate.

CDC should take the necessary actions to enhance infectious disease reporting by medical health care and veterinary health care providers. Innovative strategies to improve communication between health care providers and public health authorities should be developed by working with other public health agencies (e.g., the Food and Drug Administration [FDA], the Health Resources and Services Administration [HRSA], USDA, the Department of Veterans Affairs [VA], state and local health departments), health sciences educational programs, and professional medical organizations (e.g., the American Medical Association, the American Society for Microbiology, the American Nurses Association, the American Veterinary Medical Association, the Association for Professionals in Infection Control and Epidemiology, the Association of Teachers of Preventive Medicine).

CDC should expeditiously implement automated electronic laboratory reporting of notifiable infectious diseases from all relevant major clinical laboratories (e.g., microbiology, pathology) to their respective state health departments as part of a national electronic infectious disease reporting system. The inclusion of antimicrobial resistance patterns of pathogens in the application of automated electronic laboratory reporting would assist in the surveillance and control of antimicrobial resistance.

Exploring Innovative Systems of Surveillance

The ability to gather and analyze information quickly and accurately would improve the nation's ability to recognize natural disease outbreaks, track emerging infections, identify intentional biological attacks, and monitor disease trends. Surveillance systems within the United States, however, remain fragmented and have not evolved at the same rate as the electronic technological advances that could significantly improve the timeliness and integration of data collection.

Research on innovative systems of surveillance that capitalize on advances in information technology should be supported. Before widespread implementation, these systems should be carefully evaluated for their usefulness in detection of infectious disease epidemics, including their potential for detection of the major biothreat agents, their ability to monitor the spread of epidemics, and their cost-effectiveness. Research on syndromic surveillance systems should continue to assess such factors as the capacity to transmit existing data electronically, to standardize chief complaint or other coded data, and to explore the usefulness of geospatial coding; CDC should provide leadership in such evaluations. In addition, promising approaches will need to be coordinated nationally so that data can be shared and analyzed across jurisdictions.

Developing and Using Diagnostics

Etiologic diagnosis—identifying a microbial cause of an infectious disease—is the cornerstone of effective disease control and prevention efforts, including surveillance. Etiologic diagnosis has declined significantly over the past decade. A dangerous consequence of decreased etiologic diagnosis has been an increase in the inappropriate use of broad-spectrum antibiotics and the emergence of antimicrobial resistance. Improving etiologic diagnosis would be of value to human health worldwide in directing appropriate therapy, as well as informing disease surveillance and response activities.

CDC and NIH should work with FDA, other government agencies (e.g., DOD, USDA, the national laboratories), and industry on the development, assessment, and validation of rapid, inexpensive and cost-effective, sensitive, and specific etiologic diagnostic tests for microbial threats of public health importance.

Public health agencies and professional organizations (e.g., those concerned with patient care, health education, and microbiological issues) should promulgate and publicize guidelines that call for the intensive application of existing diagnostic modalities and new modalities as they are established. Such guidelines should be incorporated into continuing education programs, board examinations, and accreditation practices. Payers for health care should cover diagnostic tests for infectious diseases to increase specific diagnoses and thereby inform both public health and medical care, including monitoring of inappropriate use of antimicrobials.

Educating and Training the Microbial Threat Workforce

The workforce necessary to accomplish the needed improvement in the national capacity to respond to microbial threats must be supported with strong training programs in the applied epidemiology of infectious disease prevention and control. As a vital component of this workforce, the knowledge and skills needed to confront microbial threats must be better integrated into the training of all health care professionals to ensure a prompt and effective response to any and all infectious disease threats, whether naturally occurring or maliciously introduced.

CDC, DOD, and NIH should develop new and expand upon current intramural and extramural programs that train health professionals in applied epidemiology and field-based research and training in the United States and abroad. Research and training should combine field and laboratory approaches to infectious disease prevention and control. Federal agencies should develop these programs in close collaboration with academic centers or other potential training sites. Domestic training programs should include an educational, hands-on experience at state and local public health departments to expose future and current health professionals to new career options, such as public health.

Vaccine Development and Production

Our nation—and the world—faces a serious crisis with respect to vaccine development, production, and deployment. Concern has increased over the inadequacy of vaccine research and development efforts, periodic shortages of existing vaccines, and the lack of vaccines to prevent diseases that affect persons in developing countries disproportionately. Yet, too little has been done to resolve these issues. The evolving threat of intentional biological attacks makes the need for focused attention and action even more critical.

The challenges associated with vaccine innovation, production, and deployment are many and complex. Solutions will require a novel, coordinated approach among government agencies, academia, and industry. Issues that must be examined and addressed in a more meaningful and systematic fashion include the identification of priorities for research, the determination of effective incentive strategies for developers and manufacturers, liability concerns, and streamlining of the regulatory process. Currently, the federal government is neither addressing all of these challenges at a sufficiently high level nor providing adequate resources. Leadership, empowerment, and accountability are urgently needed at the cabinet level to ensure a comprehensive, integrated vaccine strategy that will address the following critical elements:

The U.S. Secretary of Health and Human Services should ensure the formulation and implementation of a national vaccine strategy for protecting the U.S. population from endemic and emerging microbial threats. Only by focusing leadership, authority, and accountability at the cabinet level can the federal government meet its national responsibility for ensuring an innovative and adequately funded research base for existing and emerging infectious diseases and the development of an ample supply of routinely recommended vaccines. The U.S. Secretary of Health and Human Services should work closely with other relevant federal agencies (e.g., DOD, the Department of Homeland Security, VA), Congress, industry, academia, and the public health community to carry out this responsibility.

The U.S. Secretary of Defense, the U.S. Secretary of Health and Human Services, and the U.S. Secretary of Homeland Security should work closely with industry and academia to ensure the rapid development and deployment of vaccines for naturally occurring or intentionally introduced microbial threats to national security. The federal government should explore innovative mechanisms, such as cooperative agreements between government and industry or consortia of government, industry, and academia, to accelerate these efforts.

The Administrator of USAID, the U.S. Secretary of Health and Human Services, and the U.S. Secretary of State should work in cooperation with public and private partners (e.g., leaders of foundations and other donor agencies, industry, WHO, UNICEF, the Global Alliance for Vaccines and Immunization) to ensure the development and distribution of vaccines for diseases that affect populations in developing countries disproportionately.

Need for New Antimicrobial Drugs

Drug options for treatment of infections are becoming increasingly limited, largely as a result of growing antimicrobial resistance. Many generic but essential antibiotics are in short supply, and the development of new antibiotics has been severely curtailed. In the past three decades, only two new classes of antibiotics have been developed, and resistance to one class emerged even before the drugs entered the commercial market. Only four large pharmaceutical companies with antibiotic research programs remained in existence in 2002 and not one new class of antibiotics is in advanced development. Likewise, antivirals for only a limited number of viral diseases are available, and few are in development. In the event of a natural or intentionally introduced microbial threat, antimicrobials may be the only available first line of response. A readily available supply, therefore, should be a priority of preparedness plans.

The U.S. Secretary of Health and Human Services should ensure the formulation and implementation of a national strategy for developing new antimicrobials, as well as producing an adequate supply of approved antimicrobials. The U.S. Secretary of Health and Human Services should work closely with other relevant federal agencies (e.g., DOD, the Department of Homeland Security), Congress, industry, academia, and the public health community to carry out this responsibility.

The U.S. Secretary of Health and Human Services and the U.S. Secretary of Homeland Security should protect our national security by ensuring the stockpiling and distribution of antibiotics, antivirals (e.g., for influenza), and antitoxins for naturally occurring or intentionally introduced microbial threats. The federal government should explore innovative mechanisms, such as cooperative agreements between government and industry or consortia of government, industry, and academia, to accelerate these efforts.

Inappropriate Use of Antimicrobials

The world is facing an imminent crisis in the control of infectious diseases as the result of a gradual but steady increase in the resistance of a number of microbial agents to available therapeutic drugs. The problem is of global concern and is creating dilemmas for the treatment of infections in both hospitals and community health care settings. Moreover, as noted above, the pharmaceutical industry is developing fewer new antimicrobials than in previous years. Therefore, immediate action must be taken to preserve the effectiveness of available drugs by reducing the inappropriate use of antimicrobials in human and animal medicine.

CDC, FDA, professional health organizations, academia, health care delivery systems, and industry should expand efforts to decrease the inappropriate use of antimicrobials in human medicine through (1) expanded outreach and better education of health care providers, drug dispensers, and the general public on the inherent dangers associated with the inappropriate use of antimicrobials, and (2) the increased use

of diagnostic tests, as well as the development and use of rapid diagnostic tests, to determine the etiology of infection and thereby ensure the more appropriate use of antimicrobials.

FDA should ban the use of antimicrobials for growth promotion in animals if those classes of antimicrobials are also used in humans.

Vector-Borne and Zoonotic Disease Control

Vector-borne and zoonotic diseases remain major causes of morbidity and mortality in humans living in tropical climates, and represent a large portion of newly emerged diseases worldwide. Vector-borne and zoonotic pathogens have the ability to spread rapidly across broad geographical areas, as evidenced by the spread of West Nile virus across the United States. Exacerbating the situation is the potential for many vector-borne and zoonotic agents to be weaponized and used by terrorists. The national and international capacity to address these diseases must be strengthened by rebuilding the workforce and infrastructure, and developing the tools necessary to respond appropriately to such threats.

CDC, DOD, NIH, and USDA should work with academia, private organizations, and foundations to support efforts at rebuilding the human resource capacity at both academic centers and public health agencies in the relevant sciences—such as medical entomology, vector and reservoir biology, vector and reservoir ecology, and zoonoses—necessary to control vector-borne and zoonotic diseases.

DOD and NIH should develop new and expand upon current research efforts to enhance the armamentarium for vector control. The development of safe and effective pesticides and repellents, as well as novel strategies for prolonging the use of existing pesticides by mitigating the evolution of resistance, is paramount in the absence of vaccines to prevent most vector-borne diseases. In addition, newer methods of vector control—such as biopesticides and biocontrol agents to augment chemical pesticides, and novel strategies for interrupting vector-borne pathogen transmission to humans—should be developed and evaluated for effectiveness.

CDC, DOD, and NIH should work with state and local public health agencies and academia to expand efforts to exploit geographic information systems (GIS) and robust models for predicting and preventing the emergence of vector-borne and zoonotic diseases.

Comprehensive Infectious Disease Research Agenda

To ensure that the United States is strategically poised to protect itself against the threat of infectious diseases and to maximize its assistance in global efforts to combat these diseases, further investments must be made to support a diverse array of multidisciplinary research domains. These new investments must be part of an overall strategy for improved public health preparedness and protection against infectious disease threats. A comprehensive system of accountability must be in place to ensure that no critical areas are neglected. Given that the emergence of infectious diseases is the result of a complex convergence of factors, it is clear that multidisciplinary studies are greatly needed.

NIH should develop a comprehensive research agenda for infectious disease prevention and control in collaboration with other federal research institutions and laboratories (e.g., CDC, DOD, the U.S. Department of Energy, the National Science Foundation), academia, and industry. This agenda should be designed to investigate the role of genetic, biological, social, economic, political, ecological, and physical environmental factors in the emergence of infectious diseases in the United States and worldwide. This agenda should also include the development and assessment of public health measures to address microbial threats. A sustained commitment to a robust research agenda must be a high priority if the United States is to dramatically reduce the threat of naturally occurring infectious diseases and intentional uses of biological agents. The research agenda should be flexible to permit rapid assessment of new and emerging threats, and should be rigorously reevaluated on a 5-year basis to ensure that it is addressing areas of highest priority.

Interdisciplinary Infectious Disease Centers

As noted, addressing the highly complex nature of infectious disease emergence requires the involvement of experts from a broad range of disciplines and health sectors. The present structure of academic and public health institutions, however, requires that most of these arenas operate independently of each other. Opportunities for collaboration and synergism will be enhanced if experts convene under the same roof (or on the same campus) to discuss a problem, thus avoiding lost opportunities for collaboration and reducing often unnecessary redundancies of effort and expense. Furthermore, an interdisciplinary, collaborative approach can facilitate the training of the workforce needed to address the problems of emerging microbial threats facing the world today.

Interdisciplinary infectious disease centers should be developed to promote a multidisciplinary approach to addressing microbial threats to health. These centers should be based within academic institutions and link (both physically and virtually) the relevant disciplines necessary to support such an approach. They would collaborate with the larger network of public agencies addressing emerging infectious diseases (e.g., local and state health agencies, CDC, DOD, the U.S. Department of Energy, FDA, the Food Safety and Inspection Service, NIH, the National Science Foundation, USAID, USDA), interested foundations, private organizations, and industry. The training, education, and research that these centers would provide are a much-needed resource not only for the United States, but also for the entire world.

CONCLUSION

Today's world is truly a global village, characterized by growing concentrations of people in huge cities, increasing global commerce and travel, progressive damage to natural ecosystems, poverty, famine, and social disruption. One can safely predict that infectious diseases will continue to emerge, and that we will encounter unpleasant surprises, as well as increases in already worrisome trends. Depending on present policies and actions, this situation could lead to a catastrophic storm of microbial threats.

Thus while dramatic advances in science and medicine have enabled us to make great strides in our struggle to prevent and control infectious diseases, we cannot fall prey to an illusory complacency. We must understand that pathogens—old and new—have ingenious ways of adapting to and breaching our armamentarium of defenses. We must also understand that factors in society, the environment, and our global interconnectedness actually increase the likelihood of the ongoing emergence and spread of infectious diseases. It is a sad irony that today we must also grapple with the intentional use of biological agents to do harm, human against human.

No responsible assessment of microbial threats to health in the twenty-first century, then, could end without a call to action. The magnitude and urgency of the problem demand renewed concern and commitment. We have not done enough—in our own defense or in the defense of others. As we take stock of our prospects with respect to microbial threats in the years ahead, we must recognize the need for a new level of attention, dedication, and sustained resources to ensure the health and safety of this nation—and of the world.

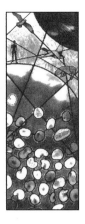

Introduction

It was "the perfect storm"—a tempest that may happen only once in a century—a nor'easter created by so rare a combination of factors that it could not possibly have been worse. Creating waves ten stories high and winds of 120 miles an hour, the storm whipped the sea to inconceivable levels few people on Earth have ever witnessed.

The Perfect Storm: A True Story of Men Against the Sea
Sebastian Junger

A transcendent moment nears upon the world for a microbial perfect storm. Unlike the meteorological perfect storm—happening just once in a century—the microbial perfect storm will be a recurrent event. The two events share a common feature; a *combination of factors* is the driving force behind each.

The increasingly interconnected and fast-paced world of transcontinental commerce and international travel has made any nation susceptible to the infectious diseases that occur incessantly outside its borders. Infectious diseases today ignore geographic and political boundaries, and thus constitute a global threat that puts every nation and every person at risk. Food products, livestock, exotic pets, and material goods—and the microbes they may carry—are exchanged as cultures from every region of the world are explored. Individuals travel to the other side of the planet in less time than it takes to manifest symptoms of disease, potentially infecting anyone they encounter along their route. Others migrate to escape the perils of war, living in poverty, and under conditions of poor sanitation, creating environments ripe for the emergence of infectious diseases. Land development for housing or use in agriculture; the creation of dams and reservoirs necessary to maintain water for agricultural use and public consumption; and outdoor recreational activities all bring humans into contact with arthropod vectors, rodents, and other animals capable of transmitting infections. Furthermore, changing climate and weather, as well as natural disasters such as floods and earthquakes, can impact on ecosystems to generate ideal conditions for the transmission of pathogens. The convergence of any number of such factors can create an environment that allows infectious diseases to emerge and become rooted in society.

Whereas the angry sea dissipates to an eventual calm, leaving few witnesses to a meteorological perfect storm, the factors creating a microbial perfect storm can perpetuate and even accelerate its effects—leaving multitudes of people to bear witness and fall victim to its destructive forces. In just two decades, for example, the world has witnessed widespread devastation due to the human immunodeficiency virus (HIV), a pathogen unrecognized before 1981. By 2001, more than 40 million people were estimated to be living with HIV, and 20 million had already died from acquired immunodeficiency syndrome (AIDS), the result of HIV infection.

In 1999, West Nile virus was isolated for the first time in the Western Hemisphere. The infection began with an epicenter in New York; by 2002, nearly 4,000 cases of West Nile encephalitis had been reported in 39 states and the District of Columbia, of which 254 were fatal. Although the first case of West Nile encephalitis was identified in Uganda in 1937, the virus was not considered to be a significant human pathogen because most infections were either mild or asymptomatic. Between 1996 and 1999, however, three major epidemics in urban areas (southern Romania, the Volga region of southern Russia, and the northeastern United States) resulted in hundreds of cases of severe neurological disease and fatal infection from West Nile virus, suggesting a change in the pathogen's virulence.

In 2001, 22 people in the United States contracted anthrax as innocent victims of an act of bioterrorism. Of these 22, 11 suffered from inhalational anthrax, the most lethal form of disease caused by *Bacillus anthracis;* 5 deaths resulted. This intentional use of a microbe to cause harm was the sobering realization of a once hypothetical factor in the emergence of a microbial threat. While the anthrax event may be more analogous to artifactual seeding of the clouds, HIV and West Nile virus have emerged as a result of microbial perfect storms—and now continue as turbulent microbial threats to health.

An infectious disease epidemic can be a major destabilizing force for any nation, and endemic infectious diseases sap strength from the population and impede national development. The economic and social instability that typically accompanies or follows in the wake of an infectious disease outbreak, including an intentional biological attack, can undermine national and international security (National Intelligence Council, 2000). Only very recently has the impact of major infectious diseases on global economic health become a central topic for discussion among world leaders, resulting in significant investments of global resources by the United Nations and major industrial nations. Although numerous infectious diseases—such as tuberculosis, malaria, cholera, plague, and infections with drug-resistant pathogens—have been major destabilizing forces (Chukwuani, 1999; Eandi and Zara, 1998), none has had a more devastating and far-reaching impact than the HIV pandemic in sub-Saharan Africa. The 28.5 million people infected with HIV in the region (UNAIDS, 2002) affect all sectors of society—from the household to industry to the broader regional economy (Dixon et al., 2002; Morris et al., 2000; Topouzis and du Guerny, 1999). With its disproportionate impact on young working adults, the pandemic has greatly intensified labor shortages, leading to catastrophic socioeconomic decline in the regions of highest incidence (Baier, 1997). It is expected that by 2010, per capita gross domestic product (GDP) in some of the hardest-hit countries will drop by 8 percent (UNAIDS and WHO, 2001); heavily affected countries could lose more than 20 percent of GDP by 2010. Decreased productivity translates into weaker prospects for economic growth and long-term development, and also means that fewer resources are available to invest in public health, thereby amplifying and perpetuating the original disease problem. The global security threat from AIDS will only increase as other densely populated nations, such as India and China, continue to struggle with the pandemic.

This report is the successor to a 1992 Institute of Medicine report, *Emerging Infections: Microbial Threats to Health in the United States*, that first examined the impact of new and reemerging infectious diseases on the United States. Ten years later, the impact of the global burden of infectious diseases on the United States has only increased. Infectious diseases unknown in this country just a decade ago, such as West Nile encephalitis and hantavirus pulmonary syndrome, have emerged to kill hundreds of Americans—and the long-term consequences for survivors of the initial illnesses are as yet unknown. Other known diseases, including measles, multidrug-resistant tuberculosis, and even malaria, have been imported and transmitted within the United States in the last 10 years. Moreover, gains made against sexually transmitted diseases have slowed or reversed in certain population groups. Compounding the threat posed by these infectious diseases is the continuing increase in antimicrobial resistance, which has become pervasive not only in the United States, but worldwide. Further exacerbating the situation is the fact that, despite the link between public health investment and infectious disease control, the United States has diminished its public health capacity to recognize and respond to infectious disease threats—particularly those originating at the global rather than the national level.

The Committee on Emerging Microbial Threats to Health in the 21st Century was charged to identify, review, and assess the current state of knowledge pertaining to the factors in emerging infectious diseases; to assess the capacity of the United States to respond to emerging microbial threats to health; and to identify potential challenges and opportunities for domestic and international public health actions to strengthen the detection and prevention of, and response to, emerging microbial threats. The scope of this report is limited to infectious diseases that have a direct effect on human health. The committee acknowledges that infectious diseases in animals and agriculture can have indirect effects on human health (e.g., reductions in available food sources, economic and psychological hardships in food animal producers due to culling), but limited the scope of the study for practical purposes. The committee's recommendations are focused on the most urgent and critical issues that need to be addressed immediately if we are to prevent and control microbial threats to human health.

Chapter 2 examines the magnitude of the problem and reviews the spectrum of microbial threats to health. Chapter 3 sets forth the major factors involved in the emergence of a microbial threat and presents a model and case example to illustrate how the complex convergence of these factors can lead to epidemics of disease. Chapter 4 presents the committee's conclusions and recommendations for improving the U.S. response to infectious agents that threaten not only the health of its citizens, but also the economy, security, and well-being of the world's population.

The primary aim of this report, therefore, is to extend understanding of the factors involved in the emergence of infectious diseases and of the global context in which this emergence occurs. Containing future epidemics of infectious disease will require that we recognize and respond to microbial threats whenever, and wherever, they occur.

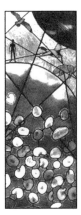

2

Spectrum of Microbial Threats

Microbial threats to health are microbes[1] that lead to disease in humans. The challenges posed by microbial threats to health are daunting. Most developing nations have not shared fully in the public health and technological advances that have aided in the fight against infectious disease in the United States—a fight that some had hoped would come close to eliminating these threats in this country (see Box 2-1). In developing countries, clean water is scarce; sewage systems are overwhelmed or nonexistent; the urban metropolis is growing exponentially as the global market economy expands and rural agricultural workers migrate to cities; and economic need, political conflict, and wars are displacing millions of people and creating growing refugee populations (see Chapter 3). Thus, infectious diseases affect poorer nations in the developing world disproportionately, and from thence become a global burden. Infectious diseases are responsible for one in every two deaths in developing countries—and are the leading cause of death for children and young adults (WHO, 1999a, 2000a). It has been estimated that every hour, 1,500 people die from an infectious disease—over half of them are children under 5 years of age. Ninety percent of deaths from infectious diseases worldwide are due to respiratory infec-

---

[1]For the purposes of this report, the term *microbe* refers to any microorganism or biologic agent that can replicate in humans (including bacteria, viruses, protozoa, fungi, and prions). The term *microbial threat* includes the agent and its associated disease. Some helminths are also embraced by the discussion.

BOX 2-1
The End of Infectious Diseases in the United States?

At the start of the twentieth century, tuberculosis, pneumonia, and diarrheal diseases caused 30 percent of all deaths in the United States. Infectious diseases resulted in such high mortality among infants and children that the average life expectancy at birth in the United States was only 47 years in 1900 (NCHS, 2001). During the first few decades of the 1900s, improved hygiene and sanitation, cleaner water and safer food, improved housing and nutrition, and advanced vector control led to a significant decline in infectious disease mortality in the United States. With the introduction of antibiotics in the middle of the century, the downward trend accelerated even further. Deaths from infectious disease, particularly tuberculosis and pneumonia, declined more than 8 percent each year from 1938 to 1952 (Armstrong et al., 1999). By the mid-1960s, effective pertussis, polio, smallpox, tetanus, and diphtheria vaccines had become widely available. As a result, deaths from numerous infectious diseases were prevented. For example, the number of cases of paralytic poliomyelitis in the United States dropped from more than 57,000 in 1952 to only 72 in 1965 (CDC, 2002a) and the last case of smallpox was documented in the United States in 1949 (CDC, 2002b; IOM, 1999a).

These exhilarating accomplishments of the mid–twentieth century were fueled by an unprecedented outlay of government resources, a vast network of field epidemiologists and research scientists, and extensive cooperation from private industry (Garrett, 1995). The eradication of smallpox in 1980 was a testament to the success of comprehensive vaccine coverage, and indeed has been praised by many as the greatest achievement in public health history. From 1900 to 1980, annual deaths from infectious disease had dropped from 797 to 36 per 100,000 persons (Armstrong et al., 1999). By the turn of the 21st century, the average life expectancy in the United States had increased to over 76 years.

As a result of this apparent reprieve from infectious diseases, the United States government moved research funding away from infectious diseases toward the "new dimensions" of public health—noncommunicable disorders such as heart disease and lung cancer. The government closed "virtually every tropical and infectious disease outpost run by the U.S. military and Public Health Service" (Garrett, 1989, p. 1). Infectious disease surveillance and control activities were deemphasized. Research, development, and production of new antibiotics and vaccines declined. The potentially devastating impact of infectious diseases was either relegated to the memory of previous generations or left to the imagination of science fiction enthusiasts. Americans could all

---

tions, acquired immunodeficiency syndrome (AIDS), diarrheal diseases, tuberculosis (TB), malaria, and measles (see Table 2-1).

This chapter begins by reviewing the global burden imposed by three of today's most devastating infectious diseases: AIDS, TB, and malaria. Other emerging infectious diseases and antimicrobial-resistant infections are discussed in the subsequent two sections. Chronic diseases with infectious etiology are then reviewed. The chapter ends with a brief discussion of microbes potentially used for intentional harm.

look forward to long, healthy lives, free from infectious disease ... or could they? The figure below suggests quite otherwise.

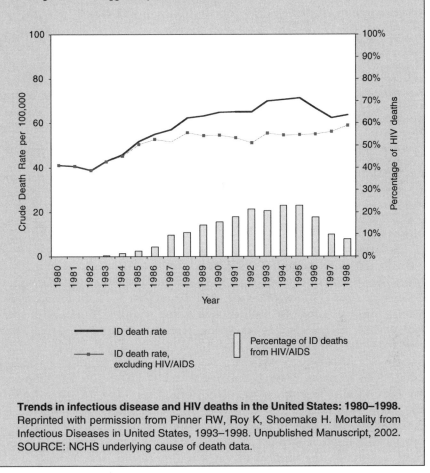

Trends in infectious disease and HIV deaths in the United States: 1980–1998. Reprinted with permission from Pinner RW, Roy K, Shoemake H. Mortality from Infectious Diseases in United States, 1993–1998. Unpublished Manuscript, 2002. SOURCE: NCHS underlying cause of death data.

THE GLOBAL BURDEN OF AIDS, TUBERCULOSIS, AND MALARIA

Efforts to reduce the global burden of infectious diseases must concentrate on AIDS, TB, and malaria. Combined, these three diseases could account for 500 million or more illnesses a year and at least 6 million deaths (WHO, 2002a).

TABLE 2-1 Leading Infectious Causes of Death Worldwide, 2001

Cause	Rank	Estimated Number of Deaths
Respiratory infections	1	3,871,000
HIV/AIDS	2	2,866,000
Diarrheal diseases	3	2,001,000
Tuberculosis	4	1,644,000
Malaria	5	1,124,000
Measles	6	745,000
Pertussis	7	285,000
Tetanus	8	282,000
Meningitis	9	173,000
Syphilis	10	167,000

SOURCE: WHO, 2002b.

Acquired Immunodeficiency Syndrome

In less than 20 years, AIDS has become a pandemic requiring an unprecedented global response (see Figure 2-1) (UNAIDS and WHO, 2001). More than 60 million people have been infected with the human immunodeficiency virus (HIV) worldwide, and 20 million have died from AIDS, leaving an estimated 40 million adults and children living with HIV. Roughly 14 million children are living bereft of one or both parents who died from the disease. In 2001 alone, it is estimated that 5 million people became HIV-positive worldwide, 800,000 of them children (UNAIDS, 2002). Nearly one-third of those living with HIV/AIDS—11.8 million—are between 15 and 24 years of age (UNAIDS, 2002). Specific projections of the number of anticipated HIV/AIDS cases are difficult because the incidence of HIV infection is declining in some populations and increasing in others, HIV-testing continues to be voluntary, and reporting may be incomplete. Generally, the number of cases is expected to rise in areas where poverty, poor health systems, poor access to health care services, and gender inequality are prevalent; where resources for health care and prevention are limited; and where a high degree of stigma and denial is associated with HIV infection (Monitoring the AIDS Pandemic Network, 2000).

In 2001, the highest incidence of HIV/AIDS worldwide was in Africa, where an estimated 3.5 million adults and children were newly infected with HIV in that year alone (UNAIDS, 2002). Of the 40 million people living with HIV/AIDS worldwide at the end of 2001, 28.5 million were in sub-Saharan Africa (UNAIDS, 2002). The majority of adults living with HIV/AIDS in Africa are women under 25 years of age, whose infection rates are astonishingly high. At the end of 2001, mean HIV prevalence rates for

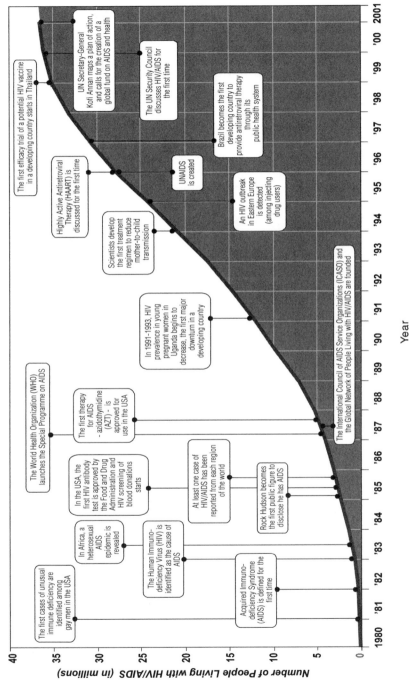

FIGURE 2-1 The first two decades of HIV/AIDS.
SOURCE: UNAIDS, 2001.

females aged 15 to 24 in sub-Saharan Africa ranged from 6.4 to 11.4 percent, as compared with 1.0 to 1.8 percent for women of similar ages around the world (UNAIDS, 2002). Ignorance of AIDS is widespread among young people, who are at the greatest risk. Half of all teenage girls in sub-Saharan Africa do not know that a healthy-looking person can be living with HIV/AIDS. A study in Mozambique found that 74 percent of girls aged 15–19 were unaware of any means to protect themselves from infection (WHO, 2002a).

An estimated 1.9 million people were living with HIV in Latin America and the Caribbean in 2002 (UNAIDS, 2002), making it the second most affected region of the world. Recent reports suggest that India, China, Russia, Ethiopia, and Nigeria each are on the cusp of an exploding epidemic. Together, these countries will account for 50 million to 75 million cases of HIV infection by 2010 (National Intelligence Council, 2002). In northeast India, the widespread use of illicit injection drugs accounts for most HIV transmission; in other parts of the country, most cases of infection appear to have been acquired through contact with infected sex workers. By the mid-1990s, approximately one-fourth of the prostitutes in cities such as New Delhi, Hyderabad, Madurai, Pune, Tirupati, and Vellore tested positive for HIV (UNAIDS, 2000). China has recognized these same risky behaviors—intravenous drug use and prostitution—as the primary modes of HIV transmission in that country (Monitoring the AIDS Pandemic Network, 2000). The number of HIV-infected persons in Russia has increased progressively, virtually doubling every year from 1993 to 1998, mainly as a result of an increase in intravenous drug use (Netesov and Conrad, 2001). Furthermore, it is estimated that the official statistics on HIV in Russia may reflect only 10 to 20 percent of the actual number of carriers, since many patients treated in private clinics are not officially reported.

Most infectious diseases have severe consequences at the two ends of the spectrum of life: infants/children and the elderly. In contrast, HIV is spread predominantly among young adults, who represent the most economically active segment of the population (United Nations Economic Commission for Africa, 2000); thus HIV infection dramatically changes a country's demographics. AIDS is erasing decades of progress made in extending life expectancy; average life expectancy in sub-Saharan Africa is now 47 years, whereas it would have been 62 years without AIDS (UNAIDS, 2002). Of the 14 million orphans resulting from the AIDS pandemic, 80 percent reside in sub-Saharan Africa (UNAIDS, 2002). By 2010, nearly 42 million children in 27 countries are expected to have lost one or both parents to AIDS (National Intelligence Council, 2000). Many countries in South and Southeast Asia are expected to undergo similar demographic changes as HIV/AIDS and associated diseases (e.g., tuberculosis) reduce human life expectancy (National Intelligence Council, 2000). The vast majority of HIV-infected people are unaware they are infected (WHO, 2002a).

The estimated number of deaths from AIDS in the United States decreased from more than 45,000 in 1993 to less than 17,000 in 1999, largely as the result of access to improved therapies for treating opportunistic infections, the development of antiretrovirals, and decreased perinatal transmission through the diagnosis and treatment of HIV-positive pregnant women (CDC, 2000a). The extent of the decrease varied among different demographic risk groups and was most dramatic from 1993 to 1997; since 1997, however, the annual count of deaths from AIDS in the United States has stabilized or increased slightly. The AIDS epidemic in the United States is not disappearing by any means; rather, it is becoming concentrated in populations who lack easy access to prevention programs and health care services (diagnosis and treatment), including racial and ethnic minorities, women, and the poor (Karon et al., 2001). In addition, increases in unprotected anal sex and in sexually transmitted diseases (STDs) in major U.S. cities among men who have sex with men indicate the potential for the resurgence of HIV infections in this population (Wolitski et al., 2001). Over half a million persons were living with HIV/AIDS in the United States as of December 2001, including the 43,000 new cases that were reported in 2001 (CDC, 2001a).

Tuberculosis

Whereas AIDS emerged only within the latter half of the twentieth century, infection with *Mycobacterium tuberculosis* has a millennia-long history as a human disease. Spinal column fragments of Egyptian mummies have provided evidence that tuberculosis has been killing humans for at least 3,000 years (Morse et al., 1964; Nerlich et al., 1997). In the early 1600s, the disease grew to epidemic proportions in Europe as cities expanded and human population densities increased. Improved socioeconomic conditions, improved public health services, and the effectiveness of the antituberculosis therapies developed in the mid-twentieth century maintained a steady decline in TB through the early 1980s.

The decreased public health focus on TB in the United States that occurred toward the end of the twentieth century, combined with increasing rates of homelessness and drug abuse, the growing HIV/AIDS epidemic, and increasing immigration rates from countries with high TB prevalence, led to a resurgence of the disease in the United States that peaked in 1992. Transmission of pulmonary TB frequently occurred within institutions such as hospitals, correctional facilities, residential care facilities, and homeless shelters. With the reinstatement of federal funding in 1992, improved casefinding, and the implementation of directly observed therapy (DOT), the prevalence of TB in the United States decreased 39 percent from 1992 to 2000 (Bloom, 2002). Today, the majority of TB cases in the United States are among foreign-born persons.

Roughly 2 million people die each year from TB worldwide (WHO, 2002c), with the vast majority of these deaths (98 percent) occurring in developing countries (Mukadi et al., 2001). In 2000, approximately 8.7 million new TB cases were reported, of which an estimated 3 to 4 percent were multidrug-resistant (Jaramillo, 2002). In most countries, the average incidence of TB has recently been increasing approximately 3 percent per year; however, the increase is much higher in Eastern Europe (8 percent per year) and those African countries most affected by HIV (10 percent per year). Twenty-three countries account for 80 percent of all new TB cases. In 2000, over half of these cases were concentrated in five countries: India, China, Indonesia, Nigeria, and Bangladesh. Although Zimbabwe and Cambodia report fewer total cases, they possess the highest global rates per 100,000 population (562 and 560, respectively) (WHO, 2001a). If present trends continue, more than 10 million new cases of TB are expected to occur in 2005, mainly in Africa and Southeast Asia; by 2020, nearly 1 billion people will be newly infected, 200 million will develop the disease, and 35 million of them will die (WHO, 2002a).

The global resurgence of TB is not confined to developing countries. From 1990 to 1995, TB rates in Russia increased by 70 percent, with more than 25,000 persons dying from the disease each year (Netesov and Conrad, 2001). The increased incidence is compounded by the spread of multiple drug-resistant TB (MDR-TB), especially in prisons, where patients typically self-administer treatment. Because most prison clinics experience massive shortages of drugs, most patients are unable to complete their full course of treatment, thus fostering the emergence of MDR-TB. Indeed, the rate of MDR-TB among TB isolates in Russian prisons is an astonishing 40 percent, compared with 6 percent in the general population. The overall rate of TB per capita in prison populations (i.e., including both MDR-TB and other forms of the disease) is nearly 100 times higher than in the Russian population at large.

TB is the leading cause of morbidity and mortality among HIV-infected people worldwide (Mukadi et al., 2001), who are at greater risk of developing the disease (Wood et al., 2000). In 1995, approximately one-third of HIV-infected people worldwide were also coinfected with *M. tuberculosis*; the vast majority of these cases were in sub-Saharan Africa (Harries and Maher, 1996). The incidence and case-fatality rate (i.e., the proportion of patients who die among those diagnosed) for TB in sub-Saharan Africa has increased dramatically since the HIV epidemic first began (Mukadi et al., 2001). In some sub-Saharan countries, the case-fatality rate for HIV-positive pulmonary TB patients can exceed 50 percent (Dye et al., 1999; Mukadi et al., 2001).

Malaria

Malaria, caused by plasmodia parasites, is responsible for 300–500 million clinical cases and 1.5–2 million deaths each year (Bloland, 2001). Malaria is the most prevalent vector-borne disease and is endemic in 92 countries (Martens and Hall, 2000). It disproportionately affects rural populations living in housing without screens and doors, children under 5 years of age, and pregnant women. Africa accounted for nearly 90 percent of new cases reported worldwide in 1998; of these, 40 percent occurred in children under 5 years of age (WHO, 1999b).

Nearly all people who live in endemic areas are repeatedly exposed to mosquitoes that carry the infective agent, and those who survive malaria develop partial immunity. Endemic areas are subject to irregular rapid increases in incidence as the warm seasons arrive, rainfall and humidity increase, and populations migrate (IOM, 1991; WHO, 1999b). In areas where the infection rate is low and people are rarely exposed to the disease, however, the population is generally much more susceptible to the devastation of epidemic malaria—and the number of malaria epidemics is growing worldwide. Between 1994 and 1996, malaria epidemics in 14 countries of sub-Saharan Africa caused a high number of deaths, many in areas previously free of the disease (Nchinda, 1998). Drug resistance has been implicated as a contributing factor in the spread of malaria to new areas and the reemergence of the disease in areas where it had previously been eliminated, leading to increased morbidity and mortality (Bloland, 2001).

In 1999, the Centers for Disease Control and Prevention (CDC) received 1,227 reports of malaria cases with onset of symptoms in 1998 among persons in the United States and its territories; 98 percent of these cases were classified as imported, primarily from Africa (60 percent), Asia (20 percent), and the Americas (19.1 percent) (Holtz et al., 2001). Western European countries are reporting similar statistics for imported malaria (Fayer, 2000). Between 1990 and 1996, malaria increased as much as 100-fold in certain southern regions of the former Soviet Union; more recently, it has begun to emerge even as far north as Moscow (Fayer, 2000). Only a few isolated cases or small outbreaks have occurred in the United States, in areas where individuals with imported disease have provided a reservoir of infection for local-vector mosquitoes that have subsequently transmitted the infection to persons from that locality (Olliaro et al., 1996). However, increasing global travel, immigration, and the presence of competent anopheline vectors throughout the continental United States all contribute to the growing threat of malaria transmission even in nontropical North

America, as well as other temperate regions of the world. Indeed, two cases of locally acquired malaria were recently discovered in Loudon County, Virginia, 30 miles from Washington, D.C. (CDC, 2002c)

EMERGING INFECTIOUS DISEASES

The emergence of a microbial threat is a phenomenon in which something has changed—either our perception of a microbial threat, our recognition of a threat, or the true biological expansion of a microbe. An emerging infectious disease is either a newly recognized, clinically distinct infectious disease, or a known infectious disease whose reported incidence is increasing in a given place or among a specific population. As illustrated in the previous section, HIV, TB, and malaria are certainly emerging infections, even though the latter two diseases have been around for centuries. Figure 2-2 and Table 2-2 provide examples of several emerging infectious diseases identified by scientists in the final decades of the twentieth century. These examples include some diseases that have been known for decades, but have reemerged in new geographic locations and/or in newer, more deadly, drug-resistant forms. These and other examples of emerging infectious diseases, including STDs, nosocomial infections, and vector-borne and zoonotic diseases, are discussed in Chapter 3, along with the major factors in their emergence.

We will inevitably see more emerging infections in the future as the factors that lead to emergence become more prevalent and converge with increased frequency. We can only guess at how many more of the microbes in the environment will eventually be found as human pathogens. Even small, isolated events cannot be readily dismissed because of their potential to expand with time. After all, when the initial handful of cases of what would later be termed AIDS first appeared, few could foresee that their affliction would soon become a global catastrophe, threatening the security of entire nations.

ANTIMICROBIAL-RESISTANT INFECTIONS

Antimicrobial resistance is a paramount microbial threat of the twenty-first century. With the presence of antimicrobial resistance may come a corresponding increase in mortality and morbidity from untreatable disease, an increased risk of the global spread of drug-resistant pathogens, a rise in the health care costs associated with the need for multidrug therapy and longer and more frequent hospital stays, and the costs of research and development of alternative drugs. For example, efforts to control each of the three major global infectious diseases discussed earlier—AIDS, TB, and malaria—are seriously thwarted by the rise of antimicrobial resistance.

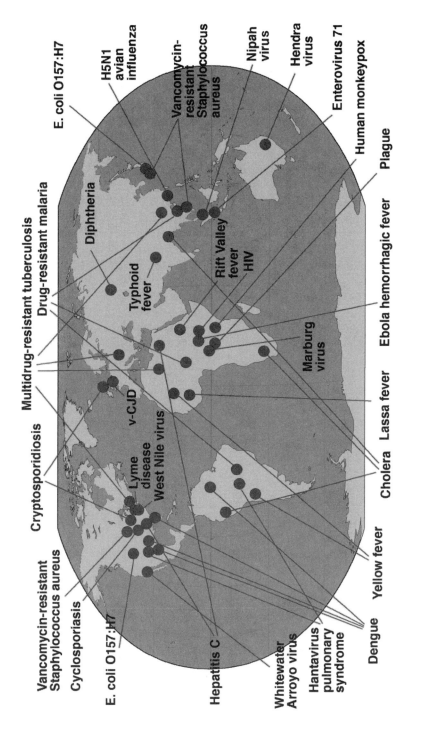

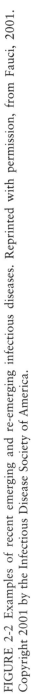

FIGURE 2-2 Examples of recent emerging and re-emerging infectious diseases. Reprinted with permission, from Fauci, 2001. Copyright 2001 by the Infectious Disease Society of America.

TABLE 2-2 Examples of Recent Emerging and Re-Emerging Infectious Diseases

Disease/Agent	Mode of Transmission	Comment
Bacteria		
Anthrax (*Bacillus anthracis*)	Inhalation of spores; via skin contact with contaminated tissues or materials; ingestion of contaminated food.	Primarily an infection of animals; long-term persistence in contaminated soil or environment; agent of bioterrorism.
Cholera (*Vibrio cholerae* O139)	Ingestion of bacteria in contaminated food or water.	Emerged in Asia in 1992–1993 in areas with poor sanitation; has caused large outbreaks in India and Bangladesh; prior infection with *V. cholerae* O1 does not protect against O139; ongoing genetic reassortment in O139.
Diphtheria (*Corynebacterium diphtheriae*)	Close contact with person who has diphtheria or who carries *Corynebacterium diphtheriae*.	Massive outbreak (>150,000 cases) in the former Soviet Union countries and Mongolia in 1990s at time of decreased vaccination, declining socioeconomic conditions, and breakdown in public health infrastructure; sporadic outbreaks elsewhere in world.
Escherichia coli O157:H7 hemorrhagic colitis (severe bloody diarrhea and kidney failure)	Ingestion of contaminated food or water; can be spread from person to person via fecal-oral route.	Healthy cattle are primary reservoir (carried in feces); bacteria survive in acidic environment; small inoculum of bacteria can cause infection; sporadic cases and large outbreaks in U.S. and other countries; vehicles of transmission have included meat, milk, fresh produce, cider, contaminated water ingested during swimming, other; mass processing and wide distribution of contaminated foods has led to widely dispersed outbreaks.
Lyme disease (*Borrelia burgdorferi*)	Bite of infective tick.	Zoonosis; rodents and deer maintain transmission cycle; common in parts of North America, Europe; also found in Asia, Australia; increase in human cases attributed to reforestation and expansion of deer populations; increased human-tick contact.
Plague (*Yersinia pestis*)	Bite of infective flea; inhalation of airborne bacilli; close contact with infected animal or tissues.	Primarily a zoonosis; rodents are reservoir host; most sporadic cases and outbreaks occur in Africa but infections also occur in the Americas (including the U.S.), Asia, and Europe; outbreak in India in 1994; possible agent of bioterrorism.

Staphylococcus aureus, vancomycin-resistant	Contact with infected person.	First emerged in U.S. in 2002; consequence of intensive use of antimicrobials; can be spread from patient to patient in health care settings; risk of spread into the community.

Protozoa

Cryptosporidiosis (*Cryptosporidium parvum*)	Fecal–oral spread; may be food or water borne.	Massive outbreak in Milwaukee in 1993 (estimated >400,000 cases) linked to contamination of municipal water supply; oocysts are resistant to chlorine and other chemicals used to purify drinking water; infection may be severe in persons with AIDS or otherwise immunocompromised because of drugs or disease.
Cyclospora (*Cyclospora cayetanensis*)	Ingestion of contaminated food or water.	Multiple outbreaks in North America in 1990s linked to imported raspberries from Guatemala; endemic in many countries.
Malaria	Bite of infective mosquito.	Increasing morbidity and mortality in many areas, especially in Africa; increase linked to poor vector control and rising resistance to inexpensive antimalarial drugs, lack of resources for other drugs and other control measures.

Viruses

Dengue fever (and dengue hemorrhagic fever and shock syndrome); dengue viruses, serotypes 1,2,3,4	Bite of infective mosquito, usually *Aedes aegypti.*	Found in most tropical and subtropical areas worldwide, including urban areas; outbreak in Hawaii in 2001–2002; epidemics are increasing in size and severity, especially in Asia and Latin America; factors in worsening situation include poor mosquito control, abundant mosquito breeding sites in growing tropical cities, travel of humans who carry the virus, and wide circulation of more than one serotype of virus.

continues

TABLE 2-2 Continued

Disease/Agent	Mode of Transmission	Comment
Ebola hemorrhagic fever	Spread from person with acute infection by contact with blood, secretions, or other material.	Repeated outbreaks with high mortality in sub-Saharan Africa; secondary spread of infection has occurred in health care settings and in households in Africa; reservoir for the virus not yet identified.
Enterovirus 71	Direct contact with material from infected persons (nose/throat discharge or droplets, feces).	Multiple outbreaks documented since 1974; major epidemic in Taiwan, 1998, with highest incidence in children <1 year, and again in 2000; virus highly mutable.
Hantavirus pulmonary syndrome (Sin Nombre and multiple other hantaviruses)	Presumed aerosol transmission of excreta from infected rodents.	Zoonosis; rodent reservoir host; sporadic cases and outbreaks especially in North and South America; rise in reported human cases linked to factors that lead to expansion of rodent population (e.g., rainfall, weather conditions), increased human–rodent contact (changes in land use), and increased recognition.
Hendra virus (related to Nipah virus)	Humans infected by direct contact with infected horses.	Zoonosis; 3 human cases in Australia in 1994–1995; fruit bats may be reservoir host.
HIV	Person to person via blood and body fluids.	Continued spread and rising rates of infection in some areas; emergence of resistant strains related to antiviral therapy; resistant strains can be transmitted; infected persons can be infected with second strain; HIV-associated immunosuppression contributes to increase in multiple other infections, including TB.
Influenza, avian H5N1	Presumed direct spread from chickens or other birds to humans.	Major epizootics of influenza H5N1 in avian species in Hong Kong in 1997 and spread of avian virus to humans; millions of chickens killed to halt spread of infection to humans; virus infected multiple avian species; no or limited spread of H5N1 from human to human.

Monkeypox (human) Orthopoxvirus related to smallpox virus	Close contact with infected animal or person.	Zoonosis; several generations of person-to-person spread documented; outbreaks in central and western Africa; vaccination with vaccinia virus, which is protective, may have limited spread in the past; possible confusion with smallpox.
Nipah virus	Human cases resulted from close contact with infected, sick pigs.	Zoonosis; fruit bats are probable reservoir host; outbreaks in Malaysia started in 1996, in areas with intensive pig farming and movement of pigs; large-scale culling of pigs was used to halt outbreaks.
Noroviruses (formerly Norwalk-like viruses, caliciviruses)	Person to person; food or waterborne; airborne droplets	Multiple large outbreaks, especially in institutions and shared environments, including nursing homes, schools, cruise ships; multiple modes of transmission, stability of virus in environment and low infectious dose favor transmission; recently emerged strain may be more transmissible.
vCJD (new variant Creutzfeldt-Jakob)	Presumed via consumption of flesh from cattle with bovine spongiform encephalopathy (BSE).	A transmissible spongiform encephalopathy; human cases first appeared in UK in 1996 following an epizootic of BSE in cattle in the UK (by 1997, >170,000 head of cattle had been diagnosed with BSE); feeding ruminant animal proteins to animals was thought to have key role; more than 100 human cases of vCJD have been diagnosed, the majority in the UK.
West Nile virus	Bite of infective mosquito.	First outbreak in U.S. in 1999 with epicenter in New York. Has subsequently spread through most of the U.S. and into Canada and Mexico; virus infects many species of birds and other animals; migratory birds have facilitated spread of virus.
Whitewater Arroyo virus (an arenavirus)	Inhalation of virus in aerosolized rat urine	Presumed zoonosis with rodent reservoir host; caused human deaths in California in 2000.
Yellow fever	Bite of infective mosquito.	Recent spread into some urban areas of Africa and South America; poor vector control; increase in urban tropical areas infested with mosquitoes competent to transmit virus increases risk of introduction by infected traveler; many at-risk populations not vaccinated with highly effective vaccine.

Despite the steadily increasing availability of new drugs against HIV, the management of drug-resistant HIV poses a serious worldwide challenge. Drugs that mitigate opportunistic infections have also encountered an increase in resistance, with a profound effect on the remaining life expectancy of HIV-infected individuals, as well as their quality of life.

Antimicrobial resistance may represent a more profound hindrance to TB prevention and control efforts than is the case with HIV, in that antituberculin drugs can cure the infected individual and also prevent subsequent infection of others. In 1997 more than 50 million cases of TB worldwide were resistant to one or more drugs (WHO, 1998a). Developing countries in which TB is rampant often have limited laboratory resources to test for drug resistance. Individuals infected with drug-resistant strains, therefore, are often treated inappropriately, thus compounding the spread of MDR-TB.

As with the thwarting of efforts to control TB, drug-resistant malaria continues to expand and impair control efforts. Multiple drug-resistant strains of *Plasmodium falciparum*, the malaria with the highest fatality rate, are common in many parts of the world. Resistance of *P. vivax* to certain antimalarials has also been described. The spread of resistance results from numerous factors, including incomplete courses of therapy, changes in vector and parasite biology, pharmacokinetics, and economics (Bloland, 2001).

The health challenges created by antimicrobial resistance extend far beyond the management of these three major killers. For example, *Staphylococcus aureus* was the most common cause of nosocomial infections in the 1990s (Rubin et al., 1999). *S. aureus*, often referred to simply as "staph," is normally found on the skin of healthy individuals, but occasionally enters the body to cause infections ranging from minor problems, such as pimples and boils, to life-threatening septicemia or pneumonia. Methicillin or related drugs (i.e., oxacillin, nafcillin) have become the antibiotics of choice for treating serious staph infections, since more than 95 percent of staph-infected patients worldwide fail to respond to first-line antibiotics such as penicillin and ampicillin (Neu, 1992). In 1990, however, 15 percent of all *S. aureus* isolates were reported to be resistant to methicillin; in critical care units, 22 percent of all nosocomial *S. aureus* isolates were methicillin-resistant (Wenzel et al., 1991), and this figure had jumped to over 55 percent by 2000 (National Nosocomial Infections Surveillance, 2001). CDC estimates that as many as 80,000 hospital patients are infected with methicillin-resistant *S. aureus* (MRSA) each year in the United States. Thus MRSA, which first emerged as a nosocomial infection in the early 1960s (shortly after methicillin was introduced to the market), has been increasing in incidence worldwide ever since (O'Brien et al., 1999; Simor et al., 2001; van Belkum and Verbrugh, 2001).

As of this writing (2003), vancomycin remains the mainstay for treatment against staph infection. Yet extensive transfer of antimicrobial resistance can occur among MRSA pathogenic bacteria and normal flora residing in the human colon (Shoemaker et al., 2001). Since 1989 vancomycin resistance has been increasing substantially in enterococci (*Enterococcus faecium*) isolated from hospitalized patients, and vancomycin resistance is threatening to become a problem in *S. aureus* as resistant genes can be transferred to *S. aureus* through horizontal spread. In 1996, the first case of *S. aureus* infection with intermediate resistance to vancomycin was reported in Japan (CDC, 1997a); the following year, the United States reported two additional cases (CDC, 1997b). In 2002, the first case of vancomycin-resistant *S. aureus* was isolated from a 40-year-old Michigan resident with diabetes. This newly identified strain underscores the urgent need to prevent the spread of antimicrobial resistance through the appropriate and controlled use of antimicrobials, as well as the need to develop new classes of antibiotics (CDC, 2002d).

Although MRSA infections are much more likely to develop in hospitals and long-term care facilities than in the general healthy population, several recent deaths due to MRSA infection in previously healthy children show that the condition is now circulating outside of hospitals (Groom et al., 2001). Moreover, the incidence of MRSA in prison populations is unexpectedly high for non–health care settings (CDC, 2001b). Public health officials recently reported a foodborne outbreak of community-acquired MRSA infection, which is believed to have been caused by a food handler who had recently been exposed to MRSA while visiting an elderly relative in a nursing home (Jones et al., 2002).

A dramatic increase in resistance among community-acquired bacteria (i.e., pathogens that normally circulate in the general community and outside of hospital settings), including streptococci, pneumococci, and gonococci, has occurred. For example, evidence indicates a very clear relationship between erythromycin use and resistance among Group A streptococci; when erythromycin use is controlled, the prevalence of erythromycin-resistant isolates declines dramatically (Seppala et al., 1997). Resistance to penicillin among isolates of *Streptococcus pneumoniae* increased from 5 percent in 1991 (Spika et al., 1991) to 24 percent in 1998 (Whitney et al., 2000). Many penicillin-resistant pneumococci are now resistant to multiple other drugs as well; for example, fluoroquinolone-resistant pneumococci emerged as recently as the late 1990s (Chen et al., 1999) (see Figure 2-3). Over the past decade, several countries—including the United States (Kilmarx et al., 1998), Denmark (Su and Lind, 2001), and Greece (Mavroidi et al., 2000)— have reported fluoroquinolone-resistant gonococci as well. The regional surveillance program in the Western Pacific WHO Region documented increases in the proportion of quinolone-resistant gonococci in Hong Kong (from 3.3 percent in 1994 to 49 percent in 1998), in Singapore (from 0.3 percent in 1993 to 7 percent in 1998), and in Australia (from less than 0.1 percent in 1993 to 5.6 percent in 1997) (WHO, 2001b). Quinolone-resistant gonococci are now highly common (greater than 80 percent) in most large cities in the Peoples Republic of China (Su, 2002). More than 20 percent of gonococci in Hawaii are quinolone-resistant, and similar resistant organisms are being reported in California (see Figure 2-4) (CDC, 2002e). The emergence of fluoroquinolone-resistant gonococci in the Pacific rim, Hawaii, and California is a particularly bad sign because of the historical trend for resistant gonococci to move from those areas across the United States.

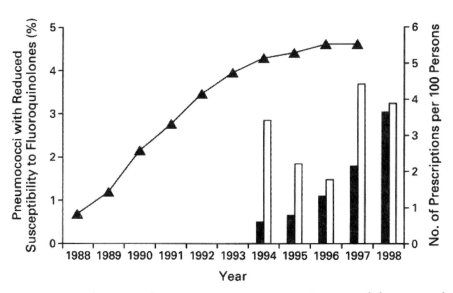

FIGURE 2-3 Fluoroquinolone prescriptions per capita (curve) and frequency of pneumococci with reduced susceptibility to fluoroquinolones in Canada according to the patient's age (bars). No isolates with reduced susceptibility were identified for persons who were younger than 15 years. Solid bars indicate an age of 15 to 64 years, and open bars an age of 65 years or older. Data on per capita fluoroquinolone prescriptions were obtained from 1988 through 1997, and data on the frequency of pneumococci with decreased susceptibility to fluoroquinolones in each age group were obtained in 1988 and in 1993 through 1998. No isolates with reduced susceptibility were identified in 1988 or 1993. Reprinted with permission, from Chen et al., 1999. Copyright 1999 Massachusetts Medical Society.

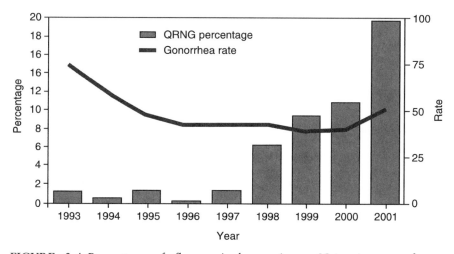

FIGURE 2-4 Percentage of fluoroquinolone-resistant *Neisseria gonorrhoeae* (QRNG)* among tested gonococcal isolates and gonorrhea rate,[†] by year[§]—Hawaii, 1993–2001.

*Defined as *N. gonorrhoeae* resistant to ciprofloxacin (minimal inhibitory concentration [MIC] ≥ 1.0 µg/mL or disk diffusion zone size ≤ 27 mm) or ofloxacin (MIC ≥ µg/mL or disk diffusion zone size ≤24 mm) by the Committee on Clinical Laboratory Standards.

[†]Per 100,000 population.

[§]Data for 1993–2001 include Gonococcal Isolate Surveillance Project (GISP) and non-GISP isolates.

SOURCE: CDC (2002e).

CHRONIC DISEASES WITH INFECTIOUS ETIOLOGY

A growing body of evidence supports the hypothesis that infectious agents cause or contribute to many chronic diseases and cancers previously thought to be caused by genetic, environmental, or lifestyle factors (see Table 2-3) (Cassell, 1998; Pisani et al., 1997). Specific microbes claimed to be associated with chronic conditions may be cofactors with other microbes or other etiologic factors in the disease, sometimes being necessary but perhaps not sufficient elements in the causation pathway. The era of molecular biology and intensive research efforts in the field of AIDS have led to powerful advances in technology for the sensitive detection of infectious agents. These diagnostic tools, plus the realization that organisms of otherwise unimpressive virulence can produce slowly progressive chronic disease with a wide spectrum of clinical manifestations and disease outcomes, have resulted in the discovery of new infectious agents and new concepts in the understanding of infectious diseases.

TABLE 2-3 Infections Associated with Chronic Conditions

Infectious Agent	Chronic Condition
Bacterial	
Campylobacter jejuni	Guillain-Barré syndrome
Borrelia burgdorferi	Lyme arthritis
Helicobacter pylori	Peptic ulcer disease
	Gastric adenocarcinoma
	Gastric lymphoma
	Immunoproliferative small intestinal disease
	Mucosa-associated lymphoid tissue lymphoma
Chlamydia trachomatis	Infertility
Chlamydia pneumoniae	Atherosclerosis
Enteric bacteria (*Shigella, Salmonella, Yersinia, Campylobacter*)	Arthritis
	Reiter's syndrome
E. coli O157:H7	Hemolytic uremic syndrome
Viral	
Varicella-zoster	Post-herpetic neuralgia
	Congenital mental retardation
Cytomegalovirus	Congenital mental retardation
Human herpesvirus-8 (HHV-8)/Kaposi's sarcoma-associated herpesvirus (KSHV)	Kaposi's sarcoma
	Primary effusion lymphoma
	Castleman's disease
Hepatitis B	Hepatocellular carcinoma
Hepatitis C	Hepatocellular carcinoma
Human papilloma virus (HPV-16, 18, 31, 45)	Genital carcinomas (cervical, penile, vulvar, anal)
Epstein-Barr virus (EBV)	Burkitt's lymphoma
	Nasopharyngeal carcinoma
	Hodgkin's lymphoma
Human T-cell lymphotropic viruses (HTLV-1 and -2)	Adult T-cell leukemia
	T-cell lymphoma
Human immunodeficiency viruses (HIV-1, HIV-2)	Lymphoma
	Kaposi sarcoma
	Genital carcinomas related to HPV
Simian virus (SV-40)	Mesothelioma
	Ependymomia
Coxsackievirus	Myocarditis

TABLE 2-3 Continued

Infectious Agent	Chronic Condition
Helminth	
Schistosoma haematobium	Urinary bladder carcinoma
Schistosoma japonicum	Colonic carcinomas
Schistosoma mansoni	Colonic carcinomas
Opisthorchis viverrini	Cholangiocarcinoma

SOURCES: Campbell et al., 1998; Danesh et al., 1997; de The, 1995; Epstein et al., 1999; Humphrey et al., 1998; Klein et al., 2002; Persing and Prendergast, 1999; Roivainen et al., 2000.

Cases in point are the proof that many stomach ulcers are due to the bacterium *Helicobacter pylori* (Parsonnet, 1998; Marshall, 1989; Moller et al., 1995), and the demonstration that at least one form of chronic arthritis and neurologic disorders can be caused by *Borrelia burgdorferi*, most likely through induction of autoimmunity (Danesh et al., 1997). Recent data obtained in humans and animal models also suggest that mycoplasmas may cause some cases of chronic lung disease in newborns (Cassell et al., 1994; Dyke et al., 1993; Valencia et al., 1993) and chronic asthma in adults (Sabato et al., 1984; Seggev et al., 1986; Yano et al., 1994; Henderson et al., 1979). It has been estimated that more than 15 percent of cancers—including more than 50 percent of stomach and cervical cancers and 80 percent of liver cancers—could be avoided by preventing the associated infectious diseases (WHO, 1996).

Findings such as these raise the possibility that other chronic conditions may also have infectious etiologies. Many of these culprit microbial agents are potentially treatable with existing antibiotics (Cassell, 1998), and they may even be vaccine preventable. For example, the realization that *H. pylori* causes ulcers revolutionized ulcer treatment. In addition to its causal role in the development of peptic ulcers and gastritis, *H. pylori* appears to play a role as well in the development of gastric maltomas (i.e., low-grade B-cell gastric lymphomas of mucosa-associated lymphoid tissue); eradication of the underlying *H. pylori* infection has been shown to result in tumor regression (Wotherspoon et al., 1993).

The basic biology of those organisms implicated in chronic diseases and cancer is relatively obscure. With rare exceptions, the means by which pathogens suppress, subvert, or evade host defenses and establish chronic and/or latent infection have received little attention. Given that many of these diseases are among the most common in the world, a substantial impact on improving health and reducing health care costs could be achieved even if only some cases were proven to be of infectious origin, and effective therapies and/or vaccines could be developed. Major advances could be made through the application of functional genomics and integrative biological technologies.

Cardiovascular Disease

Whereas a number of infectious agents—including herpes simplex virus (HSV) and cytomegalovirus (CMV)—have been implicated as causal agents of cardiovascular disease, *Chlamydiae pneumoniae* has been identified most frequently as a causal infectious agent (Saikku et al., 1988; Campbell et al., 1998). *C. pneumoniae* is better known for its causal role in community-acquired pneumonia; an estimated 26 percent of all community-acquired pneumonia cases in patients over 65 years of age are due to chlamydial infection (Gant and Parton, 2000). *C. pneumoniae* infections are usually mild or asymptomatic, but they can be severe, especially in the elderly (Peeling and Brunham, 1996). Prevalence rates of *C. pneumoniae* antibodies increase from about 50 percent in young adults to 75 percent in the elderly, suggesting that most individuals are infected and reinfected with the bacterium throughout their lives (Kenny and Kuo, 2000).

Compelling evidence of a link between *C. pneumoniae* and heart disease has been accumulating from a variety of sources, including polymerase chain reaction (PCR), immunocytochemical (ICC) staining, and electron microscopy studies (Campbell et al., 1998). Seroepidemiologic studies have revealed consistent associations between *C. pneumoniae* antibodies and both coronary heart and cerebrovascular disease, independent of other artherosclerosis risk factors (i.e., hypercholsterolemia, cigarette smoking, hypertension, diabetes, and family history) (Saikku et al., 1992). Insofar as infection does predispose to the development of atherosclerosis, the risk of coronary artery disease is related to the aggregate number of potentially atherogenic pathogens to which an individual has been exposed (Epstein et al., 1999). In addition, infectious agents lead to an increase in other factors, such as C-reactive protein, that may play a causal role in atherosclerosis.

Human Papillomaviruses and Cervical Cancer

Cervical cancer is one of the most common malignant diseases of women. In the United States each year there are approximately 12,800 new cases of invasive cervical cancer and 4,600 deaths due to the disease (CDC, 2001c). Worldwide, an estimated 190,000 deaths occur from cervical cancer, over three-fourths of these in developing countries (Pisani et al., 1999). Fewer than 50 percent of women affected by cervical cancer in developing countries survive longer than 5 years, whereas the 5-year survival rate in developed countries is about 66 percent (Pisani et al., 1999). Cervical cancer generally affects multiparous women in the early postmenopausal years, although prominent risk factors include the number of sexual partners and age at first intercourse (Brinton, 1992; Herrero, 1996; Schiffman and Brinton, 1995), as well as the sexual behavior of the woman's male partners (Brinton et al., 1989a).

Human papillomavirus (HPV) is one of the most common causes of STD in the world. Health experts estimate that there are more cases of genital HPV infection than of any other STD in the United States (NIH, 2001). An estimated 5.5 million new cases of sexually transmitted HPV infection occur every year, and at least 20 million Americans are already infected (American Social Health Association, 2001). Scientists have identified more than 100 types of HPV, most of which are not known to cause harm. About 30 types are spread through sexual contact. Some types of HPV that cause genital infections can also cause cervical cancer and other genital cancers. Genital warts (condylomata acuminata, or venereal warts) are the most easily recognized sign of genital HPV infection. Many people, however, have a genital HPV infection without genital warts.

Today, it is well established that infection with certain HPV types is the central causal factor in cervical cancer (Franco et al., 2001; Holly, 1996; International Agency for Research on Cancer Working Group, 1995; Koutsky et al., 1992; Nobbenhuis et al., 1999; Shah, 1997). Relative risks for the association between HPV and cervical cancer are in the 20–70 times range, which is among the strongest statistical relations ever identified in cancer epidemiology. Both retrospective (Munoz et al., 1992; Ylitalo et al., 2000; Zielinski et al., 2001) and prospective (Liaw et al., 1999; Moscicki et al., 2001) epidemiologic studies have demonstrated the unequivocally strong association between infection with the virus and the risk of malignancy, as both cervical intraepithelial neoplasia (CIN) and invasive disease. However, not all infections with high-risk HPVs persist or progress to cervical cancer, thus suggesting that, albeit necessary, HPV infection is not always sufficient to induce cancer; other factors, environmental or host-related, are also involved. Among these cofactors are smoking (Ho et al., 1998); high parity (Brinton et al., 1989b); use of oral contraceptives (Pater et al., 1994); a diet deficient in vitamins A and C (Potischman and Brinton, 1996); and genetic susceptibility traits, such as specific human leukocyte antigen (HLA) alleles and haplotypes (Maciag et al., 2000) and polymorphisms in the p53 gene (Klug et al., 2001). Understanding the role of these cofactors is the objective of much ongoing research on the natural history of HPV infection and cervical cancer.

Scientists are doing research on two types of HPV vaccines. One type would be used to prevent infection or disease (warts or precancerous tissue changes); the other would be used to treat cervical cancers. Both types of vaccines are currently undergoing clinical trials. Vaccine-induced protection against cervical HPV 16 infection appears to prevent early precancerous changes (Koutsky et al., 2002).

MICROBES INTENTIONALLY USED FOR HARM

Since the terrorist events of September 11, 2001, and the subsequent anthrax attacks through the U.S. mail system, the threat of terrorism has been a prominent subject in the national news. Bioterrorist attacks could occur again at any time, under many circumstances, and at a magnitude far greater than has already been witnessed (IOM, 2002a) (see later discussion in Chapter 3). The knowledge needed for developing biological weapons is accessible to individuals through the open literature and the Internet; the technology is readily available and affordable; and, perhaps most alarming, as the field of molecular genetics advances, an increased capability exists to bioengineer vaccine- or antimicrobial-resistant strains of biological agents. Currently, many terrorist-sponsoring nations or states are suspected of having active bioweapons programs in place.

The United States has been rather complacent about the threat of bioterrorism until recently. A number of factors could account for this complacency, including insufficient intelligence concerning which nations and states have weaponized infectious agents, a naivete regarding the ease with which biological agents can be obtained and weaponized using today's molecular and biological technology, a general lack of familiarity and skepticism with regard to the dangers of biological weapons, the unpredictable nature of a bioterrorist attack, and little supporting evidence that biological weapons have been widely used thus far. Recent reports have reviewed the threat of bioterrorism (e.g., National Commission on Terrorism, 2000), and in November 2001, the Institute of Medicine (IOM) convened a workshop on *Biological Threats and Terrorism: Assessing the Science and Response Capabilities* (IOM, 2002a). Experts agree that the United States is vulnerable to bioterrorist attacks and that the likelihood of such an event is increasing. Several agents have been identified and categorized as to their threat potential (see Box 2-2).

The anthrax attacks of 2001 increased awareness that the threat of bioterrorism is real and capable of producing widespread disruption, damage, disease and death. Anthrax is a proven risk and of immediate concern. Smallpox is an equally urgent concern because of its capability for person-to-person transmission and the large numbers of completely susceptible individuals in the United States and worldwide. Three other high-priority potential bioterrorist agents are plague, tularemia, and botulinum toxin. However, these are not the only credible bioterrorist agents. For example,

BOX 2-2
Diseases/Agents of Biological Warfare

Category A Diseases/Agents

The U.S. public health system and primary health care providers must be prepared to address various biological agents, including pathogens that are rarely seen in the United States. High-priority agents include the following organisms that pose a risk to national security because they can easily be disseminated or transmitted from person to person, result in high mortality rates, could cause public panic and social disruption, and require special action for public health preparedness:

- Anthrax (*Bacillus anthracis*)
- Botulism (*Clostridium botulinum* toxin)
- Plague (*Yersinia pestis*)
- Smallpox (variola major)
- Tularemia (*Francisella tularensis*)
- Viral hemorrhagic fevers (filoviruses [e.g., Ebola, Marburg] and arenaviruses [e.g., Lassa, Machupo])

Category B Diseases/Agents

Agents with the second-highest priority include those that are moderately easy to disseminate, result in moderate morbidity rates and low mortality rates, and require specific enhancements of CDC's diagnostic capacity and enhanced disease surveillance:

- Brucellosis (*Brucella* spp.)
- Epsilon toxin of *Clostridium perfringens*
- Food safety threats (e.g., *Salmonella* spp., *Escherichia coli* O157:H7, Shigella)
- Glanders (*Burkholderia mallei*)
- Melioidosis (*Burkholderia pseudomallei*)
- Psittacosis (*Chlamydia psittaci*)
- Q fever (*Coxiella burnetii*)
- Ricin toxin from *Ricinus communis* (castor beans)
- Staphylococcal enterotoxin B
- Typhus fever (*Rickettsia prowazekii*)
- Viral encephalitis (alphaviruses [e.g., Venezuelan equine encephalitis, eastern equine encephalitis, western equine encephalitis])
- Water safety threats (e.g., *Vibrio cholerae*, *Cryptosporidium parvum*)

Category C Diseases/Agents

Agents with the third-highest priority include emerging pathogens that could be engineered for mass dissemination in the future because of availability, ease of production and dissemination, and potential for high morbidity and mortality rates and major health impacts:

- Emerging infectious disease threats, such as Nipah virus and hantavirus
- Influenza viruses, such as H5N1

SOURCE: CDC, 2003a.

the former Soviet Union is known to have weaponized at least 30 biological agents, including several vaccine- or drug-resistant strains.

Many bioterrorist scenarios are possible; two examples are aerosol and foodborne attacks. Aerosols exhibit wide-area coverage, and their small particle size allows them to deposit very deeply in the lung tissue, which is where many agents, including anthrax, induce maximal damage (see Chapter 3). A large amount of agent disseminated under ideal meteorological conditions over a city of substantial size could have considerable downwind reach, resulting in large numbers of casualties. Foodborne bioterrorism, which could encompass a variety of agents, must also be considered a likely threat. Agents that cause foodborne illness are easy to obtain from the environment and often have very low-dose requirements. Foodborne pathogens may in fact be the easiest bioterrorism agent to disseminate.

Consideration of the various bioterrorism agents and some of their properties is the first step in prioritizing defenses against them. Each has unique properties as we see them today, and thus each presents a distinct threat with different opportunities for control.

Anthrax

Bacillus anthracis is a highly stable organism because of its ability to sporulate. Most naturally occurring anthrax cases are cutaneous and are transmitted from agricultural or other occupational exposure. Under natural circumstances, humans become infected through contact with infected animals or contaminated animal products. The incidence of infection is unknown; most cases occur in developing countries.

Several characteristics of *B. anthracis* make it a potentially very lethal bioweapon (Inglesby et al., 2002). Most important are its stability and infectivity as an aerosol and its large footprint after aerosol release. Anthrax is also widely distributed in nature and thus readily available to terrorists in virulent form. The spores are extraordinarily stable, making them relatively easy to store or transport as an aerosol. An aerosol release of anthrax could potentially affect millions of individuals.

Currently, three types of preventative or therapeutic countermeasures exist against anthrax: vaccination, antibiotics, and various adjunctive antitoxin treatments. Since the late 1930s, attenuated strains of *B. anthracis* have been used throughout the world as live veterinary vaccines and have proven to be highly effective in controlling disease in domesticated animals. Since the 1950s, one of these strains has been used as a live attenuated vaccine in humans in countries of the former Soviet Union. An inactivated cell-free product is currently used in the United States to vaccinate military personnel and laboratory workers. The molecular pathogenesis of anthrax, including the exact target of its lethal factor, is largely unknown. However, enough is known that we can begin to predict where second-generation vaccines and various antitoxin modalities might work.

Smallpox

Unlike anthrax, smallpox is a contagious disease with fairly high rates of human-to-human transmission. Consequently, smallpox is considered to pose an even greater threat as an agent of biological terrorism than anthrax (Henderson et al., 1999). Smallpox represents a threat whose consequences are potentially catastrophic; hence it requires careful attention, regardless of the probability of its use. Several features make it an attractive bioterrorist agent: it is moderately stable; it is infectious by droplets and aerosol; it is moderately contagious; and, because vaccination against smallpox ceased after eradication in 1980, most of the world's population is highly susceptible to infection.

While a smallpox vaccine exists, several bioterrorism-related issues regarding prophylactic smallpox vaccination are unresolved (IOM, 2003). Therefore, we must develop clinician awareness, diagnostic systems, and stockpiles of existing vaccine that will give us a validated countermeasure to deploy in case of the intentional use of this biological agent.

Plague

Yersinia pestis poses a risk to national security because this pathogen can be disseminated by aerosol and/or transmitted from person-to-person, could cause high mortality, and requires special action for public health preparedness (CDC, 2000b). Plague was weaponized in the former Soviet Union for aerosol delivery, and engineered for antimicrobial resistance and possibly enhanced virulence (Inglesby et al., 2000). Plague cultivation in virulent form and its dissemination in stable aerosols, however, are more difficult than is the case for anthrax. Plague generates special concern because of its potential to cause panic, its contagiousness in the pulmonary form, its fulminating clinical course and high fatality, and the possibility that it could be engineered for plasmid-mediated resistance to multiple antimicrobial agents (Galimand et al., 1997). In the WHO modeling scenario that was developed in 1970, a 50 kg release over a city of 5 million would cause about 150,000 cases and 36,000 deaths in the first wave (WHO, 1970). A secondary spread would cause a further 500,000 cases and 100,000 deaths. Plague requires intensive medical and nursing support and isolation for at least the first 48 hours of antibiotic treatment, followed by 2 to 3 weeks of slow convalescence. The hospitalization and isolation that would be required for this number of people in a single city is nearly unimaginable. Pneumonic plague's contagiousness would require isolation and possible quarantine, which would complicate medical and public health management.

Currently in the United States, there is no available plague vaccine. The live vaccines that are sometimes used in other countries have unacceptable adverse effects. However, a number of laboratories are attempting to develop a new-generation vaccine, as well as new delivery methods. Several different types of antibiotics that can be used to treat plague are included in the national pharmaceutical stockpile. Antibiotic treatment must be instituted early in the course of infection; otherwise death occurs in 3 to 6 days.

Tularemia

Francisella tularensis was weaponized as an aerosol in both the United States and the former Soviet Union, where it was also engineered for vaccine resistance (Dennis et al., 2001). In the WHO modeling scenario of 1970, a 50 kg release over a city of 5 million would incapacitate 250,000 people and cause 19,000 deaths (WHO, 1970). Tularemia is highly infectious but not contagious. Treatment is similar to that for plague but more extensive, as is the post-prophylaxis to prevent relapse. The tularemia vaccine is a live attenuated vaccine that was previously available as an investigational drug through the U.S. Department of Defense and is now being investigated by the Joint Vaccine Acquisition Program. However, it does not offer full protection against inhalational transmission, and about 14 days is required for protection to develop. The vaccine has been recommended for use in people who work routinely with the organism in the laboratory, but how useful it would be among first responders at high risk for exposure is unknown.

Botulinum Toxin

Botulinum toxin has several features that make it an attractive bioweapon, including its extreme potency and lethality; the ease of its production, transport, and misuse; and its profound impact on its victims as well as the health care infrastructure. Botulinum toxin is readily available as a bioweapon because of the relative ease with which its source, *C. botulinum*, can be isolated from nature or otherwise obtained. A minimal amount of laboratory equipment and microbiological expertise is needed to cultivate *C. botulinum* and concentrate its toxin to weaponized material for oral intake. Like tularemia, botulinum toxin can be transmitted through diverse modes: it can spread through foods or beverages or as an aerosol. The toxin, of which there are seven serotypes, kills by paralyzing its victims' ability to carry out normal respiratory function and is the most poisonous substance known. One gram, evenly aerosolized and inhaled, could generate more than 1 million lethal doses; 100 grams, evenly distributed in a food or beverage and ingested, could kill a million victims (Arnon et al., 2001).

An investigational vaccine exists, but immunization is really not a viable option for bioweapon defense: the vaccine is still only investigational after 10 years; its components are aging and losing potency; it protects only against serotypes A, B, C, D, and E, and not F and G; it is very painful to receive; it requires a booster at 1 year; and its use deprives the recipient of access to medicinal botulinum toxin for life.

The army has developed an equine antitoxin that provides coverage against all seven serotypes, but the supply is limited, and the drug carries the risk of serious allergic reaction. However, equine antitoxin is inexpensive to produce and could be made in large quantities if a specialized facility were available. A human-derived botulinum antitoxin has been developed as an orphan drug, but is difficult to produce in large quantities and is of limited use because it protects against only five serotypes.

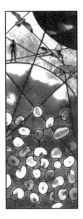

3

Factors in Emergence

Six factors in the emergence of infectious diseases were elucidated in a 1992 Institute of Medicine (IOM) report, *Emerging Infections: Microbial Threats to Health in the United States*. A decade later, our understanding of the factors in emergence has been substantially influenced by a broader acceptance of the global nature of microbial threats. As a result, this report expands the original list, identifying thirteen factors in emergence (see Box 3-1). These thirteen factors are reviewed in turn in this chapter. The chapter ends with a case example—influenza—illustrating the interaction among the factors in the emergence of an infectious disease.

Future scientific discoveries and an increased understanding of the complexity of the emergence of infectious diseases will no doubt add to the list of factors identified in this report. In this light, the committee developed a model for conceptualizing how the factors in emergence converge to impact on the human–microbe interaction and result in infectious disease (see Figure 3-1). This model organizes the various factors into four broad domains: (1) genetic and biological factors; (2) physical environmental factors; (3) ecological factors; and (4) social, political, and economic factors. As we examine the individual factors, envisioning each as belonging to one or more of these four domains may simplify the understanding of the complex dynamics of emergence.

MICROBIAL ADAPTATION AND CHANGE

Microbes live on us and within us and inhabit virtually every available ecological niche of the external environment, and they will expand into new

---

BOX 3-1
Factors in Emergence

1992

- Microbial adaptation and change
- Economic development and land use
- Human demographics and behavior
- International travel and commerce
- Technology and industry
- Breakdown of public health measures

2003

- Microbial adaptation and change
- Human susceptibility to infection
- Climate and weather
- Changing ecosystems
- Human demographics and behavior
- Economic development and land use
- International travel and commerce
- Technology and industry
- Breakdown of public health measures
- Poverty and social inequality
- War and famine
- Lack of political will
- Intent to harm

---

niches that occur as we continue to alter the environment and extend our contact with the microbial world. Most of the microbes that live on or inside humans or exist in the environment do not cause disease in humans (see Box 3-2). These microbes may appear to be unimportant. However, they are often crucial to the human ecosystem. Moreover, microbes that have heretofore not affected humans directly may still represent a potent threat. Microbes that are pathogenic to the animals and plants on which we depend for survival, for example, are an indirect threat to human health. Other microbes live in apparent harmony with animals but can be pathogenic for humans, as evidenced by the number of emerging zoonotic diseases that are transmitted to humans from animals. Microbes are also adept at adaptation and change under selective pressures for survival and replication, including the use of antimicrobials by humans. Microbial adaptation and change continually challenge our responses to disease control and prevention. For example, the influenza virus is renowned for its ability to continually evolve so that new strains emerge each year, giving rise to

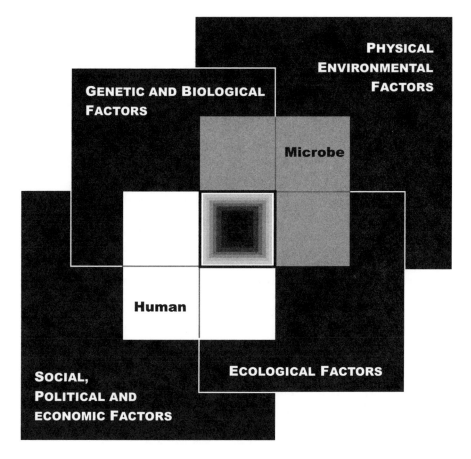

FIGURE 3-1 The Convergence Model. At the center of the model is a box representing the convergence of factors leading to the emergence of an infectious disease. The interior of the box is a gradient flowing from white to black; the white outer edges represent what is known about the factors in emergence, and the black center represents the unknown (similar to the theoretical construct of the "black box" with its unknown constituents and means of operation). Interlocking with the center box are the two focal players in a microbial threat to health—the human and the microbe. The microbe–host interaction is influenced by the interlocking domains of the determinants of the emergence of infection: genetic and biological factors; physical environmental factors; ecological factors; and social, political, and economic factors.

annual epidemics and necessitating the ongoing development of new influenza vaccine strains.

When the "germ theory" of disease was born in the late nineteenth century, Robert Koch and his contemporaries were convinced that diseases were caused by invariant, monomorphic microbial species. Early microbiologists dismissed the variants seen in petri dishes as mere contaminants—foreign entities that had floated into the culture medium from the atmosphere. Now, of course, the inherently variable nature of these early microbial species is well known. Microbes have enormous evolutionary potential and are continually undergoing genetic changes that allow them to bypass the human immune system, infect human cells, and spread disease. They may also traverse an alternative pathway that is a symbiotic accommodation to their hosts (see Box 3-2).

Numerous microbes have developed mechanisms to exchange or incorporate new genetic material into their genomes; even unrelated species can exchange virtually any stretch of DNA or RNA. Genomic sequencing of pathogens made possible by technological advances shows that horizontal movement, or lateral transfer, of DNA is common and may be responsible for the emergence of many new microbial species. Lateral transfer can involve the exchange of virulence genes (genes that confer pathogenicity) and/or other genes required for adapting to a particular host or environment. Indeed, the exchange of virulence genes is so pervasive among bacterial pathogens that species-specific chromosome regions containing virulence genes have inspired their own name—"pathogenicity islands" (Ochman and Moran, 2001; Groisman and Ochman, 1996; Hacker et al., 1997; Hacker and Kaper, 2000). Some pathogenicity islands encompass very large genetic regions, as many as 100 kilobases long. The transfer of just a single pathogenicity island in *E. coli* is sufficient to convert a benign strain into a pathogenic one (McDaniel and Kaper, 1997).

Pathogens have devised other means of adapting rapidly to new circumstances in their environment. RNA viruses, and retroviruses in particular, can mutate at very high rates, allowing them to adapt rapidly to changes in their external environment, including the presence of therapeutic drugs. Because microbes reproduce so quickly—as often as every 10 minutes—even very rare mutations build up rapidly in viral and bacterial populations. Many pathogenic bacteria have short runs of identical bases ("repeats") in their DNA; very minor changes in these repeats occur commonly and result in changes in gene expression. Moreover, many bacteria and viruses can sense changes in the external environment, and depending on what they sense, their genes can enable virtually instant changes in the regulation of certain sets of other genes, thus allowing the microbe to adapt to the new environment.

The more we learn about microbial genetics, structure, and function, the more we marvel at the sophistication of the survival strategies of microbes. Their mechanisms of survival are many and varied, and specific pathogens are generally tailored to flourish in particular niches. Many viruses and bacteria use our own cellular receptors to attach to and enter human cells; others utilize various human proteins for their own essential needs. Microbes use several means to defend themselves from being disabled or destroyed by the human immune system, including the rapid evolution of new antigenic variants, the masking of crucial surface antigens, inhibition of the immune system, and escape from the immune system by "hiding" inside human cells. Some microbes coat their surfaces with mimics of human tissue to prevent recognition by their human host as "nonself." As a result, the human immune response is not activated, and the microbe is ignored and left to survive and reproduce at will. Some microbes have evolved mechanisms to downregulate the human innate immune system, which would otherwise serve as the human body's first line of defense. Others stimulate an immune response that is injurious to the human host; for example, a sustained anti-self response may be triggered by viral or bacterial antigens that are molecular mimics of human antigens leading to chronic inflammation. Other strategies for survival include the ability to cause latent infections that can reactivate years later at a time when the host's immune responses are blunted. Clearly, pathogens are extraordinarily adept (and successful) in carrying out their game of survival of the fittest.

The development of preventive vaccines and antimicrobial therapies is among the greatest achievements of modern medicine. Unfortunately, the tremendous evolutionary potential of microbes empowers them with adeptness at developing resistance to even the most potent therapies and complicating attempts to create effective vaccines. In some cases, the antimicrobial drug target on the microbe mutates in such a way that binding of the antiviral or antibiotic no longer inhibits the virus or bacteria. For example, one of the major obstacles to the development of an effective vaccine against HIV is the very rapid antigenic change that the viral surface proteins undergo regularly. In fact, their mutation rate is so high that almost every retroviral particle is genetically different from every other particle by at least one nucleotide substitution. In other cases, bacteria have evolved enzymes that modify or destroy the antibiotic before it can reach its target inside the bacterium, or they "pump it back out" before it can do any damage to the microbe. Many genes for resistance can be transferred readily among different bacterial species; resistance can easily spread through multiple populations of species that occupy the same host environment.

Acquisition of genes for resistance is advantageous for the microbe only when it is under attack by therapeutics. The adapted microbe may be slightly less fit in the absence of antimicrobial therapy, and thus the organ-

BOX 3-2
The Microbiome

Medical science is imbued with the Manichaean view of the microbe–human host relationship: "we good; they evil." Indeed, the ascription of microbes to pathology has pervaded the teaching of biomedical science for over a century and consequently has left us with certain blind spots in our biological perspective of the pathogen–human host relationship. Obviously, microbes do have a knack for making us ill, killing us, and even recycling our remains to the geosphere. Nevertheless, in the long run, microbes have a shared interest in our survival. After all, if a pathogen does too much damage to its host, it will kill off not only the host but itself as well. "Domesticating" the host is a much better long-term strategy, and thus natural selection tends to favor less virulent pathogens that do not cause quite so much harm. Most successful parasites likely travel a middle path with regards to the amount of damage they do to their host; they need to be aggressive enough to enter the body surfaces and toxic enough to counter their host's defenses, but once established they also do themselves (and their hosts) well by moderating their virulence.

A better understanding of the host–pathogen relationship might be achieved by thinking of the host as a superorganism—or "microbiome"—with the host's genome and those of all of the host's indigenous microbes yoked into a chimera of sorts (Lederberg, 2000; Hooper and Gordon, 2001). The microbiome refers to the small biotic community that defines each of us as individuals, as well as the collective set of genomes that inhabit our skin, gut lumen, mucosal surfaces, and other body spaces. For the most part, the microbiome is a poorly catalogued ensemble, of which the majority of entries have yet to be cultivated and characterized, let alone understood with regard to their pathogenicity. Indeed, from a microbiome perspective, the mitochondria—which provide the oxidative metabolism machinery for every eukaryotic cell, from yeast to protozoa to multicellular organisms—can be regarded as the most successful of all human microbes. Mitochondria derive from an ancient lineage within the proteobacteria (Gray et al., 1999) and illustrate just how far the genomic collaboration between a host and a member of its indigenous microbial community can evolve.

Until recently, infectious disease research has given sparse attention to how microbes have evolved adaptations for sustaining themselves as chronic inhabitants or "domesticators" of their human hosts. The evolutionary rate of large, complex multicellulars such as ourselves is, for the most part, simply too slow to evolve their own resistance and keep pace with the rapid evolution of microbes. A year in microbial history matches all of primate, perhaps mammalian, evolution. Not only do microbes evolve much more quickly than humans, but their enormous evolutionary potential is further enhanced by their sheer numbers as well as their many ingenious mechanisms of gene exchange (e.g., conjugation and plasmid interchange).

Microbes can go beyond inhabiting our body space to completely set up genetic shop. Retroviruses, for example, are unable to replicate until they have become integrated into the host DNA; thereafter, their replication involves simply the fairly standard transcription of host chromosomal DNA into RNA copies. Indeed, it appears that some of the so-called HERVs (human endogenous retroviruses), with which the human genome is so heavily populated, have evolved so far as to participate in the physiology of our placenta and in our gustatory behavior. We have no idea what pathways HERVs have used to reach their target, nor can we predict the long-term consequences of their further evolution. But experience has shown we have every reason to expect that our most notorious retrovirus, HIV, will find a way to lodge itself in the germ line as well. The human genome encodes some 223 proteins with significant homology to bacterial proteins, suggesting that they were acquired from bacterial sources via horizontal transfer (Lander et al., 2001). These apparent insertions from microbial sources serve as further evidence of a historic host–microbe collaboration among the various components of the microbiome.

Our focus on "conquering" infectious disease may deflect from more ambitious, yet perhaps more pragmatic, aims; little consideration has been given to the notion that perhaps we could learn to live with a pathogen instead of being so insistent on getting rid of it. Natural history abounds with infections that have, over the course of evolutionary history, achieved a mutually tolerable state of equilibrium with their host. Genetic variation of the influenza A virus, for example, has remained stable in its wild aquatic bird reservoir, and infected avians often show no sign of disease. Although the recognition of AIDS in 1981 has inspired the most intense biomedical research program in history, the incidence of disease is only increasing. Would this trend reverse if, instead of focusing exclusively on ways to conquer HIV, we were to give equal weight to developing therapeutic measures that nurtured the immune system that HIV erodes?

Indeed, consider that many of the microbes that reside in our gut—such as *Lactobacillus* spp.—actually serve a protective, not a pathogenic, role. In fact, their protective advantage is currently being exploited in so-called "probiotic" therapy—the administration of live, benign microbes that benefit the host and aid in the treatment of disease (Hooper and Gordon, 2001; IOM, 2002b). Although scientists have known about the health benefits of lactic acid bacteria in particular for more than a century, the broader concept of probiotic therapy is a recent one (IOM, 2002b; Fuller, 1989). In addition to *Lactobacillum*, other probiotic preparations have contained *Bifidobacterium*, *Streptococcus* spp., and *E. coli*. Thus far, probiotic therapy has proven most beneficial in treating active ulcerative colitis, as well as complications following surgical intervention for that condition (Gionchetti et al., 2000; Rembacken et al., 1999). Probiotic lactobacillus may even prove useful in strengthening immune responses in persons infected with HIV. Normal bacterial flora are altered in HIV infection, as evidenced by the frequency of bacteremia associated with altered gastrointestinal function, diarrhea, and malabsorption; and failure-to-thrive, which is linked to altered gastrointestinal function, is relatively common in congenital HIV infection. Recent studies have shown that the effect of *L. plantarum* 299v, a specially developed probiotic lactobacillus, has a generally beneficial effect on the immune response in HIV-infected children (Cunningham-Rundles and Nesin, 2000).

The concept of probiotic therapeutics extends even beyond simply introducing a living microbe. Recent studies have demonstrated that genetically engineered gut commensal bacteria can be used as drug delivery platforms to treat infectious disease (Steidler et al., 2000; Beninati et al., 2000; Shaw et al., 2000). Other possible uses of probiotic therapy include using microbial products that target specific disease processes, such as weakened epithelial barriers or reduced activity of the mucosal immune system (Hooper and Gordon, 2001); using microbes that bear relevant cross-reacting epitopes instead of vaccines; and using them as optional food additives (Lederberg, 2000).

The rewards of a microbiomal perspective on infectious disease could be great. Not only would we achieve new insights with regard to how we and the microbes around and within us adapt to each other, and thus how pathogens emerge, but we would likely develop new approaches to preventing and treating infectious diseases.

ism may slowly revert to a sensitive state when therapy is withdrawn. Thus, the frequency of antimicrobial use is key; less use results in less resistance, while more use leads to more resistance. Unfortunately, antibiotics are frequently used when they are not truly needed (see the discussion of inappropriate use of antimicrobials in Chapter 4).

HUMAN SUSCEPTIBILITY TO INFECTION

Many properties of the human body—from its genetic makeup to its innate biological defenses—affect whether a microbe will cause disease. The body has evolved an abundance of physical, cellular, and molecular barriers that protect it from microbial infection, beginning with the skin. Even minor breaks in the skin increase susceptibility to infection. The normal bacterial flora of the gut and inner mucosal surfaces serve a protective role; not only do they occupy receptors to which pathogenic bacteria would otherwise attach themselves, but they produce antimicrobial substances that inhibit the growth of their pathogenic competitors. When these normal bacterial flora are reduced, as happens when a broad-spectrum antibiotic is used to treat an infection or when acidity in the stomach is reduced through various medications, the body is more susceptible to pathogens. Another protective defense mechanism is seen with the enzyme lactoferrin, which is plentiful in breast milk and on mucosal surfaces. Lactoferrin serves a protective role by sequestering iron, thereby making the mineral unavailable to invading pathogens that need it to reproduce. Susceptibility to infection can result when these normal defense mechanisms are altered or when host immunity is otherwise compromised as a result of impaired immune function; genetic polymorphisms; and other factors, such as aging and poor nutrition.

Impaired Host Immunity

The innate or nonspecific immune response is the body's initial inflammatory reaction to any kind of injury or microbial invasion. Innate immune defenses are believed to have first evolved in insects and other lower organisms that lack the ability to produce antibodies and thus depend entirely on this primitive but effective system for their protection against infection. In humans, more than a dozen different so-called TLRs (TOLL-like receptors)[1] have been found on cells that make up the mucosa and skin (including macrophages and dendritic cells), which is where pathogens first encounter their human host. When foreign molecules, such as bacterial DNA

---

[1]TOLL is a gene first discovered in *Drosophila*.

or flagella, bind to TLRs, they trigger a complex set of responses that leads to the production of inflammatory cytokines and local antimicrobial peptides. When the inflammation is inadequate to deal with an injury or microbial invader, the so-called adaptive or acquired specific immune response kicks in. This mechanism encompasses both cell-mediated and humoral responses. The former involves the production of antigen-specific T cells, which, depending on their surface protein makeup, serve a variety of functions, such as influencing the activities of other immune cells; the latter involves the production of antigen-specific B cells, which produce humoral antibodies.

New knowledge about the innate and specific immune responses is being used to develop potential therapies for infectious disease control. For example, the key to a good innate immune system defense is a balanced, regulated production of inflammatory cytokines. Otherwise, microbial infection can provoke such a massive release of inflammatory cytokines as to seriously damage and even kill their host. Researchers are exploring ways to interrupt the TLR pathways in order to either downregulate overly active inflammatory responses or upregulate weak responses. These could be useful strategies in the treatment of infectious diseases for which no otherwise effective specific therapies exist.

Genetic Polymorphisms

J.B.S. Haldane (1949) was among the first to suggest that pathogens serve as potent natural selective forces that have helped shape the evolution of human defenses against infection (Hill, 1998; Weatherall, 1996a; Lederberg, 1999). In particular, Haldane predicted that people who live in historically malaria-laden areas may have evolved genetic polymorphisms—in particular, heterozygous hemoglobinopathies—that increase their ability to survive infection with malaria.

Hemoglobinopathies are a group of diseases caused by or associated with the presence of abnormal hemoglobin in the blood; they are one of the most common single-gene disorders in humans. The hemoglobin gene has several allelic variants, including hemoglobin S, which, if homozygous, causes sickle cell disease. Hemoglobin S heterozygotes have the sickle cell trait and are virtually asymptomatic; however, they exhibit 80 to 95 percent protection against *P. falciparum* infection (Weatherall, 1996b). Hemoglobin S homozygosity exacts a cost in adverse health effects (as many persons of African descent have sickle cell disease), but clearly the protective power of this particular allelic variant is still under major selective pressure. Indeed, in areas free of malaria, sickle cell trait and sickle cell disease are very rare, or generally found only in lineages who have migrated from malaria-laden areas. Another structural hemoglobin variant, hemoglobin E, occurs at high frequencies throughout the Indian subcontinent, Burma, and Southeast Asia; in some areas, carriers make up as much as 50 percent of the population. Like hemoglobin S, hemoglobin E protects against *P. falciparum* (Flint et al., 1993; Weatherall, 1996b). More common than the structural variants hemoglobin S and E are a group of anemias known as thalassemias, which result from a defective production rate of either the alpha or the beta chain of the hemoglobin polypeptide. Again, heterozygotes are usually asymptomatic, and protection against malaria appears to have been the major selective force responsible for the more than 120 different beta thalassemia mutations, as well as the many different alpha thalassemia mutations (Weatherall, 1996b). The biological mechanism underlying the protective power of the heterozygous hemoglobinopathies is still unclear.

The presence of malaria in a population does more than modify hemoglobin. Several other malaria-related balanced polymorphisms, many of which involve the red blood cell structure and metabolism, have likewise evolved in response to the tremendous selective force exerted by the disease. Glucose-6-phosphate dehydrogenase deficiency (an X-linked chromosomal disorder), for example, serves a protective role in heterozygous female carriers and hemizygous males (Ruwende et al., 1995). Heterozygous carriers of a mutation in band 3 of the red blood cell membrane, which in its homozygous state causes the potentially lethal melanesian ovalocytosis, may also have a protective advantage. Finally, different blood group antigens may have evolved in response to past exposure to malaria (Miller, 1994). Racial differences in the distribution of certain red blood cell receptors for malaria parasites have been observed, possibly as a result of evolutionary genetic selection (IOM, 1991; Barragan et al., 2000; Hamblin et al., 2002). The Duffy antigen (a name taken from the hemophilia patient in whom it was first identified) is a parasite receptor on red blood cells that is recognized by certain forms of malaria, including *P. vivax* and *P. knowlesi*. Many persons of African descent lack the Duffy gene and therefore cannot be infected by either of these malaria parasites.

Other balanced polymorphisms have apparently evolved in response to malaria. For example, the tumor necrosis factor alpha gene and the HLA-DR class II genes both have polymorphic systems that have been linked to malaria (Hill et al., 1991). The remarkable human genetic diversity that has evolved in response to malaria, and that scientists have only just begun to uncover, suggests that other less common or less studied infections have probably generated extraordinary diversity as well. Fortunately, knowledge gleaned from the human genome project and its technological offshoots is leading to a dramatic explosion in new understandings of polymorphisms in a variety of genes that alter the response to infection. One of the most recently reported links between infection and natural selection is a deletion in the host-cell chemokine receptor CCR5, which reduces the risk of acquiring HIV infection after exposure (Sullivan et al., 2001). As another example, certain major histocompatibility complex class I molecules have been shown to reduce the risk of dying from HIV infection (Kaslow et al., 1996; Gao et al., 2001). Likewise, several different mutations or polymorphic systems influence the susceptibility to or likelihood of death from meningococcal infection (Read et al., 2000; Nadel et al., 1996; Westendorp et al., 1997). Numerous other examples exist of genetic associations with diseases, including cancers and chronic diseases, and the list is growing rapidly (Hill, 2001; Topcu et al., 2002; Chen et al., 2002a; Calhoun et al., 2002; Helminen et al., 2001; Pain et al., 2001).

Malnutrition

Host susceptibility to infection is aggravated by malnutrition. A strong and consistent relationship has been found between childhood malnutrition and increased risk of death from diarrhea, acute respiratory infection, and possibly malaria (Rice et al., 2000). Conversely, infectious processes, especially those associated with diarrhea, drive malnutrition in young children (Mata, 1992; Mata et al., 1977), so that diarrheal illness is both a cause and an effect of malnutrition (Guerrant et al., 1992; Wierzba et al., 2001; Lima et al., 1992). Clinically, malnutrition is characterized by inadequate intake of protein, energy, and micronutrients and by frequent infections or disease (WHO, 2002d). Malnutrition has been associated with 50 percent of all deaths among children worldwide (Rice et al., 2000). In 2000, an estimated 150 million of the world's children under age 5 were malnourished on the basis of low weight for age (WHO, 2002d). More than two-thirds (70 percent) of these children were in Asia, especially southern Asia. The number of malnourished children living in Africa—26 percent of the world's malnourished children—has risen as a result of population growth in the region, as well as natural disasters, wars, civil disturbances, and population displacement (WHO, 2000b).

Malnutrition diminishes host resistance to infection through a number of mechanisms. Virtually all bodily processes and physical barriers that keep infectious agents from invading the host are affected. These include the skin, mucous membranes, gastric acidity, absorptive capacity, intestinal flora, cell-mediated immunity, phagocyte function, and cytokine production (Chandra, 1997; Levander, 1997). Although multiple-nutrient deficiencies are much more common than single-nutrient deficiencies, lack of even one vitamin or mineral (e.g., zinc; selenium; iron; copper; vitamins A, C, E, B-6, and folic acid) can impair the immune response. For example, vitamin A deficiency significantly increases the risk of severe illness and death from common childhood infections, such as diarrheal disease and measles, by diminishing the host's resistance to infection. For children deficient in vitamin A, the periodic supplying of high-dose vitamin A has reduced mortality by 23 percent overall and by up to 50 percent for those who suffer from acute measles (WHO, 2002d). The relative risk of measles mortality in children younger than 2 years of age has been shown to be significantly reduced when the children's diets are supplemented with vitamin A for only 2 days (Barclay et al., 1987; West, 2000). Consequently, WHO recommends treating children who have measles, prolonged diarrhea, wasting malnutrition, or other acute infections with vitamin A (IOM, 2002c; WHO, 1997). Furthermore, studies have suggested an association between maternal vitamin A deficiency and an increased risk of vertical HIV transmission from mother to child (Semba et al., 1994; Greenberg et al., 1997). It is not yet clear, however, what role vitamin A supplementation has in the management of HIV infection.

CLIMATE AND WEATHER

Many elements of the physical environment influence the host directly; determine the survival of agents that exist outside the host; and mediate the transmission of agents between hosts, including the movement from animal to human hosts. Viewed in this light, the physical environment takes on considerable importance in determining the epidemiology of infectious diseases (Wilson, 2001). The interactions among vectors, animal reservoirs, microbes, and humans present many opportunities for changes in the physical environment to influence transmission dynamics. Many of the factors that affect the abundance, survival, activity, or feeding behavior of vectors also impact on the reproduction, survival, and abundance of animal reservoirs. For example, elevated rainfall often creates new breeding habitats for mosquitoes, leading to an increase in mosquito population density. Increased levels of precipitation can also lead to decreased marsh salinity, which in turn may increase the survival rates of certain toxic aquatic bacteria. Likewise, these same factors can affect human behavior or exposure to infection by impacting outdoor activities, housing, the quality and quantity of food, and agricultural or other uses of the environment.

Among the numerous elements of the physical environment that influence the emergence of infectious diseases, climate and weather[2] have received a great deal of attention in recent years. Many infectious diseases either are strongly influenced by short-term weather conditions or display a seasonality suggesting that they are influenced by longer-term climatic

---

[2]Weather refers to short-term fluctuations in the atmosphere, such as changes in cloudiness or temperature, whereas climate usually refers to average weather over a period of time.

changes (Patz et al., 2000). Climate can directly impact disease transmission through its effects on the replication and movement (and perhaps evolution) of disease microbes and vectors; climate can also operate indirectly through its impacts on ecology or human behavior (NRC, 2001). To be transported over relatively large distances from one host to another, many microbes must be borne passively through moving air or water. Some pathogenic microbes, such as those causing coccidiomycosis (see Box 3-3), are picked up from the soil and carried by dry, dusty winds (Schneider et al., 1997); some opportunistic human pathogens can apparently survive transoceanic transport in dust clouds (Griffin et al., 2001); and others, such as cryptosporidiosis, may be washed by heavy rains into reservoirs of drinking water (Alterholt et al., 1998) (see Box 3-4). The 1993 hantavirus outbreak in the southwestern United States, due to an El Nino event, is an example of how climatic factors have contributed to the emergence of infectious disease (see the later discussion of hantavirus). Likewise, higher water temperatures in the Pacific Northwest resulting from a 1997 El Nino event provided unusual conditions favorable to the growth of *Vibrio parahaemolyticus*, which led to a shellfish-associated outbreak of disease (CDC, 1998a).

The fact that local and regional climatic factors clearly influence disease emergence has led scientists to suggest that projected global climate changes will have an impact on infectious disease emergence. Climatologists project upward trends in global temperatures and estimate that by 2100, temperatures will have increased by 1.4–5.8°C (Intergovernmental Panel on Climate Change, 2001a). Climate change has already been detected, and impacts from such change are sure to follow. Arthropod-borne diseases, such as malaria, yellow fever, and dengue, are expected to be affected more readily than other types of diseases by climate change since arthropod transmission patterns are highly sensitive to changes in ambient temperature. Waterborne diseases, such as cryptosporidiosis, may also be affected (Patz et al., 2001). However, to fully assess the effects of climate change, both confounding factors (e.g., drug resistance, crop yields, population migration) and the adaptive capacity of a population must be considered. Many argue that at present, other factors—including human population density and the capacity of the public health system to prevent and control infectious disease outbreaks—affect disease risk more than does global climatic change. Indirectly, if global climatic change were to result in reduced food availability, thereby producing undernourished human populations more vulnerable to disease, its impact on infectious disease could be dramatic (Intergovernmental Panel on Climate Change, 2001b). Likewise, if social disruption, economic decline, and displaced populations were to emerge as a result of reduced food availability due to global climate change,

BOX 3-3
Fungal Threats

In 1994, a major earthquake shook Ventura County, California, generating massive landslides in the Santa Susana Mountains just north of Simi Valley. These landslides resulted in the formation of large dust clouds that were dispersed into nearby valleys by northeast winds. Within the dust clouds were tiny arthrospores of the fungus *Coccidioides immitis*. As the dust clouds settled over Ventura County, residents of the area inhaled the contaminated air; the result was 203 cases of coccidioidomycosis (also known as Valley fever and San Joaquin Valley fever), including three fatalities associated with this event (Schneider et al., 1997).

The dimorphic fungus *Coccidioides immitis* that causes coccidioidomycosis, grows in topsoil layers in the southwestern United States, Mexico, and parts of Central and South America. It is transmitted through the air following the disturbance of contaminated soil, as in the case of dust storms, earthquakes, and excavations. It is not transmitted from person to person. Although 60 percent of infected individuals are asymptomatic, the remainder can develop a range of infirmities, from influenza-like illness, to pneumonia, to severe pulmonary and extrapulmonary disease in immunocompromised individuals (CDC, 1994a). Simple environmental measures, such as planting grass and paving roads, can lower the risk of airborne dispersion of *C. immitis*. As of 2002, however, no practical method for eliminating the organism had been developed. National surveillance for coccidioidomycosis began through the National Electronic Telecommunications System for Surveillance (NETSS) in 1995; the disease is reportable in California, New Mexico, and Arizona.

In addition to dissemination by dust clouds, fungal infections can be a health threat for travelers to regions of the world where these infections are endemic (Panackal, 2002). Travelers have developed fungal infections as a result of a wide range of recreational and work activities. For example, an outbreak of coccidioidomycosis occurred in a church group from Washington State upon returning from Tecate, Mexico, where these members of the congregation had assisted with construction projects at an orphanage. Following the outbreak, *Coccidioides immitis* was isolated from soil samples taken from Tecate (Cairns et al., 2000). College students visiting Acapulco, Mexico, were diagnosed with histoplasmosis, an infection caused by the soil-inhabiting fungus *Histoplasma capsulatum*, after staying at a beach resort hotel (CDC, 2001d). Similarly, Italian spelunkers returning from Mato Grosso, Peru, displayed signs and symptoms consistent with histoplasmosis (Nasta et al., 1997). Other potential mycotic disease threats include blastomycosis, which is endemic to parts of the south-central, southeastern, and midwestern United States, as well as Central and South America and parts of Africa; cryptococcosis, the fungal agent of which has been isolated from soil worldwide, usually in association with bird droppings; aspergillosis; candidiasis; and sporotrichosis (CDC, 2001e).

BOX 3-4
An Outbreak of Cryptosporidiosis

Cryptosporidiosis, a waterborne intestinal infection caused by *Cryptosporidium* spp., produces potentially life-threatening disease in those who are immunocompromised and mild to chronic diarrhea in others (Fayer and Ungar, 1986). In 1993, an estimated 403,000 crytposporidiosis infections occurred among residents of and visitors to Milwaukee, Wisconsin (MacKenzie et al., 1994). Cryptospordium oocysts in untreated water from Lake Michigan had apparently been inadequately removed by the coagulation and filtration process in a portion of the Milwaukee water treatment plant. The source of the oocysts leading to the outbreak remains speculative. Possible sources include cattle along two rivers that flow into the Milwaukee harbor, slaughterhouses, and human sewage. Various vertebrates (e.g., cows and wild deer) are naturally infected by *Cryptosporidium* spp. (Navin and Juranek, 1984; Simpson, 1992; Tzipori et al., 1981). Perhaps considerable rainfall, combined with a high concentration of animal runoff near the municipal water supply, triggered this transmission event. Genotypic and experimental infection data may suggest a human rather than bovine source (Peng et al., 1997). In the 2 years following this contamination of the water supply, it was estimated that 54 deaths (85 percent among people with AIDS) may have resulted from the 1993 outbreak (Hoxie et al., 1997). In addition to contaminated drinking water, outbreaks of cryptosporidiosis in the United States and abroad have been linked to chlorinated and unchlorinated recreational water facilites, such as public swimming pools, water parks, lakes, and rivers (Carpenter et al., 1999).

the emergence and spread of infectious disease would likely be substantially impacted. A recent National Research Council (NRC) report, *Under The Weather: Climate, Ecosystems, and Infectious Disease*, addresses the impact of climate and weather change in further detail (NRC, 2001).

CHANGING ECOSYSTEMS

The abundance and distribution of plants and animals can, conversely, impact on components of the physical environment. Forest growth, for example, usually reduces evapotranspiration; cropping often increases local relative humidity; and the development of large urban areas generally leads to an accumulation of atmospheric particulates and warmer air temperatures. Even very minor ecological changes, such as implementing a new farming technique, can confront pathogens with new environments and significantly alter the transmission patterns of infectious diseases. Of course, the pathogens must have sufficient genetic variation to adapt to such ecological changes and new environments. But most pathogenic evolutionary changes that result in a potentially new disease still require an ecological cofactor for the disease to actually take root (Stephens et al., 1998). In other words, regardless of its genetic prowess, the pathogen still must be able to reach its animal (or human) host or vector.

Given today's rapid pace of economic development and enormous scale of ecological changes, understanding how environmental factors are impacting on the emergence of infectious diseases has assumed an added urgency. To the pressing issues of environmental conservation, natural resource utilization, population growth, and economic development can be added the need to understand the interplay of these processes with the emergence of infectious diseases. Such environmental and ecological factors are playing an increasingly important role in disease emergence. In general, changes in the environment tend to have the greatest influence on the transmission of microbial agents that are waterborne, airborne, foodborne, or vector-borne, or that have an animal reservoir.

Vector Ecology

Pathogens transmitted by mosquitoes and their arthropod allies sicken millions of people each year, cause inestimable morbidity in humans and animals around the globe, and remain major barriers to social and economic development in much of the tropical world. Of the ten diseases targeted by WHO for special control programs, seven have arthropod vectors (WHO 2003a). Many of these diseases—for example, dengue, yellow fever, and malaria—which were controlled to a substantial degree, are now resurgent in many formerly endemic areas. Malaria continues to afflict much of the tropical world and causes an estimated 1.5 million to 2 million deaths per year. More than 2.5 billion people are at risk for dengue virus infection; 100 million cases of dengue are estimated to occur annually, and the incidence of dengue hemorrhagic fever is increasing rapidly throughout the tropics. Yellow fever virus has recently caused major epidemics in Africa and South America (Gubler, 2001; Monath, 2001), and sylvatic reservoirs in these areas provide an ongoing threat for its reintroduction into *Aedes aegypti*–infested metropolitan areas throughout the world. *Ae. aegypti* is also the principal vector of the dengue viruses. Vector-borne diseases continue to emerge in new areas and/or to resurge throughout the world, even in areas where they were previously controlled. Many newly emerged pathogens and diseases, including Sin Nombre and Andes viruses (and a plethora of other newly discovered hantaviruses), Guanarito, Lyme disease, and ehrlichiosis all have rodent hosts and/or arthropod vectors (Mills et al., 1999; Gubler, 1998; Gratz, 1999). Others, such as the Seoul, dengue, Japanese encephalitis, West Nile, and Rift Valley fever (RVF) viruses (see Box 3-5), have demonstrated their ability to emerge in new or

BOX 3-5
Rift Valley Fever

Rift Valley fever (RVF) provides an excellent example of how ecological conditions determine pathogen transmission. In Saudi Arabia, 453 individuals with suspected hemorrhagic fever required hospitalization from August to October 2000 (WHO, 2000c). The case-fatality rate was 19 percent, with a median age of 47 years and an age range of 1 to 95 years. In Yemen, 1,087 similarly suspected case-patients were identified from August to November 2000; 121 of them died (CDC, 2000c). The mean age of suspected cases was 32.2 years, with an age range of 1 month to 95 years. Symptoms included low-grade fever, abdominal pain, vomiting, diarrhea, and jaundice with liver and kidney dysfunction, often progressing to death. Three out of 4 case-patients reported being exposed to sick animals, handling an abortus, or slaughtering animals in the week before the onset of illness. Using diagnostics, including antigen and antibody detection, polymerase chain reaction, virus isolation, and immunohistochemistry, the CDC confirmed the diagnosis of RVF. Satellite images and aerial surveys revealed numerous areas throughout the coastal plain and adjacent mountains that would be conducive to transmission of the RVF virus. Entomologic studies revealed large numbers of two species of mosquitoes—*Culex tritaeniorrhynchus* and *Aedes caspius*—in the flood irrigation farming areas where most of the human cases were reported. The mechanism of virus trafficking is not clear; however, it is thought that animal relocation from Africa may have resulted in introduction of the virus into Saudi Arabia. It is now believed that the RVF virus may be able to establish itself almost anywhere in the world, given the availability of potential permissive vectors and animal reservoirs.

RVF virus was first recognized and isolated as the agent of a zoonotic disease in Kenya in 1930. The disease is now widespread throughout much of the African continent. RVF virus is transmitted mainly by floodwater *Aedes* spp., which feed primarily on animals. Mosquitoes may be infected transovarially, but domestic ungulates (cattle, sheep, goats, etc.) amplify transmission and become sufficiently viremic to infect other "bridge" mosquitoes (e.g., *Culex* spp.), which can then infect humans (Wilson, 1994). Virus transmission is linked to periodic heavy rainfalls that fill shallow depressions called dambos, where mosquitoes, such as *Ae. macintoshi*, lay their eggs. This vector has been associated with vertical transmission of the virus to progeny, thereby providing a mechanism for the virus to survive adverse climatic conditions. When the dambos are flooded, infected mosquitoes can emerge to initiate the transmission cycle. The local abundance of ungulates, their movement while searching for forage, and their proximity to humans are important in the epidemiology of the disease. Thus, complex ecological factors impact on where, when, and with what intensity RVF emerges (Linthicum et al., 1999). Outbreaks outside of sub-Saharan Africa occurred in Egypt in 1977–1978 and again in 1993; the identification of RVF in Saudi Arabia and Yemen in 2000 (Ahmad, 2000) was the first confirmation of its occurrence beyond the African continent.

previously endemic regions, thereby causing significant morbidity and mortality.

Arthropod-borne parasitic diseases, such as malaria, filariasis, onchocerciasis, trypanosomiasis, and leishmaniasis, remain major human threats. An estimated 120 million people suffer from lymphatic filariasis, and approximately 18 million people are afflicted with onchocerciasis, of whom about 340,000 are blind and an equal number visually impaired. More than 10 million people are afflicted with leishmaniasis, and 50,000 to 100,000 individuals die of visceral leishmaniasis each year in India alone. In Latin America, an estimated 20 million people have Chagas disease. In Africa, approximately 45 million people are at risk for African trypanosomiasis, which has virtually precluded domestic livestock production in a geographic region of Africa larger than the United States and now is tragically resurgent in humans in areas in East Africa.

Ecological and environmental conditions are key determinants of the transmission and persistence of vector-borne pathogens. Ecological conditions can increase the risk of infection by altering human exposure to vectors or changing their distribution, abundance, longevity, activity, and habitat associations, and thereby increasing or decreasing the overall potential for the vector population to transmit the pathogen to humans. Mosquito abundance and transmission of pathogens are typically associated with rainy seasons, since juvenile mosquitoes develop in aquatic habitats. Dengue transmission, for example, typically occurs during the rainy season, although the prior month's temperature has been shown to affect transmission during the rainy season (Focks et al., 1995). Populations of floodwater- and container-breeding mosquitoes (e.g., *Ae. aegypti*) are dramatically affected by environmental conditions; their abundance is directly linked to rainfall (or snowmelt for temperate-zone mosquitoes), which induces the eggs to hatch. In contrast, transmission of Saint Louis encephalitis virus may be greatest in relatively dry periods after the rainy season (Shaman et al., 2002). The preferred breeding site of the principal vector, *Culex quinquefasciatus*, is stagnating pools of water with concentrated nutrient materials, and thus mosquito abundance increases during drier conditions, which favor the formation of such breeding sites. The emergence and re-emergence of vector-borne pathogens are linked to changes in temperature (which determines how long it takes the parasite to develop), wind speed, and relative humidity (all of which affect vector feeding frequency); the amount and diversity of vegetation; and the presence of alternative hosts (which can alter the rate of blood feeding on humans). In particular, as previously discussed, global warming could theoretically result in dramatic alterations in the incidence and distribution of vector-borne diseases.

The movement of goods and people can also support the movement of vectors, allowing them to become established in new areas (see the later discussion of international travel and commerce). This is certainly not a recent development. Probably the most notable public health example of such events is the dissemination of *Ae. aegypti* throughout the world (Tabachnick et al., 1985). After domestication and adaptation to humans and human environments, *Ae. aegypti* apparently spread to coastal areas of Africa, and was then transported throughout the world in sailing ships. Presumably *Ae. aegypti*, as well as yellow fever virus, was introduced into the New World on slave ships. *Ae. albopictus*, the Asian tiger mosquito, likely entered the United States via shipping (Moore, 1999). *Aedes* spp. eggs can easily be transported in such objects as waterlogged tires to new areas and hatch upon exposure to water. The large shipping containers used to transport so many products provide excellent environments for the transport of mosquito eggs. This presumably occurred recently as well with *Ae. japonicus* (Fonseca et al., 2001). Adult mosquitoes can be spread much more quickly throughout the world in the cabins or other areas of airplanes (Lounibus, 2002). Traveling mosquitoes can also rapidly introduce new genes, leading to the emergence of epidemiologically important vector phenotypes in new areas. Jet transport has been postulated as a mechanism for the rapid dissemination of an esterase mutation conferring pesticide resistance to organophosphates on *Culex pipiens* populations throughout the world (Raymond et al., 1998).

Traveling viremic humans can easily disseminate dengue virus to new areas via jet travel, and with the establishment of the mosquito *Ae. aegypti* in tropical and subtropical areas, can readily introduce new and perhaps virulent virus genotypes into susceptible populations. These same areas are also at risk for introduction of yellow fever virus, which is likewise transmitted by *Ae. aegypti*. Between 1970 and 2000, seven cases of yellow fever in unvaccinated travelers from the United States and Europe were reported (Monath and Cetron, 2002). It would appear to be inevitable for yellow fever to be introduced into new areas, such as Asia, with potentially catastrophic results.

Reservoir Abundance and Distribution

It has been estimated that 75 percent of all emerging infections are zoonotic, i.e., they can be transmitted from animals to humans (Taylor et al., 2001a). In some cases, the mechanisms of transmission of a pathogen from animals to humans has been identified, but the transmission of the same pathogen between various animal reservoirs remains a mystery (see Box 3-6). Pathogens transmitted to humans directly from rodents (e.g., rodent-borne viral diseases) or maintained in nature by rodents and transmitted to humans by arthropods (e.g., Lyme disease, erhlichiosis, plague)

Box 3-6
Nipah Virus

Between September 1998 and June 1999, an outbreak of a Japanese enceph-alitis-like illness occurred among people from several pig-farming villages in Malaysia; 265 cases of febrile encephalitis were reported to the Malaysian Ministry of Health, including over 100 deaths (Chua et al., 2000; Goh et al., 2000; WHO, 2001e). The majority of illnesses were characterized by 3–14 days of fever and headache, followed by drowsiness and disorientation that progressed to coma within 24–48 hours. In other cases, however, the infection was mild or inapparent. Most of the affected individuals were adult men who had histories of close contact with swine. During March of the same year, nine similar cases of encephalitis and two cases of respiratory illness that resembled some of what had been seen in the Malaysia outbreak were reported in Singapore; all eleven had handled swine im-ported from Malaysia. Concurrent with the human cases, many pigs in the regions were also becoming ill and dying.

Tissue culture isolation from human and swine central nervous system speci-mens resulted in the identification of a previously unknown infectious agent, later named Nipah virus after the village of Sungei Nipah where it is believed the out-break originated through infected bats that frequent the fruit trees near the pig farms. These fruit bats are distributed across northern, eastern, and southeastern areas of Australia, Indonesia, Malaysia, the Philippines, and some of the Pacific Islands. Infected bats appear to be asymptomatic reservoirs; it is unknown how the virus is transmitted from the bats to pigs. More than 900,000 pigs were culled in response to the outbreak (Uppal, 2000).

Transmission of the Nipah virus to humans is primarily through direct contact with infected pigs or contaminated swine tissue; no evidence has been found for any person-to-person transmission. Although pigs are the only source of human infection identified thus far, they may not be the only one. For example, dogs infected with the Nipah virus have also shown a distemper-like illness, although no epidemiological link has been found between their infection and human disease; likewise, horses have shown serological evidence of infection, which again does not appear to be linked to human disease. The apparent ability of Nipah virus to infect a wide range of hosts and the fact that it causes a fatal and untreatable disease in humans have made this emerging infection an important public health concern.

make up a significant proportion of emerging and resurging diseases (Mills and Childs, 1998). Epidemics of plague, tularemia, relapsing fever, and typhus have all occurred in recent years. Exacerbating the situation is the potential for many of these agents to be weaponized and used intentionally for harm. Rodent-borne viral diseases have been unusually refractory to control or eradication programs and continue to emerge as significant pathogens of human and animal populations. Many newly emerged viruses (e.g., Sin Nombre virus and other hantaviruses, and Guanarito and other arenaviruses) have rodents as primary hosts. The high mortality rates associated with these rodent-borne hemorrhagic fevers and hantavirus pulmonary syndrome generate great concern in the medical, scientific, and public health communities—and among the general public. Rodent-borne diseases will undoubtedly continue to emerge and increase in medical significance in many areas of the world.

Ecological and environmental conditions determine the epidemic potential of pathogens transmitted by animal reservoirs. Transmisson of arenaviruses—such as Junin virus (found in the corn mouse, *Calomys musculinus*) in Argentina, Machupo virus (in *Calomys calosus*) in Bolivia, and Lassa virus (from multimammate rats [*Mastomys spp.*]) in Africa—has strong environmental determinants. Transmission of each of these pathogens occurs via contact with rodent urine, feces, or tissues; the stability of the pathogens is influenced by humidity and sunlight. A strong link exists between the density of rodent reservoirs and arenaviral diseases in humans. For example, a longitudinal study of *C. musculinus* populations in an area in which Argentine hemorrhagic fever was endemic demonstrated a dramatic increase in the density of rodents immediately preceding an outbreak of human disease (Mills et al., 1992). During an outbreak of Bolivian hemorrhagic fever in San Joaquin, nearly 3,000 rodents (*C. callosus*) (about 10 per household) were removed during a 3-week period, apparently contributing to the rapid decline in new cases (Mercado, 1975). Changes in resources and predators that affect the abundance of rodents, combined with patterns of agricultural production and land use, appear to be the major determinants of risk for many arenaviral diseases.

The emergence of Sin Nombre virus and other hantaviral agents provides a textbook example of the effect of ecological forces on rodent distribution and abundance (Nichol et al., 1993). In 1993, an outbreak of acute respiratory distress disease occurred in the southwestern United States, with the initial cases occurring predominantly among Native Americans. The case fatality rate was approximately 60 percent, causing widespread anxiety and enormous media interest in this newly emerged disease. Sin Nombre virus (genus *Hantavirus*, family Bunyaviridae) was identified as the etiologic agent of this disease, designated hantavirus pulmonary syndrome (Nichol et al., 1993; Elliott et al., 1994). This finding was unexpected; the only other hantaviruses known in the United States at that time were Prospect Hill virus, which was not known to cause human illness, and Seoul virus, which had been associated with mild renal illnesses in humans in the eastern portion of the country (Glass et al., 1994). Thus, no a priori reason existed to associate the acute respiratory disease outbreak in 1993 with hantavirus infection.

Hantaviruses are found worldwide and are major causes of morbidity and mortality in Asia and Europe (Schmaljohn and Hjelle, 1997). In Eurasia, Hantaan virus infections have been associated with illnesses causing significant mortality following acute, systemic disorders characterized by fever, hemorrhagic manifestations, and renal failure. These illnesses have usually been clinically diagnosed as hemorrhagic fever with renal syndrome (HFRS) or Korean hemorrhagic fever. Several other viruses, including Dobrava-Belgrade virus, Puumala virus, and Seoul virus, cause similar diseases. Renal involvement, rather than respiratory symptoms, is the hallmark of these diseases.

Hantaviruses are transmitted directly between rodents and to humans via excreta (dried saliva, urine, feces). Human-to-human transmission of Sin Nombre virus has not been reported, although there is evidence from Argentina for direct human-to-human transmission of Andes virus, which is very closely related to Sin Nombre virus (Padula et al., 1998). The rodent reservoir of Sin Nombre virus has been identified as the deer mouse, *Peromyscus maniculatus*, one of the most commonly occurring and widely distributed mammals in North America (Childs et al., 1994). Hence, Sin Nombre virus shares a similar widespread distribution, but prevalence rates of the virus in this rodent reservoir can differ temporally and spatially (Mills et al., 1999).

Identification of a hantavirus as the etiologic agent of the hantavirus pulmonary syndrome epidemic prompted increased surveillance for these agents in the Western Hemisphere that has revealed an array of heretofore unrecognized hantaviruses. Cases of hantavirus pulmonary syndrome have now been documented in 31 states, Canada, and Central and South America, and serologic evidence has demonstrated the presence of hantaviral infections in Mexican rodents. More cases of the syndrome are now recognized to occur in South than in North America (Calisher et al., 2002). Of the 39 hantaviruses now recognized (CDC, 2002v), 25 have been identified since 1994, 11 occur exclusively in the United States, and many new ones have been identified in Central and South America (see Figure 3-2). Each hantavirus is associated with a primary rodent reservoir host, suggesting that more hantaviruses will be discovered as new rodent hosts are assayed for these pathogens (Monroe et al., 1999).

Data from the National Science Foundation's Long-Term Ecological Research Site at Sevilleta in Central New Mexico reveal that *P. maniculatus* densities increased dramatically beginning in the early 1990s and were highest in 1993 (Yates et al., 2002a). These conditions may have resulted from an El Nino Southern Oscillation event in previous years, which had caused ample rainfall, warm winters, dramatically increased plant productivity, and abundant forage for *P. maniculatus*. In an area of southwestern Colorado near hantavirus pulmonary syndrome cases, *P. maniculatus* abundance was estimated to be as high as 50 per hectare, and Sin Nombre virus antibody prevalence rates exceeded 50 percent (Childs et al., 1994). These areas have subsequently been monitored continuously in long-term longitu-

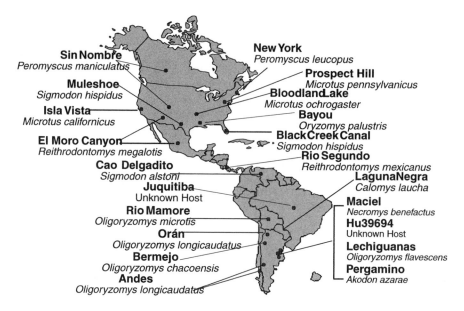

FIGURE 3-2 New world hantaviruses (bold) and their rodent reservoirs (italics). SOURCE: CDC, 2002x.

dinal studies of hantaviruses in rodent reservoirs in the southwestern United States as part of a landmark effort by the CDC to understand the environmental and epidemiologic determinants of hantavirus emergence and to develop predictive models for risk assessment (Boone et al., 1998; Glass et al., 2000; Hjelle and Glass, 2000). Rodent population densities and seroprevalence rates have not been as high in Sin Nombre virus–endemic areas since the 1993 outbreak. However, an additional El Nino Southern Oscillation event in 1997 resulted in an increased number of human hantavirus pulmonary syndrome cases and a growth in rodent populations; a more refined model for Sin Nombre virus emergence was subsequently developed (Yates et al., 2002a).

ECONOMIC DEVELOPMENT AND LAND USE

The physical environment is constantly being modified by human activities. Most economic development activities, including the consumption of natural resources, deforestation, and dam building, have some intended or unintended impact on the environment, or both. In the present context, it is important to note that a growing number of emerging infectious diseases arise from increased human contact with animal reservoirs as a result of changing land use patterns. A recent example of this phenomenon is Venezuelan hemorrhagic fever, a new disease that was identified in 1989 and emerged following the transformation of forest to agricultural land, which provided a highly favorable environment for the probable reservoir host, the cane mouse *Zygodontomys brevicauda* (IOM, 2002d). Other examples include increases in malaria following the clearing of land for rubber plantations in Malaysia; increases in schistosomiasis, malaria, and other infectious diseases following the Volta River project in Africa; increases in vector-borne diseases after the construction of new transportation routes in Brazil; and the emergence of Lyme disease in the United States after the reforestation of abandoned farmlands in the northeast (Mayer, 2000). Even the emergence of HIV is believed to have been due to increased contact with nonhuman primates infected with the related simian immunodeficiency viruses (SIVs); exposure to infected blood during the hunting and field dressing of animals and the preparation of primate meat for consumption may have led to human infection. Indeed, compelling evidence indicates that SIV counterparts of HIV, specifically SIVcpz from chimpanzees and SIVsm from sooty mangabeys, have been introduced into the human population on multiple occasions, generating HIV types 1 and 2 (HIV-1 and HIV-2), respectively (IOM, 2002b).

Reforestation and Lyme Disease

Lyme disease is a classic example of a microbial threat influenced by multiple environmental determinants. The principal vector in North America is the deer tick, *Ixodes scapularis*, which must take blood meals as larva, nymph, and adult to survive and reproduce. Wild rodents, especially *Peromyscus* spp. in the northeastern and midwestern United States and *Neotina* spp. in the western United States, serve as reservoirs for the bacterial agent of Lyme disease, *Borrelia burgdorferi*, but white-tailed deer are the definitive hosts for the adult ticks. The emergence of the disease has been linked in part to the reforestation of former farm land, which led to a dramatic increase in the distribution and abundance of white-tail deer populations (Barbour and Fish, 1993). People become infected when they encounter the tick vector, usually during outdoor recreation or near residences in wooded areas. Prior to the reforestation of land formerly cleared for farming, Lyme disease was unrecognized. Lyme disease has increased in incidence and geographic distribution in the past 10 years in the continental United States, and as people continue to build homes and expand their neighborhoods even farther into reforested areas, the number of cases continues to rise. The preservation of vertebrate biodiversity and community composition may help reduce the incidence of Lyme disease (LoGiudice et al., 2003).

Dam Building and Schistosomiasis

Environmental changes resulting in the creation of standing water, such as dam building or the diversion of water by canalization and irrigation, have been implicated in the reemergence of infectious diseases transmitted by mosquitoes and other arthropod vectors. For example, the incidence of Japanese encephalitis, which accounts for approximately 7,000 deaths annually in Asia, is closely associated with the increase in mosquitoes that reproduce as a consequence of flooding fields for rice growing (Morse, 1995). Outbreaks of RVF in some parts of Africa have been associated with increased mosquito density as a result of dam building, as well as periods of heavy rainfall (Monath, 1993).

Environmental changes involving dam-building and irrigation projects appear to be allowing the spread of schistosomiasis to new areas. More than 200 million people worldwide are infected by and up to three times as many are at risk of this parasitic worm disease which causes chronic urinary tract disease and often results in cirrhosis of the liver and bladder cancer (WHO, 1999a). The development of dams in the Senegal River basin, for example, is among the major factors leading to a significantly increased prevalence of schistosomiasis over a period of only 3 years (Gryseels, 1994). Similarly, the Aswan High Dam has been implicated in increased rates of schistosomiasis in Egypt (El Alamy and Cline, 1977; Abdel-Wahab, 1982). The potential for the Three Gorges Project in China to create conditions conducive to schistosomiasis transmission concerns many scientists.

Schistosomiasis is caused by trematode worms or blood flukes of the genus *Schistosoma*. Transmission is primarily in tropical or subtropical regions and involves certain snail species, primarily of the genera *Biomphalaria*, *Bulinus*, and *Onchomelonia*, that serve as a host for the development of one stage of the parasite's life cycle. Humans become infected as they work or bathe in water infested with *Schistosoma* larvae released by snails. These larvae penetrate the skin and travel to internal organs, where they mature to adult worms that mate and reproduce. Human disease is a consequence of reaction to the eggs deposited in tissues by adult worms that live for years inside chronically infected people. The eggs are released when people urinate or defecate, and if they do so into snail-infested waters, more snails become infected, hence perpetuating the cycle. Thus, both people and snails are important to *Schistosoma* biology, and environmental changes that affect either can increase the risk of infection. The rise in water levels and change in flow rates that result from dam building may increase the contact between snails and parasites, as well as create fertile soil and sand beds that propagate the development of snails.

HUMAN DEMOGRAPHICS AND BEHAVIOR

The opportunity for transfer of a microbe from one human to another has grown with the explosion of the world's population. People are also rapidly moving to urban settings by choice or circumstance, leading to close contacts conducive to the spread of infection. Increases in life expectancy have also increased the proportion of elderly among the population, who are at greater risk of infection by virtue of the natural decrease in immune function with age. At the opposite end of the age spectrum, the epidemiology of childhood infections has been altered by the numbers of children in day care centers, often the result of maternal employment (see Box 3-7). Yet another factor in the spread of infection is the growing number of immunocompromised individuals due to the use of steroids and other immunosuppressives, cancer chemotherapy, and HIV infection. Finally, these groups, and potentially all humans, place themselves and others at risk of infection through various behaviors.

Population Growth

The explosive growth of the world's population is illustrated in Figure 3-3. At the beginning of the twentieth century, the world's population was approximately 1.5 billion. By 1960 it had doubled, and by late 1999 it had quadrupled to 6 billion (United Nations Population Fund, 1999). The world population is growing at an annual rate of 1.2 percent, or 77 million people, per year (United Nations Population Division, 2001); six countries (India, China, Pakistan, Nigeria, Bangladesh, and Indonesia) account for half of this annual growth. International migration is projected to remain high during the twenty-first century. The more developed regions are expected to continue being net receivers of international migrants, with an average gain of about 2 million persons per year over the next 50 years (United Nations Population Division, 2001).

Like the rest of the world, the United States has seen a steady increase in its population; by 2000, the U.S. population had reached 281,421,906 (U.S. Census Bureau, 2002a). During the 1990s, every state gained in population for the first time in the twentieth century (U.S. Census Bureau, 2001). It is estimated that 852,000 more people came into the United States than left between July 1998 and July 1999. The nation's foreign-born population grew from 10 million in 1970, to 14 million in 1980, and 20 million in 1990. By March 2000, the estimated foreign-born population in the United States was 28 million. The largest-growing share of foreign-born U.S. residents between 1970 and 2000 came from Latin America.

BOX 3-7
**The Changing Demographics of Child Care
in the United States**

Although child day care establishments have existed in the United States since the first known facility opened in Boston in 1828, changes in maternal employment during the past three decades have dramatically increased the percentage of children enrolled in out-of-home child care. This increase has in turn significantly altered the epidemiology of childhood infectious diseases. Among women with children under age 5, the proportion working outside the home increased from 30 percent in 1970 to 75 percent in 2000. Estimates of the number of children attending out-of-home day care in the United States range from more than 5.3 million (Osterholm et al., 1992) to more than 11 million (Klein, 1986). About 65 percent of 4-year-old children attended organized day care or nursery schools in 1995 (Ball et al., 2002).

Several studies conducted during the last 15 years have shown that exposure to other children through nonparental child care arrangements increases the likelihood of contracting an infectious disease, including respiratory illness, ear infection, diarrhea, and skin disease. Of particular interest are epidemics of diarrhea in day care centers, caused by organisms believed to be rare 20 years ago, including the intestinal parasites *Cryptosporidium* (CDC, 1984) and *Giardia lamblia* (Sealy and Schuman, 1983).

The risk of infection does not end with the child. Day care providers, family members, and even the community at large are all potentially at risk for infectious diseases that occur in day care centers. In one study, for example, the rates of gastrointestinal infection brought into the home by a child in day care were 26 percent for *Shigella* infection, 15 percent for rotavirus infection, and 17 percent for *G. lamblia* infection (Pickering et al., 1981). More recently, 34 percent of reported cases of a 1997 community-wide hepatitis A epidemic were associated with contact with child care centers; people who had direct contact with child care were 6 times more likely to become infected than people who did not have such contact (Venczel et al., 2001).

Many more studies are needed to better evaluate which particular infectious diseases pose an increased risk among children who attend child care centers and how these risks can be decreased. Compulsory hand washing after handling infants, blowing noses, changing diapers, or using toilet facilities is believed to be one of the most important preventive measures (Klein, 1986). Other measures include ensuring that facilities have adequate light and ventilation, space for play and rest, and an appropriate number of toilet and wash areas; that toilet facilities are separated from areas where foods are prepared and eaten; that sinks, soap dispensers, and paper towels are plentiful and appropriately placed; that surfaces, toys, and materials are regularly cleaned; and that staff members are well trained with regard to hygiene. Indeed, it has been recommended that national regulations and standards be developed and enforced to ensure infection control in out-of-home child care centers and homes.

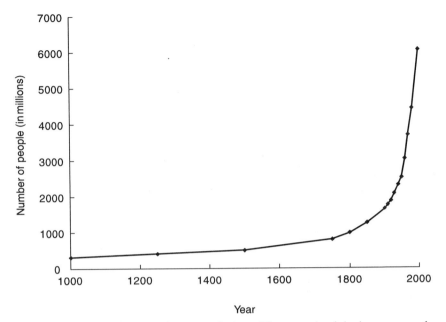

FIGURE 3-3 The human population explosion. The growth of the human population since 1000 is called the population explosion.
SOURCE: United Nations Population Division, 1999.

Aging

The global population is aging at an unprecedented rate (see Figure 3-4). Lower fertility rates, reduced death rates, and improved health have led to growing proportions of elderly people worldwide. As previously noted, aging increases susceptibility to infection even in the absence of other underlying health conditions. This is likely due to a number of factors, including senescence of gut-associated lymphoid tissue (Morris and Potter, 1997), a reduction in gastric acid secretion (low stomach pH serves as protection from enteric pathogens) (Feldman et al., 1996; Haruma et al., 2000), and diminished cell-mediated immunity and impaired host defenses (Strausbaugh, 2001). The efficacy of immunizations also decreases with advancing age (Bernstein et al., 1999). Some elderly are more vulnerable to infectious disease because of a breakdown in host defenses due to chronic disease, use of medications, and malnutrition.

Virtually all nations are experiencing growth in their elderly populations in absolute numbers (Kinsella and Velkoff, 2001). Developing countries have seen the most rapid increase, accounting for 77 percent of the world's net gain of elderly individuals from July 1999 to July 2000 (615,000 people monthly). Despite this increase, Europe remains the region with the highest proportion of population aged 65 and over (15.5 percent in 2000), while sub-Saharan Africa has the lowest proportion (2.9 percent).

Life expectancy has increased enormously in the United States since the beginning of the twentieth century (see Figure 3-5). In developed countries, the average national gain in life expectancy at birth was 66 percent for males and 71 percent for females between 1900 and 1990 (Kinsella and Velkoff, 2001). Increases were more rapid in the first half than in the second half of the century because of the expansion of public health services and infectious disease control programs that greatly reduced death rates, particularly among infants and children in developed countries. Estimates of life expectancy in developing countries in the early part of the 1900s are generally unreliable. Since World War II, changes in life expectancy in developing regions have been fairly uniform. Some exceptions include Latin America and, more recently, Africa as a result of the HIV/AIDS epidemic. In 2000, life expectancy in developing countries ranged from 38 to 80 years, as compared with 66 to 81 years in developed nations.

Urbanization

The mass relocation of rural populations to urban areas is one of the defining demographic trends of the latter half of the twentieth century. The world's cities are currently growing at four times the rate of their rural counterparts, and at least 40 percent of their expansion is the result of migration rather than natural increase. Each day about 160,000 people move from the countryside to metropolitan areas, and almost 50 percent of the world's population lives "in town" for significant periods (United Nations Population Fund, 2001; United Nations Population Division, 2002). The movement of people to cities has accelerated in the past 50 years (see Figure 3-6). The world's urban population was 2.9 billion in 2000 and is expected to climb to 5 billion by 2030. Urbanization is greater in the more developed regions of the world, where 75 percent of the population lived in urban settings in 2000. Although the percentage of urban dwellers in less-developed regions had increased to 40 percent in 2000 from 18 percent in 1950, the level and pace of urbanization differed markedly among the major constituent areas. Latin America and the Caribbean as a whole became highly urbanized, with 75 percent of their populations living in urban settlements in 2000. Conversely, only 37 percent of the populations of Africa and Asia lived in urban areas in 2000; however, this number is expected to increase more than 50 percent for both continents by 2030. With 26.5 million inhabitants, Tokyo was the most populated urban agglomeration in the world in 2001 (see Table 3-1).

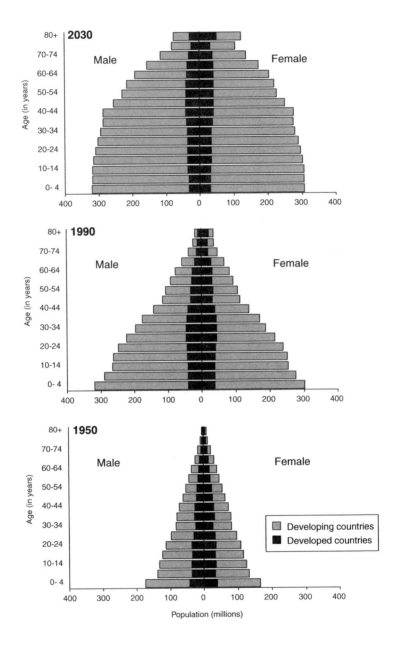

FIGURE 3-4 The world's population by age and sex: 1950, 1990, and projections for the year 2030.
Reprinted with permission, from Kinsella and Velkoff, 2001.

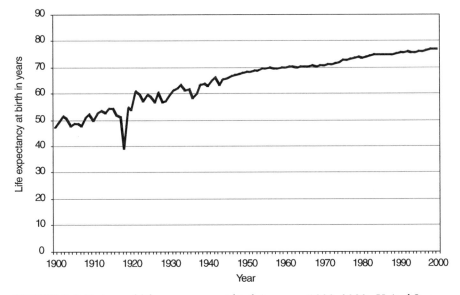

FIGURE 3-5 Estimated life expectancy at birth in years: 1900–2000, United States. Death-registration states, 1900–1928 and United States, 1929–2000.
SOURCE: National Center for Health Statistics, 2002.

Rural-to-urban migration in cities without adequate infrastructure has serious health consequences, not the least of which is the spread of infectious diseases. Many recent arrivals live in dire circumstances and suffer serious environmental health problems due to inadequate infrastructure and poor access to health services (WHO, 2001c). Impoverished rural migrants typically live in unusually crowded living conditions as a result of housing costs and relatively large family sizes, which further contribute to the spread of communicable diseases (United Nations Population Fund, 2001). Infants in poorer and more crowded portions of cities are at least four times more likely than infants in more affluent neighborhoods to die from diseases such as tuberculosis and typhoid. Moreover, many young women who migrate to cities in search of economic opportunity are able to gain economic security only through the commercial sex trade (Asthana and Oostvogels, 1996), and men often travel far from home to seek work in cities, where their reliance on the commercial sex trade increases the risk of HIV and other sexually transmitted diseases. Migrants who contract HIV in urban areas generally return to their villages to be cared for by their families, often perpetuating transmission (Adeyi et al., 2001). Other health concerns associated with increased urbanization include lack of access to clean water and sanitation, absence of adequate shelter (e.g., screens on

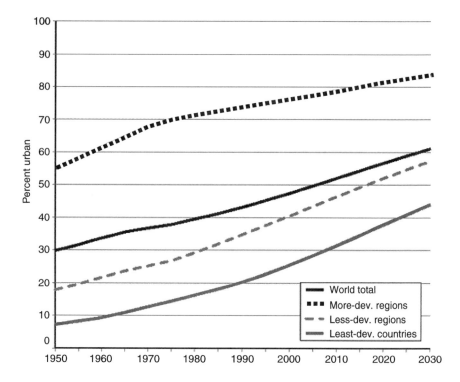

FIGURE 3-6 World Urbanization Trends, 1950–2030.
Reprinted with Permission, from UNFPA (1999), Copyright 1999.

windows), and health hazards posed by open sewers and people living in close association with animals.

Urbanization is closely tied to other demographic trends as well. Links among megacities,[3] smaller urban areas, and the surrounding rural hinterland are accelerating with the integration of all segments of society into the global economy. This increasing social, economic, and physical mobility has serious epidemiologic consequences. In recent decades, the incidence of several vector-borne diseases has increased dramatically, partly as a result of changing patterns of settlement (Gratz, 1999). Increased transport to centralized markets has helped spread emerging infections between rural and urban areas; an example is the movement of leishmaniasis to urban

---

[3]In the 1970s, the United Nations coined the term "megacities" to describe cities with 10 million or more residents.

TABLE 3-1 World Megacities, 1975, 2000, and (Projected) 2015: Population in Millions

1975	2000	2015
Tokyo (19.8)	Tokyo (26.4)	Tokyo (26.4)
New York (15.9)	Mexico City (18.1)	Mumbai (26.1)
Shanghai (11.4)	Mumbai (18.1)	Lagos (23.2)
Mexico City (11.2)	Sao Paolo (17.8)	Dhaka (21.1)
Sao Paolo (10)	Shanghai (17)	Sao Paolo (20.4)
	New York (16.6)	Karachi (19.2)
	Lagos (13.4)	Mexico City (19.2)
	Los Angeles (13.1)	New York (17.4)
	Kolkata (12.9)	Jakarta (17.3)
	Buenos Aires (12.6)	Kolkata (17.3)
	Dhaka (12.3)	Delhi (16.8)
	Karachi (11.8)	Metro Manila (14.8)
	Delhi (11.7)	Shanghai (14.6)
	Jakarta (11)	Los Angeles (14.1)
	Osaka (11)	Buenos Aires (14.1)
	Metro Manila (10.9)	Cairo (13.8)
	Beijing (10.8)	Istanbul (12.5)
	Rio de Janeiro (10.6)	Beijing (12.3)
	Cairo (10.6)	Rio de Janeiro (11.9)
		Osaka (11.0)
		Tianjin (10.7)
		Hyderabad (10.5)
		Bangkok (10.1)

SOURCE: United Nations Population Fund, 2001.

areas in South America (Jeronimo et al., 1994). Ease of transport also allows pathogens and microbial genetic material to travel between regions or continents within human hosts, vectors, animals, sources of food (plants), or cargo (Wilson, 1995).

Immunocompromised Populations

Advances in medicine, science, and technology have led to an increase in the number of people who are immunocompromised. The number of cancer patients has grown steadily during the past two decades, and cancer patients are surviving longer than ever before. The highly infectious disease-susceptible population of transplant patients has also been increasing. Likewise, the widespread use of potent antiretroviral combination therapy has led to a growing population of people living with HIV, who retain a potentially lifelong risk of spreading this infection to others.

The emergence of fungi, such as *Aspergillus* spp., and other opportunistic agents that were previously uncommon or unrecognized as human pathogens is related primarily to an increase in infection-susceptible populations, such as those having undergone cancer chemotherapy, organ and tissue transplantation, or having become infected with HIV (Dixon et al., 1996). In some oncology and transplant hospital units more than 10 percent of patients are colonized or infected with vancomycin-resistant enterococci (Morris and Potter, 1997). Moreover, under such conditions of poor host immunity, latent infections that have been lying dormant for decades, such as tuberculosis, leishmaniasis, and histoplasmosis, can be reactivated.

High-Risk Behaviors

Human behavior, both individual and collective, plays a critical role in disease emergence. Behavioral interventions to stop the spread of disease have a long history in public health. For example, a century before the rat-flea vector of bubonic plague was discovered, European travelers were advised not to wear the fur robes often bestowed upon guests of the Ottoman sultan in Istanbul (De Tott, 1973) because this action was known to cause illness. Even after the availability of effective antibiotics, behavior modification continued to be considered an invaluable strategy in the prevention of infectious disease; for some diseases, it is the only option.

The prevention of new cases of HIV is dependent on human behavior strategies; with respect to HIV, of course, such strategies must exist in a sociopolitical climate often characterized by a taboo on discussion of risky behaviors, including use of illicit drugs and unprotected sex (Coughlan et al., 2001; Holtgrave and Pinkerton, 2000; Hearst et al., 1995). The behaviors that put individuals at greater risk of contracting infection, however, do not exist in a vacuum. A network of actors encompassing conjugal, family, neighborhood, national, and regional relationships defines the economic, social, and political influences on the choices of individuals. Although changes in human behavior are difficult to achieve and maintain, in the case of HIV, such changes are the only effective prevention strategy to date.

Illicit Drug Use

Infectious diseases have a long history of being associated with illicit drug use. In the 1920s, drug users were often infected with malaria and syphilis as a result of sharing unsterilized syringes while injecting heroin or opium. When dealers started diluting heroin with quinine in the 1930s, the problem of malaria among drug users virtually disappeared as a result of the antimalarial properties of quinine (Frank, 2000). Illicit drug use also increases the risk for infection with hepatitis A, B, and C, as well as *Staphylococcus aureus* (Lange, 1989; Kapadia et al., 2002; Chambers, 2001; Ribera, 1998; Tuazon and Sheagren, 1974). The introduction of crack cocaine into New York City in 1985 and the increasing intravenous use of heroin played important roles in the emergence of a variety of infectious diseases, notably tuberculosis and HIV (Garrrett, 1998).

HIV has arguably had the greatest impact on awareness of the dangers of illicit drug use with regard to infectious diseases. People who share drug injection equipment, those who have unprotected sex with injection drug users, and children born to mothers who contracted HIV by sharing needles or having unprotected sex with an illicit drug user are at increased risk for HIV infection. In the United States, injection drug use has been responsible directly or indirectly for more than one-third of all AIDS cases since the epidemic began (CDC, 2002f). More than half of all AIDS cases among women in the United States have been associated with illicit drug use, compared with one-third of cases among men.

Noninjection drug use contributes indirectly to increased transmission of STDs, including HIV, when users trade sex for drugs or money. In addition, crack cocaine use and heroin sniffing have been associated with high-risk sexual behaviors among both men and women (Campsmith et al., 2000; Sanchez et al., 2002). Gay and bisexual men engage in riskier sexual behavior after taking popular club drugs such as methylenedioxymethamphetamine (Ecstasy), ketamine (Special K), and volatile nitrates (poppers) (Mattison et al., 2001; Mansergh et al., 2001). The resulting high-risk sexual behaviors have accounted for the greater prevalence of HIV infection among crack smokers and gay men (Edlin et al., 1994; Schwarcz et al., 2002).

The association between illicit drug use and HIV/AIDS is a worldwide problem. In 1992, only 52 countries reported HIV infection associated with illicit drug use. By the end of 1999, that number had jumped to 114. The most affected regions are Southern and Eastern Europe, Central Asia, North America, East Asia, and Latin America. Up to 90 percent of the registered HIV infections in the Russian Federation have been attributed officially to injection drug use (UNAIDS and WHO, 2002). Even Africa, where injection drug use was once believed not to be a problem, is showing an increased incidence of HIV infection associated with illicit drug use. In a 2000 study of drug injection in Lagos, Nigeria, that was presented at the XIIIth International AIDS Conference, 20 percent of 400 interviewed drug users reported having injected either heroin (63 percent) or cocaine (19 percent); 35 percent of the illicit drug users had initiated at least one person into drug injecting within the past 6 months. Among the illicit drug users, 9 percent were HIV-positive, compared with a national average of 5.4 percent. Furthermore, most of the female illicit drug users were commercial sex workers, suggesting an overlap between HIV epidemics among sex workers and illicit drug users. HIV infection associated with illicit drug use has been reported in other areas of sub-Saharan Africa as well, including Mauritius, Kenya, and South Africa.

Unprotected Sex

Unprotected sex is a key factor in the persistence of sexually transmitted diseases as a major public health problem worldwide (see Box 3-8). Today, more than 25 STDs are recognized (McIlhaney, 2000). According to recent reports, 12 to 15 million Americans, including 3 million teenagers, are infected with STDs every year (American Social Health Association, 1998; IOM, 1997).

STDs are a major problem among adolescents. Several national surveys have indicated that sexual activity among American teenagers has not changed dramatically over the past decade; nearly half of all high school students have engaged in sexual intercourse by the time they graduate (CDC, 2002g). While condom use among teenagers increased significantly in the 1990s, about 40 percent still report no condom use during last sexual intercourse. Moreover, teenagers tend to have serial monogamous sexual relationships that are short-lived, thereby increasing their exposure to multiple partners and their risk of contracting STDs (Overby and Kegeles, 1994).

Teenagers are not alone in their attitudes about risky sexual behaviors, however (see Box 3-9). More than 50 percent of men who have sex with men (both HIV-positive and HIV-negative) who reported having anal sex also reported having unprotected anal sex (Ostrow et al., 2002), a trend that appears to have been increasing since 1994 (Chen et al., 2002b; Katz et al., 2002). In another study, nearly one-third of HIV-infected men who were interviewed reported having unprotected vaginal or anal sex within the past year (Simon et al., 1999).

TECHNOLOGY AND INDUSTRY

A wealth of technological advances occurring over the past century—from modern antibiotics to organ transplants to pasteurization of food products—have greatly improved health and well-being, added years to life expectancy, and eliminated many diseases that were prevalent in the nineteenth century, including typhoid, scarlet fever, and brucellosis. However, technological and industrial advances often come at a price. New infectious diseases have emerged as a direct result of changes in technology and industry; these include Legionnaires' disease (air-conditioning cooling towers),

BOX 3-8
Sexually Transmitted Diseases

Sexually transmitted diseases (STDs) remain a major public health problem in both industrialized and developing nations. If left untreated, these infections can lead to acute illness, infertility, long-term disability, and death, and nearly all STDs increase the likelihood of HIV transmission (Fleming and Wasserheit, 1999). The exact magnitude of the global STD burden is unknown (WHO, 2001d). This is due in part to poor data collection, a large number of infections that are asymptomatic, and only a portion of the symptomatic population seeking medical care are subsequently reported. The World Health Organization estimates that 340 million new cases of STDs—syphilis (12 million), chlamydia (92 million), gonorrhea (62 million), and trichomoniasis (174 million)—occurred worldwide in 1999. The largest number of new infections was seen in South and Southeast Asia, followed by sub-Saharan Africa, then Latin America and the Caribbean. Sub-Saharan Africa experienced the greatest incidence on a per thousand population basis (WHO, 2001d).

Chlamydia. South and Southeast Asia have the most new cases of infection with *Chlamydia trachomatis* (43 million) followed by sub-Saharan Africa (16 million) and Latin America and the Caribbean (9.5 million) (WHO, 2001d). Studies among pregnant women in India have shown a prevalence rate of 17 to 21 percent (Paul et al., 1999; Rastogi et al., 1999). Reported rates of chlamydia infection have increased steadily in the United States since 1984; in 2001, 278.3 cases per 100,000 people were reported. Increased reports of chlamydia infection during the 1990s reflect the expansion of chlamydia screening activities, use of increasingly sensitive diagnostic tests, increased emphasis on case reporting from providers and laboratories, and improvements in the information systems for reporting. Higher rates in the southern region of the United States likely reflect both an expansion of screening activities in the South and the high burden of disease in this region (CDC, 2002h; IOM, 1997).

Gonorrhea. The estimated number of new cases of infection with *Neisseria gonorrhoeae* among adults worldwide in 1999 was 62 million. South and Southeast Asia have the most cases (27 million) followed by sub-Saharan Africa (17 million) and Latin America and the Caribbean (7.5 million) (WHO, 2001d). A notable increase in gonorrhea rates has been seen in Eastern Europe, with the highest rates occurring in Estonia, Russia, and Belarus (111, 139, and 125 per 100,000 people, respectively). In the United States, gonorrhea rates peaked in 1975 (467.7 cases per 100,000) and declined following implementation of the national gonorrhea control program in the mid-1970s (CDC, 2001f). The 2001 rate of gonorrhea, 128.5 cases per 100,000 persons, far exceeds the Healthy People 2010 objective of 19 cases per 100,000 persons. Despite a decrease among African Americans, rates in this population remained extremely high (782.3 in 2001); rates were highest for African Americans aged 15 to 24 years (CDC, 2002h); African American women aged 15–19 years had a gonorrhea rate of 3,495.2 cases per 100,000, 18 times higher than the rate among non-Hispanic white females of similar age.

continues

BOX 3-8
Continued

Syphilis. The estimated global burden of new cases of infection with *Treponema pallidum* among adults in 1999 was 12 million (WHO, 2001d). As with other STDs, the greatest number of cases occurs in South and Southeast Asia and sub-Saharan Africa (4 million each), followed by Latin America and the Caribbean (3 million). The newly independent states of the former Soviet Union have recently seen a dramatic rise in syphilis rates, from 5–15 per 100,000 people in 1990 to 120–170 per 100,000 of population in 1996 (WHO, 2001d). Although the primary and secondary syphilis rates in the United States declined by 90 percent from 1990 to 2000, the disease remains an important problem in the South and among certain subgroups. In 2001, the rate of primary and secondary syphilis reported among African Americans (11.0 cases per 100,000 people) was nearly 16 times greater than the rate reported among non-Hispanic whites (0.7 cases per 100,000 people) (CDC, 2002h). Recent outbreaks of syphilis among men who have sex with men may indicate an increase in high-risk sexual behavior that places them at risk for all STDs (Wolitski et al., 2001; CDC, 1999a,b; Aral, 1999). Expanding partner notification to include more high-risk populations through social networks and increasing screening among high-risk populations may improve control of inner-city syphilis epidemics (Gunn et al., 1995).

BOX 3-9
A Behavior Paradox

Antiretroviral therapy is a principal factor in prolonging the life of AIDS patients in the United States and in delaying the progression of AIDS in HIV-infected individuals receiving this multidrug regimen. Ironically, however, the role played by antiretroviral therapy in decreasing the death rate from AIDS may now be a factor in the increasing rate of unsafe sexual behaviors—potentially increasing the rate of new HIV infections. For example, men who have sex with men and believe that antiretroviral therapy decreases HIV transmission are more likely to engage in unprotected anal sex (Huebner and Gerend, 2001; Ostrow et al., 2002). Risky sexual behavior has also been associated with the belief that antiretroviral therapy improves health in HIV-positive men (Ostrow et al., 2002). Other studies have revealed that similar attitudes about antiretroviral therapy have led to increased sexual risk taking among both HIV-negative and HIV-positive illicit drug users. The increased rates of unprotected sex that have been associated with the availability of antiretroviral therapy reflect an ongoing trend (Chen et al., 2002b)

BOX 3-10
E. Coli O157:H7

Escherichia coli O157:H7 rapidly emerged within a cattle reservoir to become a public health problem associated with the large-scale production and distribution of ground beef and its role in the occurrence of hemolytic uremic syndrome (HUS), a life-threatening complication that occurs primarily among young children and the elderly (Bender et al., 1997, Elder et al., 2000). *E. coli* O157:H7 has a global distribution among cattle and a genomic diversification that suggests the pandemic spread of several clones over time, although the mechanisms by which it spread are unknown (Kim et al., 2001). Contact with cattle and environmental exposure to agricultural runoff likely contributes to the increased incidence of *E. coli* O157:H7 infection in the northern-tier states that have substantial dairy industries. Secondary environmental contamination from manure runoff has resulted in outbreaks associated with produce items including apple cider, lettuce, and sprouts. Outbreaks have also been associated with swimming in a crowded lake, and drinking contaminated unchlorinated municipal water (Chin, 2000).

toxic shock syndrome (super-absorbent tampons), and *E. coli* O157:H7 infection (mass production of ground meat) (Cohen, 2000) (see Box 3-10). Even the manner in which animals are raised before entering the meat processing industry, such as the use of antimicrobials for growth production, can impact on microbial threats to health.

Animal Husbandry Practices

Animal feeding operations (AFOs) are agricultural enterprises in which animals are kept and raised in confined situations (USDA and EPA, 1999). Approximately 450,000 AFOs exist in the United States. A relatively small number of these are concentrated animal feeding operations (CAFOs). These facilities either have more than 1,000 animal units, have 301 to 1,000 animal units and discharge wastes through human-made conveyances or directly into U.S. waters, or have been designated as CAFOs because of their significant pollution of U.S. waters (USDA and EPA, 1999). The total number of animal units in the United States increased by roughly 4.5 million (approximately 3 percent) between 1987 and 1992. During this same period, however, the number of AFOs decreased, indicating a consolidation within the industry overall and greater production from fewer, larger AFOs (GAO, 1995). In 1992, roughly 6,600 agricultural operations nationwide had more than 1,000 animal units (USDA and EPA, 1999).

Poultry and beef cattle feedlot sizes (animals per feedlot) have increased dramatically. Between 1960 and 1994, chicken production had to meet the demands of a tripling of chicken consumption from 24 pounds per capita to 72 pounds (Animal and Plant Health Inspection Service, 1999a). The number of farms selling broilers to meet this demand, however, dramatically decreased. Therefore, the consolidation of farms led to greater numbers of chickens per feedlot. By 2000, almost 36 percent of cattle were being fed on farms of 32,000 head or more (USDA, 2000a). Similar trends have been reported in the swine industry, where in 1995 approximately 60 percent of pigs were raised on farms of more than 1,000 head (USDA, 1997).

Serious concerns surround AFOs and CAFOs. The manure and wastewater produced in these facilities have the potential to overwhelm a watershed's ability to assimilate the nutrients (nitrogen and phosphorus) contained in the waste. Excess nutrients in water can result in or contribute to low levels of dissolved oxygen (anoxia), eutrophication, and toxic algal blooms. These conditions may be harmful to human health and, in combination with other circumstances, have been associated with outbreaks of microbes such as *Pfiesteria piscicida* (USDA and EPA, 1999; Grattan et al., 1998). Moreover, decomposing organic matter (animal waste) can reduce oxygen levels and cause fish kills. Pathogens in manure can also represent a food safety concern, especially when used as fertilizer or spread on pasturelands. *Cryptosporidium, Coccidioides, Giardia, E. coli, Salmonella, Campylobacter,* and *Listeria* have all been linked to human disease from fecal contamination of food and water, some of which has involved antimicrobial-resistant strains.

Antimicrobials are used in food animals for the treatment and prevention of infections, as well as for growth promotion and enhanced feed efficiency (Gorbach, 2001; McEwen and Fedorka-Cray, 2002). Use of antimicrobials in both swine and beef cattle at relatively low concentrations for growth promotion or disease prophylaxis appears to be a fairly common practice in the United States (USDA, 2001, 2000b; Wegener et al., 1999). Use of antibiotics in these animals has led to antimicrobial resistance (Fey et al., 2000; Aarestrup et al., 2001; Usera et al., 2002; White et al., 2001). Poultry growers, for example, use fluoroquinolone drugs for the treatment of *Escherichia coli*. When a veterinarian diagnoses *E. coli* in one bird, farmers treat the whole flock by adding the drug to drinking water (FDA, 2001). This usually kills *E. coli* in the chickens, but may cause drug resistance among other bacteria in the process. *Campylobacter*—a bacterium commonly found in poultry—does not cause illness in chickens, but can cause severe illness in humans who come into contact with it through undercooked or contaminated meat. The usual therapy for treating human camplyobacter infection—fluoroquinolones—will likely prove ineffective against a drug-resistant *campylobacter* strain. Even as the FDA deliberates banning the use of fluoroquinolones in poultry, some major fast food companies have announced they will no longer purchase poultry from suppliers who use the drug (Humane Society of the United States, 2002).

Many antibiotics used in animal agriculture are poorly absorbed in the animal gut and have been detected in groundwater near hog waste lagoons along with antibiotic-resistant bacteria (CDC, 1998b; Chee-Sanford et al., 2001). It is estimated that 25 to 75 percent of the antibiotics administered to feedlot animals may be excreted unaltered in feces. Given that the annual production of livestock and poultry waste in the United States is nearly 180 million tons, this waste is a potentially large source of antibiotics released into the environment. Lagoons and pit systems are typically used for waste disposal in animal agriculture. Seepage, runoff due to flooding, and fertilizing with liquid manure can expose fields and waterways to antibiotics, as well as antibiotic-resistant bacteria. Not surprisingly, antibiotics and drug-resistant bacteria have been detected in soil and groundwater in areas with fecal contamination (Hamscher et al., 2002; Esiobu et al., 2002; French et al., 1987; Kelch and Lee, 1978). Since the availability of monitoring data and other information about the fate and toxicity of antibiotics in aquatic areas and soil is limited, it is difficult to determine conclusively the risk posed to humans by antibiotics in the environment (Kummerer, 2000; Jones et al., 2001; Hamscher et al., 2002).

Aquaculture

Aquaculture is one of the fastest-growing food production sectors in the world (WHO, 1999c). Fish and shellfish processing increased threefold from 7 million tons in 1984 to 23 million tons in 1996 worldwide. The vast majority of global aquaculture production is in Asia, with developing countries accounting for roughly 87 percent of total production. In the United States, aquacultured species contribute up to 15 percent of the seafood supply (Garrett et al., 1997).

Various antimicrobials are licensed for use in fish and shrimp production worldwide. They are usually administered in feed, having been either added in during manufacture or surface-coated onto the feed pellets. Unfortunately, little information is available on the types and amounts of antimicrobials used in aquaculture, making assessment of associated public health risks more difficult (WHO, 2002e). Plasmid-mediated resistance to antimicrobials has, however, been identified in a number of bacterial fish pathogens (Aoki, 1988; Chandrasekaran and Lalithakumari, 1998; De Grandis and Stevenson, 1985). Because of lessons learned from antimicrobial use in species living on land, some countries have been exploring non-antimicrobial alternatives for some time. Norway, for instance, has been able to diminish antimicrobial use in aquaculture by more than 90 percent in a very short period of time by changing certain production practices and increasing the use of vaccines (WHO, 2002e).

Advances in Health Care

Advances in health care technology have led to improved survival of vulnerable populations, increased the numbers of invasive procedures performed, and prolonged the use of indwelling catheters and feeding tubes. Such advances have created new vehicles for the transfer of infections. The use of plastic catheters, artificial heart valves, and prosthetic joints carries the risk of organisms adhering to the surfaces of the synthetic materials; such infections are difficult to eradicate. Hepatitis C transmission has been well described in dialysis wards as a result of leakage or backflow of dialysate into machines used by multiple patients (Almroth et al., 2002), and the percentage of reported vancomycin-resistant enterococcus in U.S. dialysis centers increased from 12 percent in 1995 to 33 percent in 2000 (Tokars et al., 2002). Because hospitals are typical locations for vulnerable populations to seek medical care, they are perfect breeding grounds for transferring infections among patients (often through health care providers and other staff), and into long-term care facilities and even the community at large upon transfer or discharge (see the later discussions of nosocomial infections).

Blood Product Safety

Each year in the United States, approximately 23 million units of blood components are transfused into patients who have lost blood as a result of burns, injuries, or surgical procedures, as well as patients with sickle cell disease and various other disorders. The number of people who are willing to donate blood is increasing; in 2001, nearly 7.5 million potential donors participated in Red Cross blood drives across the nation, a 6.1 percent increase over the previous year. During the past decade, however, numerous infectious agents worldwide have been identified as potential threats to the blood supply (Chamberland et al., 2001). Of particular concern are the novel hepatitis agents (TT virus [TTV] and SEN virus [SEN-V]) and transmissible spongiform encephalopathies (Creutzfeldt-Jakob disease [CJD] and variant Creutzfeldt-Jakob disease [vCJD]). TTV was first detected in 1997 in sera from three Japanese patients suffering from post-transfusion hepatitis unrelated to hepatitis viruses A to G (Nishizawa et al., 1997). It is now known that TTV may be associated with post-transfusion hepatitis in patients from several parts of the world (Bez et al., 2000; Niel et al., 1999; Poovorawan et al., 1998). SEN-V has also been implicated as a possible cause of transfusion-associated non–A to E hepatitis (Umemura et al., 2001).

In preliminary, limited studies, approximately 2 percent of current and pre-1990 blood donors have tested positive for SEN-V (Chamberland et al., 2001). Testing of serum samples archived at the National Institutes of Health revealed the proportion of cardiac surgery patients with evidence of new infection with SEN-V to be 10 times higher among those who had received blood transfusions (30 percent) than among those who had not (3 percent), and a SEN-V-positive donor could be identified for roughly 70 percent of SEN-V-positive recipients (Chamberland et al., 2001).

Despite screening of all blood products for hepatitis B and hepatitis C, on rare occasions screening tests do not detect infected blood donors, and hence infections have been passed to transfusion recipients. A small number of cases of other diseases, such as malaria, American trypanosomiasis, babesiosis, Rocky Mountain spotted fever, and West Nile encephalitis, have been reported to be due to transfusions believed to have come from donors who have lived in or traveled to disease-endemic areas (Chamberland et al., 1998; CDC, 2002i). Recent concern has focused on the real or potential transmission through blood transfusions of such diseases as Lyme disease and variant Cruetzfeldt-Jakob Disease (vCJD). Although no confirmed cases of CJD or vCJD have occurred through blood transfusion, health officials are concerned about the risk because of the high degree of uncertainty associated with these agents. For this reason, restrictions on who can donate blood based on potential contact with bovine spongiform encephalopathy (BSE) have been implemented. For example, among the many FDA guidelines based on this criterion, people who spent 3 months or more cumulatively in the United Kingdom between 1980 and 1996 should not donate blood; neither should people who have received a blood transfusion in the United Kingdom between 1980 and the present.

Organ and Tissue Transplantation

In the United States, more than 23,000 human-to-human organ transplantations were performed in 2001 (see Table 3-2). The total number of single- and multi-organ transplants increased by 45 percent between 1991 and 2000. The immunosuppressive drugs used to prevent rejection of the transplanted organs weaken the body's immune system and leave the host susceptible to infectious diseases. Opportunistic infections, such as those also seen in patients with AIDS, and nosocomial infections are of serious concern in this population. Bacterial infections remain the most frequently diagnosed infections in transplant recipients, and a striking rise in antimicrobial resistance has occurred among these pathogens (Singh, 2000).

More common than organ transplantation is the use of human donor tissues. Each year between 600,000 and 800,000 allograft implantation procedures are performed in the United States (McCarthy, 2002). FDA has

TABLE 3-2 Organ Transplants Performed and Patients Awaiting
Transplants in 2001

Type of Transplant	Transplants (Number)	Wait-Listed (Number)
Kidney (5,969 living donors)	14,024	48,405
Liver	4,989	18,173
Pancreas alone	131	395
Pancreas after kidney	304	675
Kidney–pancreas	884	2,399
Intestine	40	177
Heart	2,171	4,076
Heart–lung	27	209
Lung	1,053	3,756
Total	23,848	78,265

SOURCE: University Renal Research and Education Association, United Network for Organ
Sharing, 2003.

specific regulations for the proper handling and processing of these tissues.
Nonetheless, in November 2001 a 23-year-old man from Minnesota died
after undergoing reconstructive knee surgery involving a bone–cartilage
allograft (CDC, 2001l, 2002j). The blood cultures obtained premortem
grew *Clostridium sordellii*, a potentially fatal anaerobic spore and toxin-
forming organism. A few days later, an Illinois man who had received
donor tissue from the same cadaver also became critically ill following
reconstructive knee surgery. The CDC investigators obtained 19 other un-
used tissues taken from that same donor. As of March 2002, federal officials had uncovered 26 cases of bacterial infection in otherwise healthy
patients who had received musculoskeletal tissue allograft implants (not all
from this same processor).

Xenotransplantation

The need for donated human organs and tissues far exceeds the present
supply. As of July 5, 2002, more than 80,000 persons living in the United
States were awaiting organs for transplantation. The shortage of human
donors has been increasing annually since the 1980s (Kemp, 1996) and has
sparked a renewed interest in transplantation of organs and tissues across
the species barrier (Candinas and Adams, 2000).

Xenotransplantation involves the transplantation of cells, tissues, and
whole organs from one species to another. While xenotransplantation offers potential benefit for both individual recipients and society, it also
represents a public health concern. Such procedures have the potential to

result in human recipients being infected with microbial agents that are not endemic in human populations, thereby potentially introducing new (xenogeneic) infections into the human community. This potential risk is presently unquantifiable (IOM, 2002d). Scientists and policy makers in the field must therefore deal with the challenge of weighing the uncertain collective risk of xenotransplantation against the potential benefit to both individuals and society (Chapman and Bloom, 2001). In 1999, European countries concluded that the scientific base was inadequate to permit proceeding to clinical trials, a decision that halted xeontransplantation studies there. The United States, however, decided that the only way to advance the scientific base was to proceed with caution to clinical trials (Daar, 1999; IOM, 1996).

In the United States, regulation of xenotransplantation procedures is within the purview of FDA, which has ruled that nonhuman primates should not be used as source animals for transplants until scientists have sufficient information to address the associated infectious disease risks (DHHS, 2000a). Significant concerns still remain about the possible transmission of infectious agents from nonprimates. For example, pigs harbor retroviruses that until recently have been considered a negligible risk for human disease (Blusch et al., 2002). Several reports on the infection of human cells in vitro and on the spread of porcine endogenous retroviruses from transplanted porcine islets in murine models may suggest a potential risk for xenogeneic infection. Such studies have reawakened concern regarding what clinicians and scientists do not know about interspecies transmission of retroviruses.

INTERNATIONAL TRAVEL AND COMMERCE

The potential for the rapid dissemination of pathogens, and their vectors and animal reservoirs, throughout the world is increasing greatly as the world continues to experience expanding global trade markets and increasing international travel. Infections that are carried by humans and transmitted from person to person—including influenza, measles, rubella, HIV, tuberculosis, *Haemophilus influenzae*, and *Neisseria meningitidis*—are especially amenable to being carried from one geographic area to another. Microbes that can colonize without causing symptoms (e.g., *Neisseria meningitidis*) or can infect and be transmissible at a time when infection is asymptomatic (e.g., HIV, hepatitis B and C) can spread easily in the absence of recognized infection in traveling or migrant hosts (see Box 3-11).

Airport and railroad malaria illustrate the continual movement of pathogens into new areas. Migrating humans have played a large role in the epidemiology of malaria worldwide, including the spread of drug-resistant malaria (Martens and Hall, 2000). Chloroquine-resistant *falciparum* ma-

BOX 3-11
Neisseria meningitidis: A Sacred Peril

Approximately 2 million people from about 140 countries, including about 15,000 from the United States, congregate in Saudi Arabia during the annual Hajj. In 1987, a Hajj-related outbreak of serogroup A *Neisseria meningitidis*, which then spread to other countries, led to the establishment of a requirement that all arriving pilgrims receive the meningococcal vaccine. In spring 2000, however, a similar outbreak of serogroup W135 *N. meningitidis* occurred among those who made the pilgrimage and subsequently spread to family members and other contacts who had not traveled to Saudi Arabia (CDC, 2000d, 2001g, 2001h). Serotyping, multilocus sequence typing, multilocus DNA fingerprints, and other techniques were used to identify W135 isolates in many other countries (Taha et al., 2000; Popovic et al., 2000). Many of the pilgrims in 2000 had not been vaccinated against the W135 serogroup, since the quadrivalent vaccine (A, C, Y, W-135) is available in only a few countries (including the United States); thus many pilgrims were able to receive only bivalent (A and C) vaccine.

Although the quadrivalent vaccine appeared to prevent disease in most people who had received it, they could still become carriers of W135 *N. meningitidis* and thus could still serve as sources of infection upon their return. Humans are the only important host for *N. meningitidis*, and many carry the organism in the oropharynx in the absence of symptoms. In a 2000 study, oropharyngeal cultures were obtained from 451 pilgrims departing from JFK Airport on direct flights to Saudi Arabia, and repeat cultures were taken from 727 returning pilgrims. None of the pilgrims carried W135 at the time of departure, but six of the returning pilgrims were infected (CDC, 2001h). A similar study done in Singapore showed that nearly 17 percent of 171 pilgrims carried *N. meningitidis* upon their return from the Hajj, 80 percent of which was serotype W135. (Gewolb, 2001).

laria, for example, emerged in two widely separated locations—in Columbia and at the Cambodia–Thailand border—and has subsequently spread from both of these locations to other areas (Wellems and Plowe, 2001). Occasional instances of local malaria transmission have occurred even in the United States, where during the past 10 years, approximately 1,000 cases of imported malaria have been reported to CDC annually; the imported cases are mainly in travelers, military personnel, and immigrants returning to or coming from malaria-endemic areas (Olliaro et al., 1996; CDC, 2002l). Fortunately, in most cases the factors necessary to establish a transmission cycle are not present, and few human cases typically occur subsequent to introduction. On the other hand, all of the necessary ingredients for the establishment of West Nile virus were present in New York City in 1999, and the virus is now established across the United States (see Box 3-12) (Petersen and Roehrig, 2001).

International Travel

The spatial mobility of the average human has increased more than 1,000-fold since 1800 (Gruebler and Nakicenovic, 1991). As the number of global travelers increases, so does the threat of the spread of infectious diseases. According to the World Tourism Organization (see Figure 3-7), world tourism grew by an estimated 7.4 percent in 2000, and the total number of international arrivals reached nearly 700 million; the latter figure is expected to reach the 1 billion mark by 2010 (Handszuh, 2001). Every region in the world is experiencing this increase. More than 5,000 airports worldwide have regularly scheduled international flights, allowing for quick links to urban centers across the globe. In 2000, more than 18 million commercial airline flights took off from airports around the world, carrying 1.1 billion passengers (Boeing, 2002). In 1999, 725,000 aircraft, 200,000 ships, 463,000 buses, 39,000 trains, and 125 million personally owned automobiles crossed U.S. borders, and in 2000, an estimated 400 million international travelers entered the United States by either land, ship, or air.

Not only are more people traveling, but travel is also faster and more socially widespread, and penetrates into areas of the world not readily accessible in the past. In the nineteenth century, it could take a year to circumnavigate the globe by ship. Today a person can go around the world in less than 36 hours. Roads, bridges, canals, and transport vehicles allow humans to rapidly bypass physical and other barriers that would have stopped or slowed movement in the past. Modern technologies have expanded the range of easily accessible destinations, and allow travelers to enter and survive more extreme environments and encounter more isolated human populations. Not only can infected travelers introduce new microbes into new environments, both while traveling and after having returned home, but, as adventure travelers intrude on new environments and have contact with exotic wildlife, the chance that they will come into contact with microbes that have never before been recognized as human pathogens is real. They may then bring these exotic infectious agents back home with them, where, under appropriate circumstances, an introduced pathogen may persist and spread.

Air Travel

The interactions that occur *during* travel are another important component of the travel process, with implications for the emergence and spread of infectious disease. In particular, many documented transmission incidents or outbreaks of both airborne and foodborne infections—including influenza, smallpox, tuberculosis, measles, cholera, shigellosis, salmonello-

---

BOX 3-12
West Nile Virus

On August 23, 1999, an infectious disease physician notified the New York City Department of Health and reported two patients with encephalitis in a hospital in northern Queens. An investigation of nearby hospitals quickly uncovered six additional persons with symptoms suggestive of encephalitis. Initial blood and cerebrospinal fluid tests indicated that the cause was viral. All eight patients were previously healthy persons between the ages of 58 and 87; they all lived within a 16-square-mile area in northern Queens; and none of them had recently traveled. The only exposure that all eight patients shared was that they had all engaged in outdoor activities around their homes in the evening (Nash et al., 2001). Environmental sampling revealed the presence of *Culex* mosquito breeding sites and larvae in many of the patients' yards and neighborhoods. Around the same time, local health officials observed an increase in dead birds, especially crows, in New York City. Officials at the Bronx Zoo noted that three captive-bred birds had apparently died from meningo-encephalitis. Eventually, testing of the initial human cases and the dead birds indicated that their illnesses were due to West Nile virus, which had previously never been isolated in the Western Hemisphere (Fine and Layton, 2001) By the end of 1999, 62 cases of severe disease, including 7 deaths, had occurred in the New York area. In 2000, 21 cases, including 2 deaths, were reported in New York, New Jersey, and Connecticut. By 2002, nearly 4,000 cases of West Nile encephalitis had been reported in 39 states and the District of Columbia of which 254 had died from this disease (CDC, 2003c).

West Nile virus belongs to a group of viruses that cause febrile illness usually lasting a week or less. Initial symptoms include fever, headache, malaise, arthralgia or myalgia,

---

sis, and staphylococcal food poisoning—have occurred inside airplanes, (Ritzinger, 1965; CDC, 1983; Kenyon et al., 1996). Influenza outbreaks have been known to affect more than 70 percent of the passengers on a single aircraft (Moser et al., 1979).

First, getting to the airport often involves using mass transportation (e.g., train or bus) and thus having contact with numerous people from many different areas in a small, enclosed space. At the airport, passengers are exposed to even more people in an often crowded terminal full of people from all over the world (or, in smaller airports, the region). The air inside the bus or airline terminal may have a higher level of microbial contamination than that inside the aircraft itself (Wick and Irvine, 1995). Once on the plane, passengers breathe recirculated, filtered,[4] low-humidity (10–20 percent) air. Particular aircraft vary, but generally the recirculated air is mixed with fresh air about 20 times an hour during flight, and less frequently during takeoff and landing. Transoceanic travel often involves

---

[4]High-efficiency particulate air (HEPA) filters are used on most aircraft to capture particles larger than 0.3 microns.

rash, and occasionally nausea and vomiting. Only a small percentage of cases develop encephalitis. West Nile virus has caused disease outbreaks in Egypt, Israel, France, Romania, and the Czech Republic, and is widespread in parts of Africa, the northern Mediterranean area, and western Asia. Birds are the primary reservoir of infection that is spread to humans by the bite of an infected mosquito. The occurrence of West Nile virus in New York illustrates how easily pathogens can extend their geographic range. But how the virus was introduced into New York, how long it has been in the United States, how far its geographic range extends, and what its long-term impact will be on human and animal health are still unanswered questions. West Nile virus could have been introduced through travel by infected humans, importation of illegal birds or other domestic pets, avian flyways, or unintentional introduction of virus-infected ticks or mosquitoes. Other recent outbreaks of West Nile encephalitis have occurred in regions of the world where the disease was previously not found or only rarely found. In 1999, more than 480 suspected cases, including 40 fatalities, of West Nile virus were reported in the Volgograd Region, Russia (Platonov et al., 2001). The Volgograd outbreak, as well as an earlier 1996 Romania outbreak, were both caused by viral strains that were genetically similar to the one that caused the New York outbreak, suggesting that the outbreaks were caused by close relatives and illustrating the ease with which pathogens can circumnavigate the globe and occupy new territories (Platonov et al., 2001; Platonov, 2001).

Public education is the key component to preventing West Nile virus infection. However, even after the highly publicized New York mosquito-borne outbreak, only 9 percent of those surveyed within the outbreak epicenter reported consistent use of personal prevention such as mosquito repellent; 70 percent reported never using mosquito repellent (Mostashari et al., 2001).

larger airplanes, whose passengers are exposed to even more people while in flight. When they exit the plane, travelers typically mingle with arriving passengers from multiple origins in the terminal, frequently spending minutes to hours standing in line, retrieving luggage, arranging transport from the airport, or moving on to another flight.

Cruise Ships

Cruise ship travel has increased dramatically. Nearly 7 million people took North American cruise vacations in 2001. Cruise ships bring together large numbers of both passengers and crew from diverse geographic origins, including countries with immunization requirements that often differ from those of the United States. Although a cruise may bring to mind days spent lounging on a sunny deck, many of the activities on cruise ships take place in closed spaces (e.g., dining rooms, movie theaters, lecture halls). The ships often stop at multiple ports, where passengers and crew may disembark and interact with people in the local environment before reboarding.

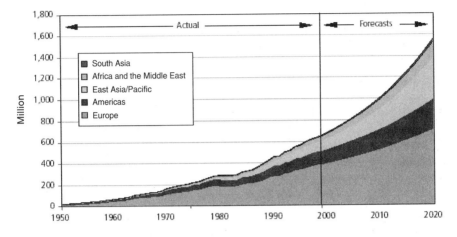

FIGURE 3-7 International tourist arrivals, 1950-2020.
SOURCE: Adapted from World Tourism Organization, 2002.

The ships may also pick up and drop off passengers along the way, thus further expanding the opportunities for mixing with microbes from other populations.

Cruise ships have a history riddled with infectious disease outbreaks, often related to contaminated food or inadequately treated water from international ports. Numerous recent reports include gastroenteritis caused by a variety of pathogens, ranging from *Staphyloccocus aureus* to *Shigella* spp. to SRSV (small, round-structured virus, formerly known as the Norwalk virus, now referred to as the norovirus). Several recent outbreaks of gastroenteritis associated with norovirus occurred on consecutive cruises on the same ship and on different ships within the same company, suggesting that environmental contamination and infected crew members can serve as reservoirs of infection for passengers (CDC, 2002m). Cruise ships also have a history of infectious respiratory illnesses, including both influenza A and B (CDC, 2001i; Miller et al., 2000), Legionnaires' disease (CDC, 1994b, 1994c), and tuberculosis (Penman et al., 1997). In 1997, rubella outbreaks occurred among crew members of two different commercial cruise lines (CDC, 1998d).

The features of cruise ships, especially ones that offer special services, such as renal dialysis or medical care, have made them highly attractive vacation options for more infection-susceptible populations. For example, on a cruise ship that experienced an outbreak of influenza while cruising from Montreal to New York in 1997, 77 percent of 1,284 surveyed passengers were aged 65 and older, and 26 percent had risk factors other than age that placed them at risk for complications of influenza. Indeed 17 percent of the passengers and 19 percent of the crew members reported experiencing an acute respiratory illness during the cruise. The etiological agent was identified as influenza A/Sydney/5/97 (CDC, 1997c).

Commerce

International trade in food and animal agriculture has increased markedly as an important aspect of globalization (see Figure 3-8). The United States and other countries now enjoy more goods from more countries than ever before. It is now possible to buy fresh produce at any time of the year, as well as a whole host of previously unattainable foods from areas around the world. Unfortunately, this wider array of product options brings with it the risk of cross-border transmission of infectious agents. Many species enter the United States each year as contaminants of commodities. Up to 70 percent of selected fruits and vegetables consumed in the United States come from developing countries during certain seasons (Osterholm, 1997). Agricultural produce, nursery stock, cut flowers, and timber can harbor insects, plant pathogens, slugs, and snails. Fish and shrimp pathogens and parasites have been introduced into the country through infected stock for

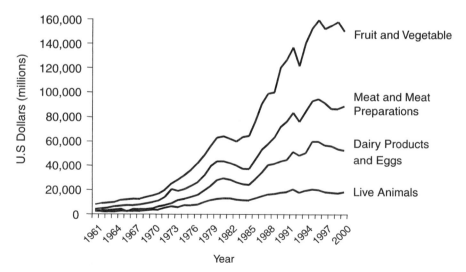

FIGURE 3-8 International agriculture trade, 1961–2000.
Reprinted with permission from Kimball, in Davis and Kimball, 2001.

aquaculture. Crates and containers are potential carriers for snails, slugs, mollusks, beetles, and microorganisms. Military cargo transport can likewise bring harmful species into new settings. Ballast water that is released from ships as cargo is loaded or unloaded has been known to carry several destructive aquatic species (Animal and Plant Health Inspection Service, 1999b). Pathogens in meat and poultry, such as the agents of BSE and foot and mouth disease, can also be delivered unintentionally across borders. This is true as well for diseases not known to affect human health directly but capable of impacting on agriculture and animal health.

Moving live animals across borders can also bring regional diseases to new areas. For this reason, pet dogs and cats are subject to inspection at ports of entry for evidence of infectious diseases that can be transmitted to humans (CDC, 2001j). Reptiles are also popular pet imports; in 1997, more than 1.7 million reptiles were imported into the United States (Humane Society of the United States, 2001). The demand for rare and exotic reptiles constitutes a significant portion of a $3 billion annual illegal trade in plants and animals in the United States. Monkeys and other nonhuman primates may not be imported as pets; however, each year approximately 9,000 primates are imported for scientific and exhibition use.

The manufacture and distribution of goods within the United States has also undergone a transformation. It is now possible to ship products from coast to coast in less than 12 hours. In addition, companies are more centralized in their production, processing, and distribution of goods. This is most evident in the food industry, with consumers now being able to enjoy fresher goods on their grocery shelves at reduced cost. Unfortunately, this rapid system of production and transport also creates a faster, more efficient delivery system for foodborne outbreaks that are more difficult to detect. In the past, such outbreaks occurred locally and could be readily identified by epidemiologic surveillance methods. A foodborne outbreak in this era of globalization is more complicated and may involve multiple states with varying times of illness onset, thus making it more difficult to trace the illness back to its origin.

Food Imports

The United States remains a consumer-driven society, with food choices motivated by competing concerns over cost, safety, nutritional value, and convenience. For example, health concerns associated with a diet rich in animal fats have changed the diet of many Americans. From 1990 to 1999, per capita consumption of whole milk decreased 67 percent and that of red meat 11 percent. In contrast, consumption of fresh fruit increased 30 percent, that of fresh vegetables increased 63 percent, and that of poultry doubled.

BOX 3-13
Shigella sonnei: **A Garnish of Parsley?**

The impact of imported produce on the occurrence of foodborne disease was demonstrated in an outbreak of multidrug-resistant *Shigella sonnei* infection among patrons of two different restaurants in Minnesota in 1998 (CDC, 1999c). Isolates were resistant to ampicillin, trimethoprim-sulfamethoxazole, tetracycline, sulfasoxazole, and streptomycin. The isolates also had the same pulse field gel electrophoresis (PFGE) pattern, which was distinct from that of the endemic *S. sonnei* strains circulating in Minnesota at the time. Epidemiological investigation implicated chopped parsley as the vehicle. Six other outbreaks linked by PFGE and parsley-use characteristics were identified in California, Massachusetts, Florida, and Canada. Trace-back of implicated parsley identified a single farm in Mexico as the likely source. Water used in cooling fresh-picked parsley had not been adequately treated and was susceptible to contamination. Two outbreaks of enterotoxigenic *E. coli* (ETEC) infection in Minnesota were also linked to parsley that may have originated at the same farm in Mexico.

Although imported parsley was the original source of contamination, handling of the produce at the restaurants contributed to the outbreaks. Each of the implicated restaurants chopped parsley, pooled it in containers, and sprinkled it over various foods and dishes as a topping or garnish. This holding of pooled, chopped parsley increased the available inoculum, making it a more efficient infective dose. In several restaurants, food workers became infected and worked while ill, providing a second amplifying mechanism. Restaurants also served to amplify source contamination through cross-contamination of ready-to-eat foods.

Just to meet today's year-round demand for fresh produce, the volume of produce imported from developing countries has increased dramatically. For example, 95 percent of green onions sold in the United States during 2000 were imported from Mexico. Green onions are susceptible to contamination by soil, water, or handling, and are typically served fresh as a garnish on salads or cooked foods. During the winter months, 25 percent of cantaloupe and 50 percent of tomatoes consumed in the United States are imported from Mexico. These examples of imported produce, as well as others, have been implicated as vehicles in foodborne outbreaks (see Box 3-13). In 1995, 1996, 1997, and 2000, outbreaks of cyclosporiasis were associated with consumption of raspberries from Guatemala. The outbreaks in 1995 were identified retrospectively, after the widespread outbreaks in 1996 had been linked to Guatemalan raspberries (Herwaldt and Beach, 1999; Herwaldt and Ackers, 1997; Koumans et al., 1998). In spite of detailed investigations, the sources of the contamination have never been identified.

Foodborne Illnesses

Overall, changes in several factors at the national level have contributed to the changing epidemiology of foodborne diseases in the United States. These include changes in diet, new methods of food production, new infectious agents, new vehicles for previously recognized pathogens, and the increasing prevalence of persons who are immunocompromised (Hedberg et al., 1994). The spectrum of illnesses caused by the consumption of contaminated foods ranges from self-limiting mild gastroenteritis to life-threatening neurologic, hepatic, and renal syndromes. Data collected by FoodNet, the active surveillance network for foodborne disease in the United States, allow comprehensive estimates of disease burden since 1996. Data from this and other surveillance systems are also being used to evaluate the public health impact of changes in food safety policies, particularly in the regulation of the meat and poultry processing industries (CDC, 2002n; Liang et al., 2001). Data from these surveillance systems indicate that contaminated foods cause approximately 76 million illnesses, 325,000 hospitalizations, and 5,000 deaths each year in the United States (Mead et al., 1999) at an estimated annual cost of $7–35 billion (Economic Research Service, 2001; Buzby and Roberts, 1997). More than 200 food-transmitted diseases are known (Bryan, 1982); in 82 percent of foodborne illnesss, however, the identity of the pathogen is unknown (IOM, 2002a). Of 1,500 deaths each year due to known pathogens, 75 percent are caused by *Salmonella* spp., *Listeria monocytogenes*, or *Toxoplasma* spp.

Expansion of the international trade in foodstuffs over the last two decades has made it difficult to screen comprehensively for the presence of dangerous microorganisms and has increased the scope and range of foodborne diseases. Theoretical concerns about the transmission of BSE prions from cattle to humans were tragically confirmed by the outbreak of vCJD in the United Kingdom (see Box 3-14). Fortunately, modern technology has made it possible to track foodborne pathogens across geographic expanses. For example, PulseNet, the molecular subtyping network for foodborne diseases, established standard protocols for pulsed field gel electrophoresis (PFGE) and enabled public health laboratories to compare molecular patterns of microbes electronically (Swaminathan et al., 2001). These methods have been instrumental in a number of investigations of multistate outbreaks of foodborne illness.

Antibiotic resistance is a serious problem among foodborne pathogens. Over the past decade, the worldwide occurrence of resistance among *Salmonella* spp., *Campylobacter* spp., and toxigenic-producing *Escherichia coli* O157 has dramatically increased (Threlfall et al., 2000). It has been estimated that 1.4 million cases of illness from *Salmonella* and 2.4 million cases of illness from *Campylobacter* infection occur in the United States every year (Mead et al., 1999); 26 percent of the *Salmonella* isolates and 54 percent of the *Campylobacter* isolates have been found to be resistant to at least one antimicrobial to which previous susceptibility was known. Although antibiotics are not always essential for salmonellosis treatment, they can be lifesaving in certain situations. Most severe *Salmonella* cases occur in children and the elderly and can be fatal. The global dissemination of the multidrug-resistant *Salmonella typhimurium* DT104 is of particular concern because of the severity of the illness it causes. Multidrug-resistant *S. typhimurium* DT104 has been associated with hospitalization rates twice those for other *Salmonella* infections, and its case-fatality rate is 10 times higher. *S. typhimurium* DT104 initially emerged in cattle in the late 1980s and can now be found in a variety of foods, including poultry, unpasteurized milk, meat, and meat products.

BREAKDOWN OF PUBLIC HEALTH MEASURES

A breakdown or lack of public health measures, such as adequate sanitation, immunizations, and tuberculosis control, has had a dramatic effect on the emergence and persistence of infectious diseases throughout the world. For example, infectious diseases have resurged in the former Soviet Union over the past decade because of the country's enormous socio-economic upheavals and the fracturing of its health services that has resulted from poor funding for treatment, vaccine prophylaxis, and health education (Netesov and Conrad, 2001; Coker, 2001). Even the United States has had difficulties maintaining adequate supplies of vaccines in recent years, and immunization rates for adults are still far below national targets. Furthermore, some public health measures, such as public health laws, need to be updated to ensure legal authority for epidemic disease control in the current political climate.

Inadequate Sanitation and Hygiene

Poor sanitary conditions and a lack of proper hygiene contribute to the transmission of many infectious diseases. To date, one of the most significant shortages worldwide is that of potable water. This shortage has implications for the transmission of numerous infectious diseases, such as cholera. Squalid living conditions with overcrowding and the presence of vermin also contribute to the spread of infections, such as plague. Even in the United States, poor infection control practices in hospitals have resulted in high rates of nosocomial infection.

BOX 3-14
Transmissible Spongiform Encephalopathies:
From Herd to Mortality

Transmissible spongiform encephalopathies (TSEs) are a family of diseases of humans and animals that are uniformly fatal, causing irreversible cumulative brain damage. In humans, the most common TSE is Creutzfeldt-Jakob disease (CJD), which was first identified in 1921; others include Gerstmann-Straussler-Scheinker syndrome, kuru, fatal familial insomnia, and now, variant Creutzfeldt-Jakob disease (vCJD). Animal TSEs include bovine spongiform encephalopathy (BSE), scrapie, transmissible mink encephalopathy, and chronic wasting disease of American mule deer, white-tail deer, and elk.

BSE, popularly known as "mad cow disease," wreaked havoc on the livestock industry in the United Kingdom when a 1986 epidemic led to the death of nearly 200,000 cattle. The outbreak is believed to have originated from an endemic spongiform encephalopathy of sheep (i.e., scrapie) that entered the cattle food chain via nutritional supplements manufactured from infected sheep carcasses. Nearly 4.5 million asymptomatic cattle were slaughtered, substantially impacting numerous industries that manufacture bovine-derived products. But perhaps most alarming, BSE has recently been associated with vCJD, a rare and fatal human neurodegenerative condition that was first described in March 1996 and linked to beef products contaminated with central nervous system tissues from BSE-infected cattle.

By 1996, 10 cases of vCJD were reported (Will et al., 1996). Early symptoms included a form of depression or a schizophrenia-like psychosis; half of the case patients experienced unusual sensory symptoms, such as "stickiness" of the skin. As the illness progressed, cases suffered various neurological problems, such as unsteadiness, difficulty walking, and involuntary movements. By the time of death, case patients were completely immobile and mute. The most notable clinical differences between the more common CJD and vCJD are that the latter affects predominantly younger people (mean age of death is 29 versus 65 with CJD) and lasts longer (median of 14 months versus

---

Cholera

Cholera is an acute intestinal infection caused by the bacterium *Vibrio cholerae,* which is spread through contaminated food and water. The infection often results in mild symptoms but can sometimes cause severe, life-threatening diarrhea. The bacterium survives and multiplies outside the human body; it can then spread rapidly in human populations where living conditions are crowded and unprotected water sources are in close proximity to fecal repositories. These conditions are not uncommon in poor countries and in many refugee camps. One refugee camp in the Democratic Republic of Congo experienced a major cholera epidemic in 1994, in which an estimated 58,000–80,000 cases and 23,800 deaths occurred within a month as a result of the consumption of untreated lake water; crowding; poor personal hygiene; and inadequate sanitation, due in part to the rocky

4.5 months for CJD). As of April 2002, 117 cases of vCJD had been reported in the United Kingdom, 6 in France, and 1 each in the Republic of Ireland and Italy (CDC, 2002w).

The nature of the causal agent for vCJD, and TSEs in general, is still a matter of debate. According to a leading theory, the disease agent is composed largely, if not entirely, of a self-replicating protein known as a prion, so that the TSEs are now sometimes referred to as prion diseases. Prions are transmissible protein particles that are devoid of nucleic acid and consist only of modified protein. According to the prion theory, the brain and other organs of mammals (at least those examined thus far) contain a normal version (PrP^C) of the pathological protein form (PrP^{SC}) that makes up a prion. When an animal or human becomes infected with PrP, the invading protein somehow converts normal protein molecules into toxic ones by causing the proteins to change shape. Despite strong evidence in support of the prion theory (Prusiner, 1995), a few scientists still believe that the ability of the TSE agent to form multiple strains is better explained by a DNA-containing, virus-like agent. To date, no such agent has been found.

Many scientists are keeping a watchful eye on chronic wasting disease (CWD), a fatal neurological illness of farmed and wild deer and elk (Animal and Plant Health Inspection Service, 2002). It was first identified in 1967, although researchers did not determine it to be a TSE until 1978. The first case was diagnosed in Colorado in 1981. By 2001, CWD had been detected in deer and elk in Wyoming, Nebraska, South Dakota, Canada, Wisconsin, New Mexico, Oklahoma, Montana, Kansas, and Illinois (Animal and Plant Health Inspection Service, 2002). Although the most obvious and consistent clinical sign of CWD is weight loss over time, many infected animals also show behavioral changes, including decreased interaction with other animals, listlessness, lowering of the head, blank facial expression, and repetitive walking in set patterns. No evidence linking CWD to any disease in humans or domestic animals had been detected as of 2002, although studies seeking such evidence have been limited.

volcanic nature of the soil in the area which made digging latrines almost impossible (GOMA Epidemiology Group, 1995). Bathing in the river, long distances to a water source, and consumption of dried fish were significantly associated with the risk of cholera during the 1997 epidemic in southern Tanzania (Acosta et al., 2001).

Cases of cholera are rare in industrialized nations, where modern sewage and water treatment systems exist. In the United States, cholera was prevalent in the 1800s but has now been virtually eliminated. Between 1965 and 1991, just 136 cases were reported to CDC. From 1992 through 1994, the number jumped to 160; half of these were among airline passengers traveling from Latin America (75) and cruise ship passengers from Southeast Asia (5) (Mahon et al., 1996). Although all regions of the world reported a reduction in the total number of cholera cases between 1999 and 2000, in 2000 WHO received reports of 137,071 cases from 56 countries, which resulted in 4,908 deaths (WHO, 2001f). Africa accounted for 87 percent of the global total. Asia, with a three-fold decrease, still reported 11,246 cases. Central and South America reported 3,101 cases and 40 deaths, these despite reportedly large decreases in Brazil, Ecuador, Guatemala, and Nicaragua. The actual number of cholera cases is believed to be higher in all countries because of alleged underreporting and other surveillance system limitations.

The sixth and most recent global cholera pandemic began in 1961 in Celebes, Indonesia, caused by *V. cholera* O1, biotype El Tor. It spread rapidly to surrounding countries of eastern Asia and reached Bangladesh in 1963; India in 1964; and the Soviet Union, Iran, and Iraq in 1965–1966 (WHO, 2000d). In 1970, cholera was found in West Africa, where it eventually proliferated and became endemic throughout most of the continent. It then spread to Latin America in 1991, and within the year had reached 11 countries in this region. By the 1990s, cholera had become endemic to Latin America, Africa, and Asia, where periodic countrywide epidemics continued into the twenty-first century.

In 1992, large outbreaks of cholera began in India and Bangledesh that were caused by a previously unrecognized serogroup of *Vibrio cholerae*, designated O139, synonym Bengal. The epidemic was widespread in the Asiatic continent, with imported cases reported from developed countries. Some regarded this as the eighth cholera pandemic, although the epidemic remained confined to Bangladesh and India. After 1992, *V. cholerae* O1 was again epidemic in that region (Seas and Gotuzzo, 2000).

Plague

Thanks to modern sanitation and the availability of antibiotics and pesticides, another occurrence of the Black Death[5] due to plague appears unlikely. However, isolated cases of plague are still reported in various parts of the world, including the United States, and plague outbreaks are still possible where wild rodent populations are persistently infected with the plague bacillus. Such regions include the western United States and parts of South America, Africa, and Asia. The last great plague epidemic occurred in the early twentieth century in India and resulted in more than 10 million deaths.

Plague is caused by the bacterium *Yersinia pestis*, which is transmitted to humans by fleas whose primary hosts are rodents; rats, ground squirrels,

---

[5]Black Death, a devastating pandemic that swept through much of Asia and Europe during the Middle Ages, killed some 20 million people, representing 20 to 25 percent of Western Europe's total populace.

and rabbits, as well as the occasional house cat, can also harbor infected fleas. Bubonic plague, the most common form of the disease, is acquired directly from the bite of an infected flea. Bubonic plague derives its name from characteristic swollen lymph nodes (called "buboes") in the groin, axilla, and neck areas. Pneumonic plague, which is less common, can develop from the bubonic form and is spread directly from person to person by the respiratory route. Untreated bubonic plague is fatal in half of all cases; untreated pneumonic plague is invariably fatal.

Crowding and poor sanitation in or near areas where rodent plague is endemic are ideal conditions for the emergence of this devastating bacterial illness. Squalid conditions were a major factor in emergence during a 1994 outbreak of plague in India (Ramalingaswami, 1996). From August to October of that year, India reported to WHO a total of 693 suspected cases of bubonic or pneumonic plague with positive test results for antibodies to *Yersinia pestis*. Nationwide, 56 of the reported plague cases were fatal (CDC, 1994d). Most of the cases were from the area of Surat, a city of 2.2 million people who generate close to 1,250 metric tons of garbage daily, 20 percent of which is left uncollected and has led to a dramatic growth in the city's rat population.

Exacerbating this problem in sanitation were two natural disasters. First, floodwaters inundated the low-lying slum areas near the river during a 1994 monsoon. Surat residents complained that nothing was done to remove the great piles of rubbish that remained after the floodwaters receded, providing an ideal habitat for rats. A year before the plague incident, an earthquake measuring 6.4 on the Richter scale had hit the adjacent state of Maharashtra, killing at least 10,000 people and causing extensive damage. Researchers believe that the disturbances and resettlement associated with the earthquake helped drive the wild rodent population inhabiting the forested area near Surat into contact with the domestic rat population, thus introducing the disease into the latter rat population (World Resources Institute, 1996). In financial terms, the plague's toll cost the Indian economy in excess of $600 million. More than 45,000 people canceled travel plans to India, and the country's hotel occupancy rate dipped by half. Many countries stopped air and ship traffic to India altogether. In total, exports from the country suffered a $420 million loss.

Nosocomial Infections

Nosocomial (hospital-acquired) infections are a serious problem worldwide. According to WHO, at any given time more than 1.4 million people worldwide suffer from infectious complications acquired in hospitals (WHO, 2002f). Nosocomial bloodstream infections are a leading cause of death in the United States (Edmond et al., 1999; Wenzel and Edmond, 2001). CDC estimates that each year nearly 2 million patients in the United States acquire infections in hospitals, and about 90,000 of these patients die as a result (CDC, 2002o).

A number of factors drive the development of nosocomial infections. Foremost in the developed world is advances in health care technology (discussed earlier), for several reasons. The first is improved survival of vulnerable populations, such as the elderly; infants of very low birth weight; and cancer, AIDS, and transplant patients. These individuals are susceptible to germs that would not be harmful to healthy people. Second, greater numbers of invasive procedures—such as placement of indwelling catheters, feeding tubes, ventilators, transplantations, and prosthetic devices—are being performed, allowing microorganisms more direct access to patients' bloodstreams. Finally, widespread use of antimicrobial drugs in hospitals is resulting in more drug-resistant organisms that are increasingly difficult to treat.

In addition, overcrowded conditions within hospitals and a lack of proper sanitation and hygiene contribute greatly to the transfer of microbes. Studies have shown that potentially pathogenic organisms can be passed on to patients from unclean stethoscopes (Marinella et al., 1997), lab coats (Wong et al., 1991), environmental surfaces, and latex gloves (Ray et al., 2002). However, cross-transmission of microorganisms by the hands of health care workers is considered the main route for the spread of pathogens in hospitals (Pittet et al., 1999). Thus, simple handwashing practices remain the most important preventive measure. Unfortunately, many hospitals are unable to maintain an adequate level of handwashing among health care workers (Vicca, 1999; Saade et al., 2001; Doebbeling et al., 1992; Jarvis, 1994).

Nosocomial outbreaks of Lassa fever and Ebola viral hemorrhagic fever in Africa illustrate the additional complexities of preventing hospital-acquired infections in developing countries. Lassa fever spread in Nigeria in 1989 because scant resources led to needle sharing and reuse of disposable equipment. Overuse of parenteral treatments, inadequate surgical facilities, and poorly trained personnel also fueled the spread of the virus among patients and health care providers (Fisher-Hoch et al., 1995). Similarly, in the absence of appropriate precautions to prevent exposure to blood and other body fluids, hospital outbreaks of Ebola viral hemorrhagic fever in Zaire in 1995 passed from patients to health care workers and to family members who provided nursing care (CDC, 1995b) (see Box 3-15).

Hospitals are perfect breeding grounds for transferring infections among patients, health care providers, and the community. Patients in intensive-care units (ICUs) are at particularly high risk for nosocomial infections as a result of their underlying illness, the multiple invasive proce-

---

BOX 3-15
Ebola Virus

The 1995 Ebola virus outbreak in Zaire is an example of the biocomplexity of the emergence of a microbial threat to health. Even though the animal reservoir for the Ebola virus has yet to be discovered, the nosocomial spread of the virus from human to human has had deadly consequences. The outbreak began on April 4, 1995, when a hospital laboratory technician in Kikwit, Zaire, experienced the onset of fever and bloody diarrhea. One week later, he underwent surgery for a suspected perforated bowel. A few days later, medical personnel employed in the hospital to which he had been admitted in Kikwit developed similar symptoms. One of the ill was transferred to a hospital in Mosango (75 miles west of Kikwit); there, several days later, personnel who had provided care for this patient began experiencing similar symptoms as well (CDC, 1995a).

On May 9, 1995, blood samples from 14 of the acutely ill persons in Zaire arrived at CDC in Atlanta and were processed in the biosafety 4 laboratory. Every sample tested positive for the Ebola virus. After sequencing the virus glycoprotein gene, CDC determined that the newly emerged virus was closely related to the Ebola virus that had been isolated during an outbreak of viral hemorrhagic fever in northern Zaire and southern Sudan in 1976 (the first time the Ebola virus had ever been isolated in humans). In 1967, an outbreak of the closely related Marburg virus had occurred in Marburg, Germany, where laboratory workers were exposed to infected tissue from monkeys imported from Uganda. Ebola and Marburg are the only two known members of the filovirus family. Other reports of filovirus infections or outbreaks have been a single case of infection from a newly described Ebola virus in Cote D'Ivoire in 1994, and a 1989 outbreak of yet another Ebola virus (not associated with human disease) in imported monkeys that had been brought into the United States from the Philippines. Among all reported human outbreaks, 50 to 90 percent of cases have been fatal.

By June 1995, public health authorities had identified 296 persons with viral hemorrhagic fever attributable to Ebola virus infection in Zaire; the case-fatality rate was 79 percent (CDC, 1995b). The median age of infected persons was 37 years, with a range from 1 month to 71 years. Transmission of the virus from person-to-person occurs through close contact with infectious blood or other body fluids or tissues; secondary cases have occurred among persons providing medical care for patients and among patients exposed to reused needles. Although aerosol spread of the virus has not been documented among humans, it has been demonstrated among nonhuman primates (Peters et al., 1991; Jaax et al., 1995).

---

dures performed on them, and their typically older ages. According to the National Nosocomial Infections Surveillance (NNIS) System, from 1997 to 1999, urinary catheter–associated urinary tract infection (UTI) rates were highest in medical (nonsurgical) ICUs (6.5 UTIs per 1,000 days a catheter was used); central line–associated bloodstream infection (BSI) rates were highest in pediatric ICUs (7.7 BSIs per 1,000 days a central line was used); and ventilator-associated pneumonia rates were highest in surgical ICUs

(13.0 cases of pneumonia per 1,000 days a ventilator was used) (CDC, 2000e).

The nosocomial transfer of antimicrobial-resistant organisms to patients remains a significant concern. Looking specifically at ICU patients with nosocomial infections in 2000, NNIS found that more than 55 percent of *Staphylococcus aureus* isolates were resistant to methicillin, oxacillin, or nafcillin. Methicillin-resistant *S. aureus* increased 29 percent in 2000 as compared with the mean of the previous 5 years (1995–1999). Resistance of *Pseudomonas aeruginosa* to quinolones increased 53 percent during the same period in the same population; vancomycin-resistant enterococci increased 31 percent (National Nosocomial Infections Surveillance System, 2001).

Immunizations

Vaccine-preventable diseases still cause millions of deaths each year, mainly in developing countries. Indeed, nearly 3 million people worldwide die annually from major vaccine-preventable diseases.

Childhood immunizations have contributed to a significant reduction in vaccine-preventable diseases, including measles, mumps, rubella, pertussis, and other potentially devastating illnesses. Yet there remains a sizable segment of the population, both in the United States and internationally, that does not receive childhood vaccinations. Several reasons may account for low vaccine rates, including misperceptions about the actual risk for a given disease, concerns about the safety of vaccines due to widely publicized but unsubstantiated claims of adverse effects, and the absence of a health infrastructure for vaccine purchase and delivery. In Africa, for example, only 55 percent of the population in the region had vaccination coverage for polio and measles in 2000 (WHO, 2001g). That same year, the Americas vaccinated 90 percent of the population against both diseases.

Even in the United States, vaccine-preventable diseases cause staggering numbers of deaths and illnesses. For example, pneumonia and influenza deaths together constitute the sixth leading cause of death in the United States. Influenza causes an average of 110,000 hospitalizations and 20,000 deaths annually; pneumococcal disease causes 10,000 to 14,000 deaths annually (DHHS, 2000b). The annual estimate of influenza vaccination for adults aged 65 and older (those at increased risk for severe disease or death from influenza) is roughly 65 percent. Moreover, the percentage of older adults reported as ever having received a pneumococcal vaccination is even lower. The Healthy People 2010 target is to increase to 90 percent the proportion of noninstitutionalized adults aged 65 and older who are vaccinated annually against influenza and who have ever been vaccinated against pneumococcal disease (DHHS, 2000b).

Measles

Reported annual measles cases worldwide declined by almost 40 percent between 1990 and 1999. Nonetheless, an estimated 30 million to 40 million cases occurred in 2000, resulting in approximately 777,000 deaths (WHO and UNICEF, 2001). Measles accounts for nearly half of the 1.7 million annual deaths due to childhood vaccine-preventable diseases. In 1999, the African continent accounted for 58 percent of all estimated measles cases in the world, 87 percent of which were located in the west and central regions (WHO, 2000g). In southern Africa, the number of reported measles cases decreased from over 50,000 annually to 100 in 1999 because of intensive vaccination campaigns (WHO, 2002k). In the Americas, countries that have adequately implemented the strategies recommended by the Pan American Health Organization/WHO have successfully inhibited measles transmission.

The number of reported cases in the United States plummeted from approximately 500,000 before vaccine introduction in 1963 to fewer than 1,500 in 1983 (Bellini and Rota, 1998). Despite these measures, however, a resurgence of measles occurred in the United States between 1989 and 1991, causing more than 55,000 cases and approximately 120 measles-associated deaths. Most of the cases occurred in children under 5 years of age. Of those who lost their lives during this epidemic, 90 percent had not been vaccinated (CDC, 2001k). As a result of successful vaccination efforts, the number of reported measles cases dropped to less than 100 in 2000 (CDC, 2002p). Although it was announced in 2000 that measles was no longer endemic in the United States (CDC, 2002q), a continued risk remains for internationally imported measles cases that could result in indigenous transmission.

Diphtheria

Diphtheria had been well controlled in Russia for two decades following the initiation of a universal childhood immunization program in the late 1950s. In the 1970s, however, the number of cases began to rise (see Figure 3-9). The epidemic of diphtheria in the Newly Independent States of the former Soviet Union in the early 1990s marked the first large-scale diphtheria epidemic in industrialized countries in three decades (Vitek and Wharton, 1998). In 1993, the number of reported diphtheria cases surged to nearly 20,000, occurring primarily throughout urban Russia, the Ukraine, Belarus, and the Baltics. By 1994, the number of reported diphtheria cases had surged to 50,412 in the Newly Independent States, with Russia accounting for 83 percent of the cases. In 1994, epidemic diphtheria was reported for

Cases per 100,000 Population

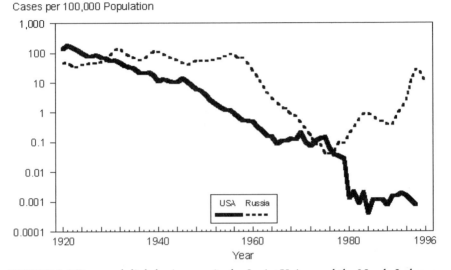

FIGURE 3-9 Reported diphtheria cases in the Soviet Union and the Newly Independent States, 1965–1996.
SOURCE: Vitek and Wharton, 1998.

all states except Estonia, where most of the adult population had been vaccinated in 1985–1987 (Vitek and Wharton, 1998).

The large increase in diphtheria cases was due mainly to low vaccination coverage for large segments of the population, which resulted from changes in vaccination policy to fewer doses of vaccine with lower antigenic content. In addition, public support for vaccination programs fell as the level of disease diminished, and a vocal anti-immunization movement received favorable press coverage in an atmosphere of increased distrust of the government. Resurgence was also associated with a change in the predominant circulating biotype of the diphtheria-causing organism, a decline in the standard of living resulting from the dissolution of the Soviet Union, and a high level of population movement. Starting in 1993, a wide-scale vaccination campaign was implemented, so that by 1999, diphtheria rates had returned to the levels recorded in the early 1990s (Netesov and Conrad, 2001).

Tuberculosis Control

The worldwide persistence of tuberculosis (TB) has been due chiefly to the neglect of its control by governments, poorly managed TB control programs, poverty, population growth and migration, and a significant increase in TB cases in HIV-endemic areas (WHO, 2002g). Lack of diagnosis of cases, together with poor adherence to antituberculosis medications among those who are diagnosed, are major barriers to eradicating tuberculosis. Insufficient treatment can lead to prolonged infection and communicability, drug resistance, and relapse of the disease, all of which pose serious health threats to those infected and their communities (Volmink and Garner, 2001).

Directly observed therapy (DOT) was introduced 40 years ago as a means of ensuring that patients with tuberculosis would complete their treatment regimens. The approach involves simply the supervised swallowing of medications. However, many DOT programs have become much more comprehensive in an effort to improve therapeutic adherence. In the United States, these programs include such services as assistance with housing, food subsidies, transportation, and social support (Volmink et al., 2000). Because programs differ with regard to the services provided and the enthusiasm of their employees, it is difficult to discern which factors account for the success of a DOT program.

WHO promotes another version of DOT called Directly Observed Therapy, Short Course (DOTS) that focuses on tropical and low-income countries. DOTS involves five elements: (1) government commitment to sustained TB control activities; (2) improved laboratory detection; (3) a standardized short course of treatment with direct observation for at least the initial two months; (4) a free, uninterrupted drug supply; and (5) a reporting system that documents patient progress and allows assessment of the program (WHO, 1999d). The number of countries using DOTS expanded from 10 in 1990 to 148 in 2000 (WHO, 2002h); however, only 27 percent of the estimated total cases of TB worldwide were treated under DOTS in 2000 (WHO, 2002i). While DOTS includes a number of useful components, the available evidence does not provide strong support for the routine adoption of this program in favor of self-administration of treatment (Volmink and Garner, 2001).

Targets for global TB control were ratified by the World Health Assembly. They include (1) successfully treating 85 percent of smear-positive TB cases and (2) detecting 70 percent of all such cases (WHO, 2002h, 2000e). These goals had not been attained by the end of 2000, so the target year was reset to 2005.

Control of Vector-borne and Zoonotic Diseases

One major factor in the resurgence of vector-borne and zoonotic diseases is the decreased support for and deterioration of public health infrastructure. Continued surveillance and control programs for these diseases are expensive. When budget shortfalls occur, these programs are especially vulnerable to funding reductions or elimination, especially when the diseases are perceived to be controlled. This is as true in the United States as it is in developing countries. The sporadic and epidemic nature of many vector-borne diseases has resulted in the closure of many state programs and laboratories. A number of states affected by West Nile virus previously had robust arbovirus programs, excellent laboratory facilities, and concomitant vector biology expertise, all of which had been dismantled. With the emergence of West Nile virus, CDC's Division of Vector-borne Infectious Diseases had to institute capacity-building programs for the states and emergency training programs in arbovirus surveillance and medical entomology (CDC, 2001m). A similar training program had to be instituted for mammalogists and field biologists following the emergence of Sin Nombre virus in the American Southwest.

Societal perceptions have also complicated the control of vector-borne diseases, especially the use of pesticides for vector control. The emergence of West Nile virus in New York resulted in a recommendation to spray pesticides to control adult mosquitoes in the face of the impending epidemic. This action was resisted by many people in the New York City area because of the perceived dangers of pesticide exposure. Public perceptions about pesticide usage may still persist from the negative consequences associated with the historical usage of DDT to control vectors. Despite this major achievement in public health to control malaria in highly endemic areas, recognition that indiscriminate DDT usage led to accumulation of the pesticide in nature and to detrimental effects on nontarget organisms resulted in a total ban on its use in many countries. Yet these environmental problems stemmed from agricultural uses of DDT, not from public health usage to treat walls in homes for vector control. New, more expensive, less stable, and less effective pesticides have replaced DDT for vector control in many countries. Unfortunately, the widespread halt in DDT usage has coincided with a resurgence of malaria in the Americas and elsewhere (Roberts et al., 1997; Attaran et al., 2000), as well as with increases in other diseases, such as leishmaniasis and dengue (see Box 3-16) (Gratz, 1999). These problems and the development of resistance to alternative pesticides in targeted vector populations have renewed the use of DDT for domicile treatment to control malaria in several countries (see the discussion of vector-borne and zoonotic disease control in Chapter 4).

Antiquated Public Health Laws

Public health laws enacted for the control of infectious diseases are rooted in colonial history. Early state and local governments recognized their responsibility to safeguard the public's health from infectious diseases (e.g., smallpox, cholera, plague) by promulgating sanitary regulations, ordering the abatement of public health nuisances (e.g., infested premises), and enforcing disease control measures (e.g., isolation, quarantine, vaccination). Shifting priorities as new diseases emerged help explain why infectious disease laws developed in piecemeal fashion. Over time, some public health laws were updated or modified as medical knowledge (e.g., testing, screening, treatment) and epidemiology advanced. Many public health laws, however, have not been regularly reviewed or revised since the middle of the twentieth century (Gostin et al., 1999).

State laws regarding infectious diseases are often fragmented and inconsistent (embodying differing approaches among the states) and inadequate (failing to provide the powers that are needed) (Gostin, 2001a). Outdated state laws do not support, and may even thwart, effective public health surveillance and interventions. Consequently, the DHHS (2000b) and the IOM (1988) have recommended reforming laws to ensure appropriate legal preparedness for naturally occurring infectious diseases and the intentional use of a biological agent. A corpus of strong public health laws is critically important to ensure such preparedness. Such laws afford public health officials essential powers, such as screening, reporting, vaccination, treatment (including DOT), and isolation or quarantine. These and other powers are constitutionally acceptable when necessary to protect the public's health if performed with procedural guarantees (Gostin, 2001b, 2002a).

Modern public health laws also enable authorities to prevent disease transmission by ensuring healthy conditions. Inspections of private premises, nuisance abatements, and business regulations can help avert and control epidemics. Legal responses to the recent emergence of West Nile virus are illustrative. Many public health authorities asked property owners to eliminate standing bodies of water that, as discussed previously, encourage the breeding of mosquitoes that transmit the virus. Inspections of public and private premises were performed. If private property owners failed to eliminate sources of standing water, authorities entered their property to abate the public health nuisance. Likewise, recognizing that stockpiles of discarded tires provide optimal conditions for breeding mosquitoes, the New York state legislature drafted regulations to require tire retailers to practice safe disposal and recycling (Hodge, 2002).

Public health laws also authorize the collection and analysis of public health information through surveillance and epidemiologic investigations. States have enacted reporting requirements for specified infectious diseases, often pursuant to guidance from CDC (see the discussion in Chapter 4). The collection and use of identifiable health data for public health purposes raise individual privacy concerns. Courts generally allow the collection of such data provided that adequate safeguards are in place. New federal privacy regulations pursuant to the Health Insurance Portability and Ac-

BOX 3-16
The Breakdown of Vector Control

The emergence of epidemic dengue and dengue hemorrhagic fever and shock syndrome (DHF-SS) in the Americas illustrates the dire consequences of the demise of public health control capacity and expertise in vector-borne diseases. More than 2.5 billion people are at risk for dengue virus infection; 50 million cases are estimated to occur annually; and the incidence of DHF-SS continues to increase throughout the world (Gubler, 2002). The major urban vector of dengue viruses is the mosquito *Aedes aegypti*, whose anthropophilic and endophilic behavior makes it an unparalleled vector. The abundance and distribution of *Ae. aegypti* are directly linked to the presence of breeding sites (e.g., water storage vessels, discarded cans, tires, or containers that hold water long enough for the vectors to hatch, develop, and emerge). This in turn greatly complicates control efforts, especially source reduction control programs designed to eliminate larval breeding sites. Increased population growth and urbanization, much of it unplanned, has contributed greatly to the dramatic increase in *Ae. aegypti* abundance (Gubler, 2002; Gratz, 1999).

The dramatic change in the epidemiology of dengue and DHF-SS in the Americas has been the subject of much speculation. Prior to the 1980s, only one or two of the serotypes of dengue circulated in the Americas, and DHF-SS was nonexistent. This was in sharp contrast to Southeast Asia, where all four dengue serotypes cocirculated, and DHF-SS was (and remains) a major public health problem. Many factors condition the differing epidemiology of dengue in the two parts of the world, including the virulence of the viruses (Gubler, 2002). However, there is no doubt that one of the major factors contributing to the emergence of DHF-SS in the Americas was the resurgence of *Ae. aegypti* in tropical and subtropical cities, concomitant with rampant and unplanned urbanization (see the accompanying figure).

In the 1950s and 1960s, the Pan American Health Organization (PAHO) and participating Western Hemisphere countries established a remarkably effective program to eradicate *Ae. aegypti* (Gubler, 2002; Gratz, 1999). The major impetus for this effort was the desire to preclude the emergence of sylvatic yellow fever into urban populations,

countability Act explicitly permit public health data collection if consistent with state law.

New and emerging infectious disease threats, especially the threat of bioterrorism, have led federal, state, and local governments to reexamine public health laws addressing infectious disease control. Antiquated laws are increasingly being reviewed and updated to eliminate inconsistencies and reflect current medical knowledge and legal and ethical norms. By 2002, thirty-six states had introduced bills and twenty states had enacted legislation based on the Model State Emergency Powers Act, which consolidates public health powers to enable authorities to respond effectively to bioterrorism and other public health emergencies (Gostin et al., 2002).

which remains a major concern today. Many countries (the United States being one notable exception) were remarkably successful in this regard. Ironically, the success of the programs led to their demise, and the resources and infrastructure needed to support these efforts were soon shifted to other priorities. Now *Ae. aegypti is* essentially hyperabundant throughout the Americas, and concomitantly all four dengue virus serotypes (including the virulent Asian genotypes which are associated with DHF-SS) are co-circulating in the region (Beaty, 2000).

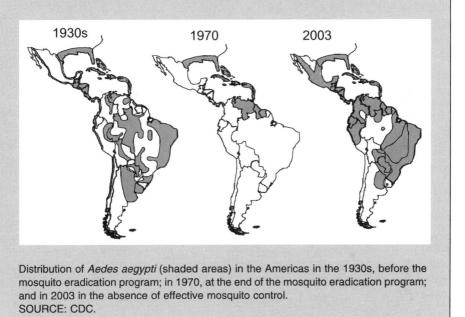

Distribution of *Aedes aegypti* (shaded areas) in the Americas in the 1930s, before the mosquito eradication program; in 1970, at the end of the mosquito eradication program; and in 2003 in the absence of effective mosquito control.
SOURCE: CDC.

Another project to develop a comprehensive model state public health act is currently under way, sponsored by the Robert Wood Johnson Foundation's Turning Point initiative. These and other legal tools may lead to significant improvements in the reformation of public health laws.

POVERTY AND SOCIAL INEQUALITY

As we enter the twenty-first century, mortality from infectious diseases is correlated more closely than ever before with transnational inequalities in income (Houweling et al., 2001). Countries throughout the developing world and the former communist bloc have been embracing the market-based policies advocated by Europe and North America. The result has been extensive privatization of state-owned banks and companies, creation of new stock and bond markets, and exposure of economies to foreign investment and capital. These global economic trends affect not only the personal circumstances of those at risk for infection, but also the structure and availability of public health institutions. The structure of health care delivery, in turn, profoundly affects the ability of high-risk populations to pursue health care. For example, the transmission of illnesses such as TB, which nearly disappeared in affluent countries after the introduction of effective antimicrobial therapy in the 1950s, has continued to rise in poor countries. It is not coincidental that many of the latter countries have been hardest hit by microbial threats to health such as HIV, dengue, drug-resistant TB, and malaria (Murray and Lopez, 1997).

The relationship between infectious diseases and economic development has been of increasing interest to scholars and practitioners in a variety of fields (Sen, 1999; Gwatkin et al., 1999; Whitehead Institute, 2002). Studies within the fields of social epidemiology and medical anthropology have illustrated the relationships between large-scale social patterns, such as poverty (see Box 3-17), and clinical, epidemiological, and even biological phenomena (Farmer, 1996; Berkman and Kawachi, 2000; Schoepf, 2001). Public health economists have also identified trends correlating health with resource distribution (Gwatkin, 2000; Gwatkin et al., 1999; Castro-Leal et al., 2000). It is important to note that the arrow points in both directions: not only do infectious diseases have significant and far-reaching economic implications, but poverty and social inequality in and of themselves are major factors in disease emergence (Bloom and Sachs, 1998; Eandi and Zara, 1998; Bhargava et al., 2001; WHO, 2002j; Dixon et al., 2002).

Socioeconomic status is often implicated in public health trends that might appear at first glance to be unrelated. For example, chronic infection with hepatitis B virus has been associated with low educational attainment, lower social stratum, and crowded urban residence. Meanwhile, hepatitis B virus has been implicated as a major etiological agent of liver cancer, suggesting that even the latter condition may have an economic determinant (Stuver et al., 1997). Socioeconomic status has been identified as a factor contributing to the escalating problem of worldwide antimicrobial resistance (Okeke et al., 1999). In 1990, developing countries spent $41 per person on health, compared with $1,500 per person in industrialized countries. This underfunding creates a chronically inadequate or erratic supply of drugs, which, combined with several other factors, such as transportation costs and the high costs of medical treatment and drugs, leads to poor patient compliance. Poor compliance, in turn, leads to the emergence of antimicrobial resistance, as has been learned all too well from the emergence of multidrug-resistant TB. Even where excellent country-level TB control programs are in place, treatment efficacy in poor communities can

BOX 3-17
World Poverty Statistics

Although extreme poverty declined worldwide in the 1990s from 28 percent in 1987 to 23 percent in 1998 (World Bank Group, 2002), 2.8 billion people are still living on less than US$2 a day and 1.2 billion are living on less than US$1 a day (see the figure below). The average income in the richest 20 countries is 37 times the average in the poorest 20, a gap that had doubled over the past 40 years (World Bank, 2001).

Within and among regions, income disparities became more pronounced during the 1990s. Countries in transition to a market economy also saw a sharp increase in inflation and poverty. Moldova, one of the poorest countries in Europe, experienced a dramatic worsening of poverty; the percentage of people living below the national poverty line increased from 35 percent in May 1997 to 46 percent in the fourth quarter of 1998. The Russian Federation similarly experienced a jump in poverty from an estimated 12 percent during the Soviet period to 43 percent by 1996. In the Kyrgyz Republic, poverty was fundamentally a rural phenomenon, whereas in Bulgaria and Hungary in 1997, the Roma population comprised a disproportionately large percentage of the poor (World Bank Group, 2002). In the United States almost 33 million people were living below the poverty level in 2001 (U.S. Census Bureau, 2002b).

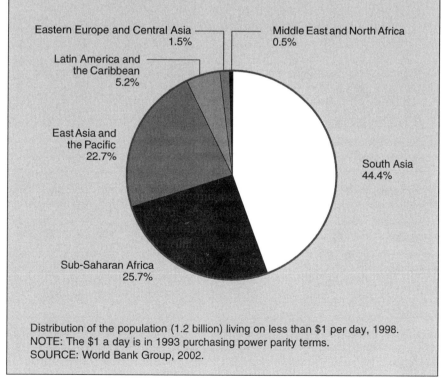

Distribution of the population (1.2 billion) living on less than $1 per day, 1998.
NOTE: The $1 a day is in 1993 purchasing power parity terms.
SOURCE: World Bank Group, 2002.

be undermined by inappropriate cost recovery policies and the remoteness of secondary or tertiary care facilities, potentially leading to the emergence or spread of drug resistance through inadequate therapy (Kim et al., 1999). The susceptibility of poor populations to disease is governed by a number of identifiable conditions, including malnutrition, lack of access to clean water and sanitation (as discussed earlier), housing conditions of poor quality, ignorance of preventive measures, absence of social agencies to teach the avoidance of risky behaviors, lack of adequate transportation to and from health care facilities, and limited funds for out-of-pocket expenditures (WHO, 2002j).

Health is closely correlated with economic productivity; indeed, recent studies indicate that disease burden and demography may be more closely correlated with macroeconomic performance than with other commonly used indicators, such as fiscal policy and political governance (Bloom and Sachs, 1998). As measured by trade and foreign direct investment, one might expect that the poorest countries would be among the world's least integrated into the global economy. However, this is not uniformly the case. While cross-border trade accounted for nearly one-fifth of the United States' and one-third of Mexico's gross domestic product in 1999, in Botswana, to take one extreme case, that figure was 44 percent (World Bank, 2002). Moreover, because of their lower overall volume and diversification of production, poor countries tend to be more sensitive to fluctuations in international commerce; shocks to commodity prices and terms of trade can drastically affect government revenues, the availability of foreign currency reserves, and economic activity in general (Diaz-Bonilla et al., 2001). Finally, the level of indebtedness in poor countries is often so high as to necessitate close coordination with outside agencies in setting fiscal policy.

The influence of the global economy is not limited to general economic function, but impacts directly on the health sector. In several relatively affluent countries with high disease burdens, increases in earnings for upper-income percentiles are leading to the formation or expansion of markets for private health services (Sbarbaro, 2000), a trend that has at times been actively promoted by development agencies (Stocker et al., 1999). Without proper planning, health-sector privatization can interfere directly with government efforts to combat emerging infectious diseases (Kim et al., 1999). Meanwhile, high levels of indebtedness in many countries with high disease prevalence can divert desperately needed funds from the health sector (Piot and Coll Seck, 2001)

Participation in the globalization process, in the worst case, can potentially further widen international health disparities, leaving the poor even more vulnerable to diseases (Diaz-Bonilla et al., 2001). Then, too, spillovers occur in the opposite direction: financial crises, environmental deterioration, and the epidemic spread of emerging infections can impact with great force far beyond their nominal zones of incidence. As a matter of both enlightened self-interest and, perhaps, a newly transnational ethical sensibility, it is essential that the United States and other developed countries incorporate in their response to emerging infectious diseases close attention to public health in the developing world.

WAR AND FAMINE

War and famine are closely linked. Not only do they both lead to severe disruptions in food distribution and consumption, but in fact a frequent causal relationship exists between the two. As of April 2001, the Food and Agriculture Organization (FAO) was tracking 16 countries with "food emergencies" (i.e., catastrophic declines in crop production) in sub-Saharan Africa; 9 of these emergencies were directly related to civil strife (FAO, 2001). So-called "complex humanitarian emergencies" provoked by the combined conditions of famine and war contribute directly to the spread of infectious diseases and have fairly consistent sequelae, including malnutrition, measles, diarrheal diseases, respiratory tract infections, and malaria (Toole and Waldman, 1990).

War

Between 1990 and 1998, 108 wars worldwide claimed 5.5 million lives (Wallensteen and Sollenberg, 1999). Conditions of armed conflict generally result in a breakdown of domestic stability, loss of food security, and destruction of the medical infrastructure. While acquiring reliable data in war-torn regions is difficult, millions of people are thought to die each year not from direct acts of violence, but from inadequate health services (Roberts, 2001; Toole et al., 1993; Toole and Waldman, 1990). According to one recent study, for example, patients with tuberculosis whose chemotherapy was disrupted because of war were three times more likely to die than those who were fully treated during peacetime (Gustafson et al., 2001). As noted, such disruption in treatment not only affects an individual's risk of death, but also increases the risk of the emergence of drug-resistant strains (Khan and Laaser, 2002; Federation of American Scientists, 2002).

The direct human cost of battle pales in comparison with the human cost of its aftermath. Of the countries in which humanitarian emergencies were designated by the National Intelligence Council in 1999, well over half were the sites of high-intensity conflict (Wallensteen and Sollenberg, 2001). These upheavals had consequences far beyond their nominal zones of incidence. A recent estimate put the number of war refugees worldwide at a full 1 percent of the global population (Summerfield, 1997). In the present context, displacement due to war can contribute significantly to the emergence and spread of infectious diseases (Kalipeni and Oppong, 1998; Murray et al., 2002). In most of these emergencies, three out of four deaths are attributable to communicable diseases. Refugee camps are usually crowded and dirty, with little or no access to medical care or protection from vectors, and full of people from many different geographic areas (and thus probably carrying a broad range of infectious agents). For example, in 1994 more than a million Rwandan refugees were sheltered in Goma, Democratic Republic of the Congo, formerly known as Zaire, when cholera and dysentery swept through the camps, killing 12,000 people in just 3 weeks. In the post-conflict phase, malaria accounted for over one-third of the total mortality among displaced populations in Central Africa in the aftermath of the Great Lakes crisis of 1994, and TB was estimated to have caused one-fourth of all deaths among refugees in Somalia in the 1990s (Connolly, 2002).

Famine

While related in some instances to large-scale environmental patterns, famine is highly correlated with factors other than the weather. Rather, it is highly correlated with social, economic, and political forces, including land tenure, deforestation, and rapid demographic change. According to one theory, a root cause of famine is ultimately a deficiency in food "entitlement," owing to political disenfranchisement (Sen, 1981); an exclusive focus on issues of food production that ignores this root condition is deeply counterproductive (Sen, 1999). During the Rwandan genocide, to take one extreme example, famine conditions in the vicinity of the refugee camps were thought to have been greatly exacerbated by the toll on household industry exacted by the shigellosis epidemic (Paquet and van Soest, 1994).

As with war, the causal chain between famine and disease is bidirectional (Topouzis and Hemrich, 2000). Emerging epidemics can severely disrupt food production, especially through high mortality and morbidity among workers in agricultural areas and the depletion of family savings to care for those stricken. The social epidemiology of HIV in sub-Saharan Africa testifies to this bidirectional phenomenon; countries that are more dependent on agriculture are affected more by HIV/AIDS (Topouzis and du Guerny, 1999). Clearly, HIV is a recipe for a catastrophic decline in food supplies; preliminary data suggest that such a decline has in fact taken place. In Zimbabwe, according to a recent report cited by FAO, communal agricultural output has declined by half over the past 5 years, almost entirely as a result of HIV/AIDS.

LACK OF POLITICAL WILL

The need for political will to fight microbial threats is still invoked frequently, more in the breach than in the observance. A global political commitment, like peace or universal love, is described in rather vague terms—an impossible goal whose absence is nonetheless to be lamented. Above all else, the notion is presented in the context of an effort to get *others* involved, parties whose intercession would presumably be decisive in a way that ours would not. Unfortunately, many possible opportunities have been lost as a result of this lack of political will and a general complacency toward infectious diseases reminiscent of the end of the twentieth century (see Box 3-18).

Vague allusions to political will have embraced, perhaps unwittingly, a rather profound concept. Such references may be traced, arguably, to Rousseau's idea of the *volonté générale*. "The problem," he wrote in 1776, "is to find a form of association which will defend and protect . . . the person and goods of each associate, and in which each, while uniting himself with all, may still obey himself alone, and remain as free as before." And the solution? "Each of us puts his person and all his power in common under the supreme direction of the general will, and, in our corporate capacity, we receive each member as an indivisible part of the whole. At once, in place of the individual personality of each contracting party, this act of association creates a moral and collective body, composed of as many members as the assembly contains votes, and receiving from this act its unity, its common identity, its life and its will" (Rousseau, 1993).

The conception of the social contract was of course a powerful one for Thomas Jefferson and other theorists of the American Revolution. In an age of rapidly increasing global integration, it takes on new resonance—and new complexity. Who would be the parties to a global social contract, and how is their will to be determined? How can the liberties of individual countries and their citizens be balanced against their collective responsibility? Is there any collective responsibility at all? Little consensus exists on these questions among the international community. What is certain, however, is that through microbial threats such as HIV, TB, and malaria, the association of human individuals is being enforced, sometimes in the most brutal possible of ways. If only in this small domain, then, it is essential that we expand our conception of political will to encompass not only governments in the regions of highest prevalence, but also corporations, officials, health professionals, and citizens of more fortunate regions that, willingly or not, share with their governments a common microbial landscape.

To proceed with any hope of success in the struggle against emerging infectious diseases, our model of political will must commit four key groups of stakeholders—donors, health professionals, country authorities, and pa-

BOX 3-18
Lost Windows of Opportunity

Emerging infectious diseases are closing, or have the potential to close, windows of opportunity for infectious disease eradication or elimination. The eradication of smallpox stands as one of the outstanding achievements in the history of public health. Eradication was achieved because of a worldwide effort that was supported by the necessary political will and human and technical resources. The world was able to take advantage of the window of opportunity for smallpox eradication because a safe vaccine was available.

In the year that smallpox was declared eradicated (1980), HIV appeared and rapidly colonized Africa and the world. Today the prevalence of HIV is greater than 25 percent in some adult populations, such as that of the Democratic Republic of Congo (formerly Zaire). In the United States, a military recruit who was immunized against smallpox developed generalized vaccinia because he was HIV-seropositive and died (Redfield et al., 1987). That tragic event highlights the fact that if the global smallpox eradication campaign had been postponed, the world would not have been able to eradicate smallpox as easily as was the case before 1980.

Many windows of opportunity have been lost. In the 1950s and 1960s, gonorrhea was highly prevalent throughout African countries. Governments did not attempt to change people's behavior to prevent its transmission. Treatment was offered either infrequently or not at all. When available, treatment for sexually transmitted diseases was many times more expensive than treatment for other diseases, especially in the private mission hospitals throughout Africa. Therefore, gonorrhea went largely untreated, and its prevalence increased to a less manageable level. Today, gonorrhea is present throughout Africa, where it causes infertility in women and is one of the major driving forces in the HIV epidemic, facilitating the transmission of the virus. Had effective public health education been in place in the 1960s to help change sexual behavior and had antibiotic treatment been used effectively, there would not be such a great problem with gonorrhea today. In this case, a window of opportunity to control one disease and reduce the rate of transmission and impact of a far more serious disease has been lost.

The prevalence of tuberculosis (TB) and multidrug-resistant TB is increasing globally. The emergence of HIV facilitated the resurgence of TB, another example of a case in which a window of opportunity has been lost. Global surveys show that there is a 1 percent prevalence of resistance to at least one TB drug. Multidrug treatment for TB costs between US$20 and US$30 for a complete cure, but treatment costs are approximately US$3,000 for multidrug-resistant TB. In many places, a window of opportunity to achieve a manageable level of TB by the proper use of drugs has been lost.

The global effort in the 1960s and 1970s to eradicate malaria succeeded in eradicating malariologists, but not the disease. Today, the malaria parasite is resistant to the

tients and civil society—to the necessity of collective action. These groups are quite interdependent in their commitments. To secure the participation of patients and community members (for example, in undergoing testing for TB or HIV), it is often necessary to convince them that treatment will be available, and then to structure their active participation through grassroots-

drugs of choice—chloroquine or pyrimethamine–sulfadoxine (fansidar), or both—because of improper treatment. Drug-resistant malaria takes longer to respond to treatment. In addition, the mosquito species that transmit the parasite are resistant to the insecticides that previously controlled them because of the improper use of the insecticides and a breakdown of public health infrastructure to monitor their appropriate use. A window of opportunity to eliminate malaria and mitigate its impact has been lost, and as a result, increasing numbers of adults are losing work and more children are dying because of the resurgence of malaria.

The spread of other infectious diseases has resulted from lost public health opportunities to prevent their spread. Poor public health practices by local hospital workers in Kikwit, Zaire, drove the 1995 Ebola hemorrhagic fever outbreak. A cycle of transmission among the patient care staff spread the virus to their families and additional patients. The international community learned of the outbreak in May 1995, nearly 20 weeks after the first case had been reported. Poor communication, poor infection control practices, and poor preventive public health measures reflect the weak public health care systems and infectious disease surveillance capacity in most of Africa. With the end of the Cold War, the end of the colonial era, and the decline of Western interest in tropical diseases, the public health infrastructure in many African countries has deteriorated. Infectious disease surveillance is nearly nonexistent, and emerging infections frequently go unrecognized and unreported.

Immunization, the vanguard of public health practice, is losing ground in both developing and developed countries. For example, the rate of immunization against yellow fever is declining in most countries of the world, particularly those in which the yellow fever virus is endemic. It is very difficult to get an African government to commit to programs of vaccination against yellow fever as part of routine immunization efforts, even though the vaccine is safe and inexpensive and confers long-lasting immunity. In addition, tourists are becoming increasingly less rigorous in obtaining vaccinations. An international alert recently occurred when a photographer returned to Germany with an unknown disease. At first it was thought to be Ebola hemorrhagic fever, but yellow fever was confirmed as the diagnosis.

The bovine spongiform encephalopathy (BSE) outbreak in cows in the United Kingdom, with the subsequent resulting outbreak among humans of variant Creutzfeldt-Jakob disease (vCJD), is an example of ignorance in animal food-handling practices and public health measures. In the late 1970s, the procedures for rendering bonemeal and other products from animal carcasses changed. The resultant food products were used in animal feed. However, infectious agents were transmitted through the animal feed from infected carcasses back into ruminants, resulting in the BSE epidemic and the transmission of the BSE agent to humans, and ultimately in vCJD.

SOURCE: Institute of Medicine (2001b).

oriented program activity. To achieve high-level cooperation in establishing those programs, it is necessary to convince country authorities that adequate and consistent funding will be available. And to secure that funding from private and public donors alike, it is necessary to convince them that interventions are reasonable in scope and have been designed appropriately and with sufficient attention to scientific and clinical safeguards; that effective public health agencies are in place to implement these programs; and, above all, that the programs will ultimately redound to the benefit of the global community as a whole.

Fortunately, much progress has been made in the last few years toward satisfying these reasonable provisions. The Global Plan to Stop TB and the WHO-led Commission on Macroeconomics and Health have each made significant strides, establishing precise estimates of resource needs for specific global interventions. The inauguration of the United Nations Global Fund provides a focal point for program activity around HIV, TB, and malaria. This useful institution has the capacity not only to direct necessary program inputs efficiently, but also to ensure that they are used in a manner consistent with best scientific practices. Structures such as the Global Fund and the MDR-TB Green Light Committee already are serving as a nexus of project activity. Given sufficient attention and resources, they have the capacity not only to turn the tide against these emerging infectious diseases, but also to build infrastructure—and perhaps more important, global consensus—sufficient to combat infections that have not yet emerged.

INTENT TO HARM

The threat of intentional attacks using biological agents on the United States and other countries has never been as serious as it is today. Even before the events in late 2001, when our nation experienced a lethal bioterrorism attack, there was reason for grave concern. Modern history confirms that biological weapons were explored by many nations, although most programs were officially terminated with the Biological Weapons Convention (BWC) treaty, developed in 1972 and now ratified by more than 140 nations. That treaty prohibited the possession, stockpiling, or use of biological weapons, although it contained no provisions for monitoring, inspection, and enforcement (Kadlec et al., 1999).

The United States abandoned its program for offensive biological warfare in 1969, but had been successful in weaponizing infectious organisms and toxins. The revelation in the mid-1990s that the Soviet state had secretly developed a similar but more extensive enterprise (Alibek, 1999) after signing on to the BWC treaty, increased alarm regarding this potential threat. Concern heightened with the disclosure of an ambitious biological weapons program mounted by Iraq (Davis, 1999; Ekeus, 1999), as well as findings that Aum Shinrikyo, the Japanese group that released nerve gas in the Tokyo subway system, had also experimented with botulin and anthrax and sent teams to Zaire in an effort to obtain Ebola for use as a weapon (Olson, 1999). Episodes in the Unites States involving extremist groups or individuals that had obtained dangerous pathogens, such as plague bacillus, for dubious purposes added to the growing perception of risk (Henderson, 1999).

Today, no one should doubt the likelihood that the development of weapons of mass destruction lies within the reach of others. Some have taken comfort in the fact that the extensive programs of the United States and the former Soviet Union are believed to have been beyond the capacity of other nations. However, we must recognize that these programs manufactured multiple agents without the benefit of today's advances in science and technology, which have significantly broadened the field of potentially capable state and nonstate actors.

Numerous commissions have reviewed the threat of bioterrorism in recent years (United States Commission on National Security/21st Century, 2001; National Commission on Terrorism, 2000; Gilmore Commission, 2000). They have uniformly concluded that the United States is vulnerable to a bioterrorist attack and that the likelihood of such an event is high. Nations suspected of having offensive biological warfare programs have been named by the Office of Technology Assessment (U.S. Congress, 1993a), and these same states are often also identified as terrorist sponsors. In light of these agreed-upon threats, why has there been so little concern about this possibility in many quarters, and why has so much surprise been expressed over the outcome of a handful of letters containing anthrax spores dispatched through the mail? One important factor is a lack of familiarity among civilian scientists with the concepts that were the pillar of the old U.S. biowarfare program as well as the Soviet program, particularly in regard to the danger of aerosols. Another reason may be the unexpected use of an envelope as the delivery mechanism for such a deadly manufactured powder as that used in the anthrax letters of 2001, instead of a more stealthy and lethal dissemination system.

Nature of the Threat

When one considers the ways in which the intentional use of a biological agent might be carried out, the first rule should be that we do not know who the possible terrorist will be, his or her motivation, or the wherewithal that may be available for the attack. Thus, attacks intended to incapacitate selected persons and thereby gain attention or to cause serious illness for revenge might employ a very different approach than attacks designed to cause mass casualties. An effort by a disgruntled clinical laboratory worker might have a very different scope from one by a well-funded nonstate organization or a state-sponsored group. Parenthetically, the failure of the Japanese Aum Shinrikyo cult to succeed with biological terrorism should not provide much comfort concerning the need for state sponsorship, given the manifest ineptitude of the perpetrators (Smithson, 2000).

A second issue is the dissemination of factual information concerning the real dangers of such an attack. Some (including members of this committee) would argue that the less is said, the better. However, American society does not respond without facts and public opinion programs. This means the actual dangers must be explained to the public and responsible political leaders without inflammatory rhetoric or disclosure of detailed methods for the assaults. In reaching a balance, we take some chance that plain speaking could motivate some to undertake the very actions we are trying to prevent. However candid discussion of the facts may help the public, the media, and health authorities respond in a calmer and more rational fashion than was observed with the aerosol anthrax attacks of 2001. The reality of those attacks is far more provocative than any abstract discussion (see Box 3-19).

Microbes could be delivered to a target population by multiple routes. Directly inoculating victims, infecting natural vectors or reservoirs and loosing them on the target population, or infecting a few people and counting on their spreading the infection even further are some possibilities. If we focus on terrorist strategies that can inflict mass casualties, however, none of these mechanisms is highly feasible today with the exception of smallpox, a virus that is well known to spread from human to human after a long and successful career in that evolutionary niche. If we conclude that other organisms must be delivered directly to the target host, we should also consider water, food, and aerosols as potential vehicles of infection. Contaminated water from wells and storage containers has been associated with outbreaks of disease, but the use of this approach for causing mass casualties is limited because of the dilution factor, chlorination, and the usual treatment of water before consumption in this country. Foodborne pathogens have caused many outbreaks in the United States and are a major cause of morbidity and mortality. Food items, however, are usually not consumed synchronously except at special events; although the extensive network of global commerce can assist in distributing an initial source over wide geographic areas. Improved surveillance of foodborne diseases and newer methods of molecular typing of offending organisms should provide a countermeasure to the possible wide dissemination of contaminated food. If a few cases are recognized and traced to a food source, warnings and recalls may serve to protect others from catastrophic harm.

The overall societal impact of any one of these dissemination methods could be considerable, regardless of the actual health damage. Case studies already exist, including nonlethal *Salmonella* infection of several hundred citizens (Torok et al., 1997); Sarin gas attacks with 12 deaths (Smithson, 2000); food tampering; and, most recently, anthrax delivered by letter and even anthrax hoaxes. Perhaps the most important route of attack, however, is aerosolization because of its ability to cause such large numbers of casu-

---

BOX 3-19
Anthrax: Postmarked for Terror

From October 4 through November, 2001, CDC, state and local public health authorities, and local health care providers identified a total of 22 cases of anthrax, including 11 confirmed cases of inhalational anthrax and 7 confirmed and 4 suspected cases of cutaneous anthrax (Jernigan et al., 2002). Five of the inhalational anthrax cases resulted in death. Most of the infected individuals were postal workers at facilities in New Jersey and the District of Columbia, where letters contaminated with anthrax were handled or processed using high-speed sorting machines. Approximately 300 postal and other facilities were tested for *B. anthracis* spores, and some 32,000 persons were administered antimicrobial prophylaxis following potential exposure at workplaces. About 5,000 persons were advised to complete a 60-day course of antibiotics. Additionally, CDC confirmed three isolates of *B. anthracis*, indistinguishable from the U.S. isolates, which had been recovered from the outer surface of letters or packages sent in U.S. State Department pouches to the United States Embassy in Peru (2) and Austria (1) (Polyak et al., 2002).

Historically, human anthrax in its various forms (i.e., inhalational, cutaneous, and gastrointestinal) has been most common in people who have regular, close contact with animals or animal products contaminated with *Bacillus anthracis* spores. Both livestock and wild herbivores are reservoirs of anthrax, which can be spread to humans during slaughtering or, less often, by human ingestion of contaminated meat. Upon exposure to air, *B. anthracis* transforms from a vegetative state to a highly resistant spore that can remain viable for years; dried or otherwise processed skins and hides of infected animals may harbor the spores and are the primary mechanisms by which the disease spreads worldwide.

Anthrax was known as "woolsorters'" disease in the 1800s, when textile workers became ill from exposure to spore-contaminated animal fibers. Although improved industrial hygiene and restrictions on imported animal products have dramatically reduced the number of cases of human anthrax in the United States in the last part of the twentieth century, epidemics occasionally occur in this country among employees who work with animal products, especially goat hair. Cutaneous and gastrointestinal outbreaks related to handling and consuming infected cattle meat occur much more regularly in other parts of the world. The estimated number of human cases of anthrax worldwide is 20,000 to 100,000 per year as a result of agricultural or industrial exposure (Braunwald et al., 2001). The largest outbreak of inhalational anthrax occurred in Sverdlovsk, Russia, in 1979, after an accidental aerosol release from a military facility; at least 66 people were documented to have died as a result (Meselson et al., 1994).

---

alties. The deficiencies of aerosols, such as dependence on meteorological conditions, the unsuitability of most organisms for airborne spread, and the technical demands involved, may be counterbalanced in the hands of skillful perpetrators by the advantages of standoff attack, the silent spread of incapacitating or lethal disease, and wide-area coverage.

Aerosol Dissemination

Aerosols and droplets have long been recognized as routes of microbial transmission. Measles, influenza, smallpox, and tuberculosis are all known to be transmissible between patients by droplets; measles can also be spread by aerosol. In the laboratory, aerosol promulgation of tularemia, rickettsiae, viral hemorrhagic fevers, and many other agents is a threat to the microbiologist (DHHS, 1999). Artificially generated aerosols of anthrax and other agents are high on the list of terrorist attack options. Decreases in human tuberculosis and virtual elimination of diseases such as measles and smallpox from common medical experience, as well as the development of enhanced methods for protecting laboratory workers (ironically using technology developed during the U.S. biowarfare program), have resulted in a loss of appreciation for this route of infection. Yet the U.S. and Soviet biological weapons programs were based largely on the properties of selected agents for causing large-scale infection of human populations under the proper meteorological conditions and with carefully developed methods of aerosol dissemination. Moreover, the terrorist could attack enclosed environments, such as stadiums or large buildings, to negate the meteorological factors that degrade a small-particle aerosol.

Biological agents have not seen widespread use in warfare, so it is not surprising that there is skepticism as to their efficacy. It is generally not appreciated that the U.S. program in offensive biological warfare (terminated in November 1969) rigorously tested each step in the link between a microorganism selected by several criteria and the delivery of a credible biological attack (U.S. Congress, 1993a, 1993b; Rosebury, 1947; Hersh, 1968; McDermott, 1987; Cole, 1997; Sidell et al., 1997; IOM, 2001c). Tularemia is an excellent example because extensive information on this agent is available in the published literature, records of congressional hearings, and the popular press. From its initial isolation (Francis, 1921) this organism was notorious for causing infections in the laboratory, a frequent hallmark of aerosol infectivity. The agent's aerosol properties were studied intensively, and methods were found to enhance its stability in storage and in aerosols. Animals and later humans were challenged with graded doses of the bacterium delivered in different particle sizes to establish the quantitative properties of these aerosols. Open-air dissemination was mimicked using a surrogate organism, *Serratia marcescens*, and this effort confirmed that an organism with the aerosol stability and infectivity of *Francisella tularensis* could cause mass casualties over large geographic areas, provided attention was given to meteorological conditions. The areas affected could reach thousands of square kilometers. The resulting environmental retransmission from the large numbers of different nonhuman mammalian and arthropod species that would be infected in a tularemia attack cannot be evaluated. Thus, little doubt exists that numerous human casualties could be caused by efficiently weaponized organisms readily available in nature.

A relatively small number of agents are suitable for causing thousands or hundreds of thousands of casualties, and this fact may provide a basis for prioritizing medical and other measures to deny the intent of terrorists. It is impossible to focus on every possible agent, and discussions persist among experts as to whether some should be added to or omitted from the list of those to be addressed. However, general agreement has been reached that those pathogens cited in Box 2-2 in Chapter 2 are the most deadly and the most likely to seriously destabilize government functioning and civil society. They grow to excellent titer for more efficient manufacture, and they are highly stable and infectious in aerosols when properly prepared. Toxins are inherently less efficient because they cannot match the killing or incapacitating power of these highly infectious organisms; the toxins must produce their effects as delivered, but the infectious agents grow and produce toxins or other effects in the recipient's body.

According to a WHO scenario, several infectious agents could be expected to produce 35,000 to more than 100,000 casualties if 50 kg were delivered in a line source and carried downwind over a populated area. In the case of some of the more stable agents, downwind reach would exceed 20 km. The Office of Technology Assessment (U.S. Congress, 1993b) has published similar figures. It must be borne in mind that the U.S. and Soviet programs prepared metric tons, not kilograms, of agent, and that appropriate devices for delivering line sources or multiple overlapping point sources were available (Alibek and Handelman, 2000; Meselson et al., 1994; Sidell et al., 1997). The impact on infected members of the population would depend on the agent used and the nature of the response (for example, the alacrity with which initial patients were recognized, public health and medical infrastructure, vaccine and antibiotic stockpiles).

The additional impact that might be possible by modifying naturally occurring organisms using methods well within the reach of simple biotechnology, including induction of antimicrobial resistance, enhancement of virulence by the addition of toxin genes, or selection of more stable or virulent organisms, is formidable. Issues surrounding the more extensive engineering of threat agents are beyond the scope of this discussion. It is important to note, however, that the potential exists.

A CASE IN POINT: INFLUENZA—WE ARE UNPREPARED

The factors that underlie the emergence of all infectious diseases are expanding in magnitude and converging at an ever more rapid pace, thus increasing individual and societal vulnerability to infection. Not only do individual factors lead to the emergence of infectious diseases, but the convergence of factors in time and space can lead to effects greater than the summing of individual factors might predict. Recognition of a convergence of factors can provide warning of an impending microbial threat, and an impetus to *act* now rather than simply *react* after an infection has become rooted in society. A better understanding of how the factors involved in emergence can converge to change vulnerability to infectious diseases would allow better preparedness for the prevention and control of microbial threats to health.

Humanity's struggle with influenza is illustrative of such a convergence of factors, which has resulted in maintaining the presence of this virus and periodically led to epidemics of the disease. Social, political, and economic factors interact with ecological factors to drive influenza viruses to respond through biological and genetic factors, thus circumventing human defense mechanisms and, in today's increasingly global society, exerting effects on economic, social, and political life worldwide (see Figure 3-1 for a visual model of this convergence of factors). The challenges to the prevention and control of influenza as a natural threat illuminate the ultimate challenge of addressing the convergence of factors that led to its emergence in the first place. Indeed, influenza is the paradigm of a microbial threat to health in which continual evolution of the virus is the main mechanism underlying epidemic and pandemic human disease. The gene pool of influenza A viruses in wild aquatic birds provides all the genetic diversity required for the emergence of new strains of pandemic influenza in humans, lower animals, and birds. A new influenza pandemic in humans is inevitable, and despite the development of pandemic plans in several countries, including the United States, we remain poorly prepared.

Epidemics and Pandemics

The highly variable nature of influenza virus permits the microbe to escape immune responses generated by previous infections and to cause annual epidemics and occasional pandemics of disease in humans (Wright and Webster, 2001). The severity of the epidemics ranges from mild to severe; on average, in nonpandemic years influenza causes 20,000 deaths in the United States. At irregular intervals—three to four times per century—human pandemics of influenza arise. The most devastating of these in recent history, the "Spanish flu" of 1918 (see Box 3-20), caused more than

BOX 3-20
The 1918 Influenza Pandemic

The 1918 influenza A pandemic claimed more than 20 million lives worldwide in less than a year and ranks among the worst disasters in human history. In the United States alone, it is estimated that 1 in 4 people became ill during the pandemic and that 675,000 people died.

Doubt remains as to whether the 1918 influenza pandemic originated in the United States, China, or France. There is agreement that a mild wave occurred simultaneously in the United States, Europe, and Asia in March–April 1918. It is postulated that genetic changes in that virus resulted in high pathogenicity in the second wave. The second wave occurred in September–November 1918 and affected one-quarter of the world's population; 500 million people were clinically affected during the pandemic.

The name Spanish flu came not from major outbreaks in Spain, but from high mortality among troops in France that for intelligence reasons were attributed to Spanish origins. The highest mortality from the disease occurred after the arrival of American troops in France. Indeed, General Erich Ludendorff, the Imperial German Army Chief of Staff, concluded that it was the virus, not the fresh troops, that ended the World War. A remarkable feature of the 1918 pandemic was that deaths were highest among young adults in the 20–40 year age range.

Molecular analysis of the hemagglutinin (HA), neuraminidase (NA), and non-structural genes from formalin-treated lung samples in paraffin blocks from soldiers that died in the second wave and from lung tissue from an Inuit woman buried in the permafrost in Alaska has provided information on the probable origin of the virus (Taubenberger et al., 2001). Phylogenetic analysis of the complete HA and NA sequences supports the hypothesis that the 1918 virus was derived from avian influenza precursors and was most closely related to classical swine influenza virus. To date, however, this analysis provides no insight into the enormous pathogenicity of the virus.

The return of military personnel throughout the world coincided with the peak of the second wave. In many cities, the disease was so severe that coffins were stacked in the streets, and the impact was so profound that it depressed the average life expectancy in the United States by more than 10 years. In spring 1919, a nasty but less lethal third wave occurred, and substantial mortality also recurred in 1920 (Kilbourne et al., 1987).

The complete sequence of the 1918 virus will be resolved in the near future, and reverse genetics technology is in place to remake this virus. If we wish to understand the molecular basis of high pathogenicity, remaking the virus may be the only option. If this is done, great care must be exercised to use the highest level of biosecurity. The available sequence information on the HA would permit us to make vaccines, and the sequence of the NA indicates sensitivity to the neuraminidase inhibitors. The precursor virus(es) of the 1918 virus still exist in nature and there is nothing to prevent it or a virus of similar virulence from re-emerging (Taubenberger et al., 2001).

20 million deaths worldwide and affected more than 200 million people. In only a few months, it killed more people than had been killed in battle during the 4 years of World War I (1914 to 1918). Viruses descended from the pandemic strain continued to cause annual epidemics from 1920 to 1956. The "Asian flu" pandemic (caused by an H2N2 virus) killed approximately 70,000 persons in the United States. The most recent pandemic, the 1968 "Hong Kong flu," killed approximately 34,000 persons in the United States. Thus, a pattern is evident: each pandemic is followed by relatively mild yearly epidemics caused by related viruses for which the populace enjoys widespread immunity. After a time, however, the evolving influenza virus gene pool inevitably produces a strain to which humans have no immunity. If we are unlucky, it is a highly transmissible and lethal strain.

Disturbingly, in 1977 an H1N1 virus similar in all respects to a virus from 1957 reappeared in humans in Northern China. This virus was not highly lethal—in fact, it caused only moderate respiratory illness in persons under 20 years of age. The cause of great concern was the possibility that this virus could have come from a frozen source, released accidentally from a laboratory. This event raises the specter of the reappearance of H2N2 influenza viruses that have been stored since the pandemic of 1957. No one born after 1957 has high-level immunity to these viruses, and the biosecurity of such agents is a matter of increasing concern. It has now been more than 30 years since a new pandemic influenza virus has emerged. The world's influenza advisory groups have warned that a new pandemic is not only inevitable, but overdue.

Impact of Influenza on Society and the Economy

The social and economic impacts of influenza are most apparent during a pandemic. During the lethal wave of the 1918 Spanish flu pandemic (October–November 1918), cities throughout the world were unable to bury their dead; in undeveloped areas, entire villages perished. The social and economic burden of influenza during interpandemic periods is less well studied, especially in tropical areas where malaria and diarrheal diseases remain major problems. However, studies in Canada, the United States, and Holland have shown that annual epidemics of influenza have a major impact on hospital costs among children and the elderly and reduce productivity. Indeed, after evaluating the economic impact of interpandemic influenza, several countries have recommended the annual use of influenza vaccine. In the United States, this recommendation has been extended to all persons aged 50 years or older and those at high risk because of underlying diseases or immunosuppression. The province of Ontario, Canada, has made the most progress in this respect; in 2002, vaccination was offered free of charge to everyone over 6 months of age. In other provinces of

Canada, vaccination is still recommended for those aged 65 and older and for all high-risk groups. Broader vaccination has not been pressed in the United States, purportedly because of limited supplies of vaccine. The result is a vicious cycle, however, as manufacturers will not produce quantities in excess of the certain demand.

Genetic and Biological Factors

Microbial Adaptation and Change

Influenza virus is ideally designed for continuous evolution. Its highly variable antigenic domains, which are situated at the outer end of the spike glycoproteins, permit maximal variability without compromising the function or assembly of the virion (see Figure 3-10) (Lamb and Krug, 2001). The virus's genome comprises eight RNA segments that can be shuffled or reassorted in cells that are coinfected with multiple viruses. Because of the lack of proofreading mechanisms, influenza virus undergoes an extremely high rate of mutation as it replicates (approximately 1.5×10^{-5} mutations per nucleotide per replication cycle). To cope with the continual genetic variation of human influenza viruses, WHO has established a worldwide network of more than 100 laboratories that isolate viruses for antigenic and molecular analysis (Cox and Subbarao, 2000). These analyses form the basis of WHO's annual recommendations for influenza vaccines for the Northern and Southern Hemispheres.

Unlike influenza viruses in humans, influenza viruses in their natural aquatic bird reservoirs appear to be in evolutionary stasis (Webster et al., 1992). Some avian influenza viruses have shown no changes in their surface glycoproteins for more than 50 years. The RNA continues to undergo mutation, but the mutations provide no selective advantage; these influenza viruses have become perfectly adapted to their natural hosts over the course of time. After transfer to a new host, however, the viruses evolve rapidly, undergoing a high rate of nonsynonymous mutation that alters their amino acid structure.

The existence of five host-specific lineages of influenza (in humans, horses, pigs, domestic poultry, and sea mammals) indicates that aquatic avian influenza viruses have adapted to these species, overcoming differences between avian and mammalian hosts in body temperature, cell surface receptors, and mode of transmission (see Figure 3-11). In aquatic birds, influenza virus is an enteric parasite that is transmitted by ingestion of fecally contaminated water. In humans, the virus replicates in the respiratory tract and is transmitted via aerosol. The available evidence suggests that the avian–human transition is accomplished via infection of pigs. Pigs possess receptors for both avian (α 2–3 terminal sialic acid) and human

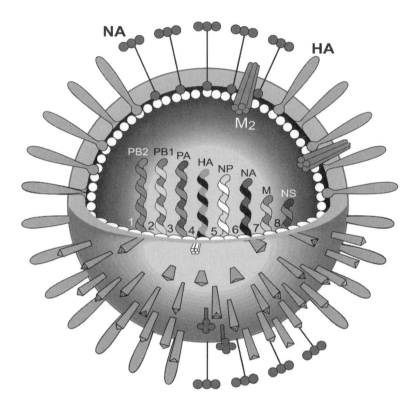

FIGURE 3-10 Diagram of influenza virus. The surface of the influenza virus particle is comprised of three kinds of spike glycoproteins—the hemagglutinin (HA) that
attaches the viruses to sialic acid residue on the respiratory tract; neuraminidase
(NA), an enzyme that releases the influenza virus from infected cells and is the
target of the anti-neuraminidase drugs; and matrix (M2) protein, which is an ion
channel and is the target for the antiviral agents amandatine and rimantadine. The
spike glycoproteins are embedded in a lipid bilayer obtained from the host cell. The
inside of the lipid bilayer is lined by the matrix protein (M1). A core of the virus
contains eight single-stranded RNA segments of negative sense that permits genetic
mixing (reassortment) when two different viruses infect a single cell. The polymerase complex (PB2, PB1, PA, NP) is involved in viral replication. The two small-
est segments (M and NS) each encode two proteins in different reading frames. The
NS gene is important in regulating the host cell response to influenza virus infection.

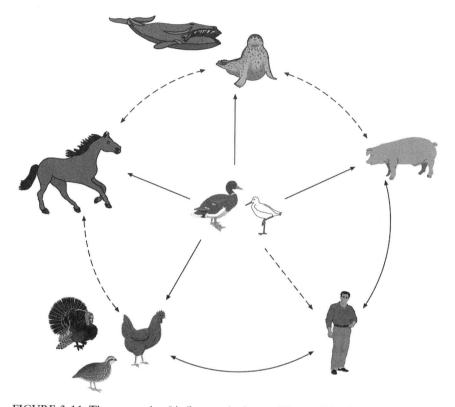

FIGURE 3-11 The reservoir of influenza A viruses. The working hypothesis is that wild aquatic birds are the primordial reservoir of all influenza viruses for avian and mammalian species. Transmission of influenza has been demonstrated between pigs and humans and between chickens and humans but not between wild birds and humans (dotted lines). There is extensive evidence for transmission of influenza viruses between wild ducks and other species (solid lines). The five different host groups are based on phylogenetic analysis of the nucleoprotein genes of a large number of different influenza viruses.

(α 2–6 terminal sialic acid) influenza viruses and thus can act as intermediate hosts. In this respect, it is noteworthy that both the 1918 Spanish and the 1968 Hong Kong pandemic viruses were isolated from pigs and from humans at approximately the same time. The interspecies transmission of influenza usually results only in transitory, localized disease that may be mild to severe. The H5N1 "bird flu" incident in Hong Kong in 1997 was such an incident. Six of eighteen infected persons died, but a stable lineage was not established (see Figure 3-12). The possibility that the virus might

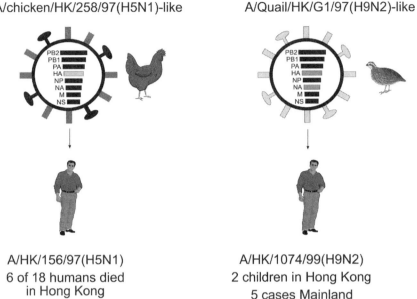

FIGURE 3-12 Direct transmission of avian influenza viruses to humans. In 1997, avian influenza viruses transmitted directly to humans in Hong Kong killed 6 of 18 persons(Left). In 1999, a quail influenza virus transmitted to humans in Hong Kong and caused mild respiratory infection in two children (Right). Five additional cases of H9N2 influenza have been reported from humans in Mainland China. It is noteworthy that the two influenza viruses from avian species that infected humans contain identical internal genes (PB2, PB1, PA, NP, M, NS—black gene segments) suggesting that these gene segments contain unique regions that facilitated transmission to humans.

adapt to humans, however, was sufficiently disquieting to prompt the wholesale slaughter of poultry in Hong Kong on two occasions.

During and after adaptation of influenza viruses to a new host, a continuing battle for supremacy occurs between microbe and host. The innate and adaptive human immune responses battle to clear the virus, while the virus evolves strategies to circumvent the immune responses. The virus stays a few steps ahead of natural or vaccine-induced human immunity by means of antigenic drift, or the accumulation of amino acid substitutions in the antigenic epitopes on the spike glycoproteins (hemagglutinin [HA] and neuraminidase [NA]) to which neutralizing antibodies bind. Genetic shift, or the acquisition of new gene segments from the aquatic bird reservoir, can completely change the epitopes that evoke humoral and cell-mediated immunity. This phenomenon may explain in part the devastation wreaked by the 1918 Spanish flu pandemic. The microbe has also developed ways to downregulate the innate immune response. One of the nonstructural proteins of influenza A viruses (NS1) is an interferon agonist that downregulates interferon—a natural inhibitor of influenza viruses (Garcia-Sastre, 2002). The yearly epidemics of influenza attest to the ongoing battle between host and virus. Human interventions—vaccines and antivirals—are efficacious on an individual basis, but have had little effect on the global spread of the disease.

Two classes of antivirals are used against influenza viruses: the adamantines, which block the ion channel formed by the influenza matrix (M2) protein, and the neuraminidase inhibitors, which prevent virus release by blocking NA enzyme activity (Hayden, 2001). The virus is able to circumvent these antivirals through the natural selection of resistant mutants. Resistance to the adamantines emerged in the first patients who were treated. However, the microbe has had less success in developing resistance to the NA inhibitors. Resistance to these agents requires mutations in both HA and NA, and the NA mutation compromises transmission of the virus. Thus, resistance can be achieved only at a price to the virus.

In summary, the challenges presented by influenza virus reflect its ability to alter itself with remarkable rapidity. This characteristic allows it to survive, to adapt to new hosts, and to evade control strategies.

Human Susceptibility to Infection

The most severe influenza virus infection experienced by most humans is the first infection acquired after the decline of maternal antibodies; the outcome depends on the competency of the individual's immune function and on the pathogenic potential of the specific variant of influenza virus. Patients who are immunosuppressed because of disease or therapy may shed influenza virus for long periods, and a greater likelihood exists in these individuals that the virus will acquire resistance to natural immune mechanisms and to antiviral therapy. The pathogenicity of influenza virus strains may also differ among host groups. Young adults were most susceptible in the 1918 pandemic, despite peak immune competence at that age. The future may reveal that the virus was able to downregulate the host immune response through as-yet unrecognized mechanisms.

Pacific Island communities also appeared to differ in their susceptibility to the 1918 Spanish flu. The death rate among the Maori population in New Zealand was 43.3 per 1,000 people—almost six times the death rate among New Zealanders of European extraction. Socioeconomic factors account for some but not all of this difference. Other possible factors include the absence of previous exposure of the Maori population to any influenza virus.

The main preventive human defense mechanism against influenza virus infection is humoral immunity (i.e., antibodies) to the highly variable HA and NA spike glycoproteins of the virus. To recover from influenza infection and remove infected cells, on the other hand, the body depends on cell-mediated immunity. Thymus-derived lymphocytes (T cells) recognize specific antigenic epitopes on the viral nucleoprotein and polymerase proteins, and they cross-react with these epitopes on other influenza virus strains. Both types of specific immune response require prior exposure to the virus. Therefore, an immune-naïve child, who has developed neither humoral nor cell-mediated immunity to the virus, may have a severe respiratory infection. On exposure to a second influenza virus that is antigenically similar to the first but has undergone antigenic drift, the child will be infected but will recover more rapidly because of the cross-reactive cell-mediated immune response. However, there is a conundrum associated with the immune response to highly variable microbes. The child's second exposure to influenza virus will induce a response directed mainly against the *first* influenza virus encountered. In this phenomenon, known as original antigenic sin, the immune system retains a lifelong memory of the first virus exposure in childhood. Thus, the antibody response is misdirected, and the efficacy of humoral immunity is reduced. This mechanism affects immunity to all infectious agents that undergo antigenic drift, including HIV.

Ecological Factors

Fifteen HA and nine NA subtypes of influenza A viruses circulate in the aquatic birds of the world. The viruses cause no apparent disease in these natural hosts, with which they appear to be in near-perfect equilibrium (Webster et al., 1992). Phylogenetically, these viruses can be divided into two clades, one in the Americas and the other in Eurasia. To date, only three of the fifteen HA subtypes have established lineages in humans. It is possible that only those subtypes have the capacity to infect humans. However, the direct transmission of avian H5N1 and H9N2 influenza viruses to humans in Hong Kong in 1997 and 1999 suggests the possibility that all subtypes can infect humans. The adaptation of influenza viruses to wild aquatic birds that migrate over vast distances (e.g., from southern South America to the North Slopes of Alaska) is an evolutionary strategy that allows the widespread fecal dissemination of the viruses at no apparent cost to the host. It is only after transmission and adaptation to mammals or domestic poultry that the virus evolves into a disease-causing microbe.

Social, Political, and Economic Factors

Animal Husbandry, Human Behavior, and Travel

The human population of the world continues to increase, as does the number of animals required to feed it. China has seen the most dramatic rise in the number of animals over the past decade. The demand for meat protein has increased strikingly as the result of socioeconomic progress, and populations of pigs and chickens have grown exponentially. Zoonotic disease potential inevitably increases in proportion to the animal population. Poultry, pigs, and people are the known hosts of influenza viruses, and most of the influenza pandemics of the twentieth century have originated in China. Substantial influenza activity has been noted in Hong Kong, which is hypothesized to be a documentable epicenter for the emergence of influenza pandemics. In 1997, avian H5N1 influenza virus was transmitted directly from poultry to humans, killing six of eighteen infected persons. In 1999, avian H9N2 influenza viruses were transmitted to two children and caused mild respiratory disease (see Figure 3-12). In 2001 and 2002, H5N1 viruses that are highly pathogenic to poultry and to mammals (as shown by testing in mice) reappeared in Hong Kong. To prevent spread to humans of the 2001/H5N1 viruses, all of the poultry in Hong Kong was killed and buried. Since 2001, all poultry markets in Hong Kong have been emptied on the same day each month to reduce the buildup of virus. Despite these precautions, however, all of the elements are in place to generate a new pandemic: vast numbers of the primary and secondary susceptible hosts on the mainland and in Hong Kong, and a constantly evolving pathogen. It is inevitable that an influenza pandemic strain will emerge from this mix.

However, the purchase of live poultry is a long-standing tradition, and thousands of people are employed in that industry. A change to the Western-style sale of chilled or frozen slaughtered poultry will meet with resistance until health authorities and the public recognize the ultimate cost of a new pandemic in Asia. Technical and political factors are also at work. The wide availability of refrigeration has now rendered the live poultry markets obsolete, but cultural preferences remain a strong political impediment to regulatory change. As a long-term solution, live poultry markets should be closed not only in Asia, but also in New York City. The markets in New York City are a factor in the emergence of the H7N2 influenza viruses that are causing great losses in the poultry industry in the northeastern United States. More than 4 million birds have had to be slaughtered, and the disease outbreak has prompted a ban on U.S. poultry in Japan. Besides the live markets, close monitoring of other crowded flocks of poultry will be needed.

Modern air travel (discussed earlier) will inevitably hasten the spread of a new pandemic of influenza. Once the virus appears in a major urban area, modern travel will allow its global distribution within a matter of days. The economic impact of an outbreak of highly pathogenic influenza was clearly seen in Hong Kong in 1997. The tourist and poultry industries collapsed because of the H5N1 "bird flu" incident, and Hong Kong suffered a severe economic downturn.

Intent to Harm

Recent advances in reverse genetics of influenza viruses now make it possible to generate influenza viruses to order (Neumann and Kawaoka, 2001). This new technology can reduce the time needed for vaccine preparation by 1 to 2 months if all other necessary resources are available. Perhaps more important, it will allow us to discover the molecular basis of the lethality of some viruses, such as the 1918 Spanish flu pathogen, and identify new targets for intervention in both the microbe and the host. Unfortunately, this new knowledge will also make it possible to generate extremely deadly agents—to recreate the 1918 Spanish flu virus, for example, or to add the H5N1 bird flu genes to a human influenza strain. Although influenza is not high on the list of bioterrorism agents, it has the potential to wreak widespread havoc on human life or to devastate important agricultural resources. Influenza is an exemplar of nature's natural biowarfare; it now has the added potential to be used by humans for intentional harm.

Pandemic Preparedness

Influenza is not an eradicable disease. It has now been more than 34 years since the Hong Kong/68 (H3N2) pandemic, and, as noted, all influenza virologists agree that a new pandemic is imminent. All of the developed countries of the world and WHO have created influenza pandemic plans to deal with such an event, and WHO is in the process of developing a Global Agenda for Influenza. Key issues in the global agenda are improvement of global surveillance, assessment of the global burden of influenza, and acceleration of vaccine development and usage.

The disturbing reality is that despite the certainty of a pandemic, even the developed countries of the world are quite unprepared for such an event. The public health infrastructure is inadequate. Hospitals lack the capacity to accommodate a surge of patients. Vaccine manufacturers had severe problems in meeting the demand in 2001 and 2002, the mildest influenza years in two decades, and the repertoire of antiviral drugs is completely inadequate. And increasing bacterial resistance to antibiotics raises questions about our ability to deal effectively with secondary pneumonia, a common cause of influenza deaths.

If a country cannot cope with interpandemic influenza, it is likely that the pandemic, when it does occur, will cause massive societal disruption. Such disruption cannot be prevented, but it can be lessened if we take action now. A minimum of 6 months is needed to prepare a new influenza vaccine. Only 11 companies worldwide manufacture influenza vaccine, and all of these companies together could not prepare a sufficient quantity even for national, let alone global needs. Therefore, the only immediately available strategy in the face of an influenza pandemic is the use of antivirals. Supplies of these agents are currently tailored to meet very low demand, and it takes an estimated 18 months to manufacture significant quantities of the drugs from the starting materials. Therefore, anti-influenza drugs will be available only if they are stockpiled in advance of a pandemic. Modeling studies are needed to plan the most effective use of such a stockpile of drugs.

The steps needed to deal effectively with interpandemic influenza can also help in preparing for an influenza pandemic. The new initiative promoting universal influenza vaccination in Ontario, Canada, can serve as a model for the world. If demonstrated to be effective, it should be expanded to other areas. Unless vaccine usage is substantially increased during interpandemic years, vaccine manufacturing capacity will be inadequate to meet the demand generated by a pandemic.

Addressing the Threats: Conclusions and Recommendations

Ten years after the 1992 Institute of Medicine report *Emerging Infections: Microbial Threats to Health in the United States* was issued, it has become even more apparent that infectious diseases continue to have a dramatic impact on the United States and the world. The response to microbial threats—from detection to prevention and control—requires a multidisciplinary effort involving all sectors of the public health, clinical medicine, and veterinary medicine communities. The committee's recommendations, which emerged from focused deliberations and the application of the criteria of urgency, priority, and amenability to immediate action, are presented in this chapter. Given that infectious diseases are a significant threat to the health of the world's population, several of the committee's recommendations could be justified solely on the basis of humanitarian need; *all* are justified as being in the best interest of the United States to protect the health of its own citizens.

ENHANCING GLOBAL RESPONSE CAPACITY

The emergence of infectious diseases reflects complex social, economic, political, environmental, ecological, and microbiological factors that are globally linked. A number of forces operating in developing countries in particular, including urbanization, deforestation, changes in land use and climate, population growth, poverty, malnutrition, political instability, and even terrorism, have created the conditions for several infectious diseases to become new or recurrent threats. To devise and implement effective prevention and control strategies, therefore, the factors influencing the emergence of infectious disease must be recognized and addressed at a global level.

Disease burdens—such as those incurred as a result of HIV, tuberculosis, and malaria—can contribute to the destabilization of nations, damaging their social and political infrastructures (National Intelligence Council, 2000; Denver Summit of the Eight, 1997). The past decade has seen the HIV epidemic besieged but entrenched in the United States, and spread globally with a catastrophic social and economic impact on many developing countries. Affecting adults in their productive years disproportionately, HIV has led to a grievous decrease in per capita gross domestic product (GDP) across Africa, resulting in a vicious spiral of decreased investment in public health and worsening of the epidemic. The resurgence of tuberculosis is devastating many countries, particularly Russia and other former Soviet republics, where tuberculosis rates have increased an astounding 70 percent in less than a decade. Antimicrobial resistance has become a major barrier to treatment of tuberculosis and malaria worldwide, threatens the effectiveness of antiretroviral therapy in persons with AIDS, and has made treatment of common bacterial infections more difficult in the United States and elsewhere. Infectious diseases are appearing abruptly in new locations and claiming hundreds of lives; a case in point is West Nile encephalitis, which spread to most parts of the United States within 3 years following its sudden appearance in the Northeast. Certain risks to health, such as contamination of food products, have resulted in enormous economic consequences, along with implications for human disease. Infectious diseases have even been used to intentionally terrorize populations, further dramatizing the need for a comprehensive assessment of and response to microbial threats.

Amelioration of major health risks and problems in any country, therefore, is a global good that may indirectly benefit the United States. Moreover, in an era of heightened concern regarding international networks of terrorism and nations with weapons of mass destruction, leadership in addressing the infectious disease problems of other countries can build trust and goodwill toward the United States. Repeatedly, U.S. efforts to monitor and address infectious disease threats in other countries have been welcomed and have increased understanding and improved relationships between countries. The need for an adequate global response to infectious disease threats, therefore, derives from the United States' humanitarian, economic, and national security interests.

According to a recent analysis by the National Intelligence Council (2000), newly emerging infectious diseases, including the intentional use of a biological agent, will pose an increasing global health threat and will complicate U.S. and global security over the next 20 years. As outlined in that report, the future impact of infectious diseases will be heavily influenced by three sets of variables: (1) the relationship between increasing antimicrobial resistance and the success of research to develop new antibiotics and vaccines; (2) the trajectory of developing and transitional economies, especially concerning the basic quality of life of the poorest groups among the population; and (3) the degree of success of global and national efforts to create public health infrastructure with effective systems of surveillance and response. The interplay among these variables will determine the overall outlook regarding the impact of infectious diseases.

In this context, it is clear that the response to emerging infectious diseases at a global level requires an investment in the capacity of developing countries to address these diseases as they arise. Such investments should take the form of financial and technical assistance, operational research, enhanced surveillance, and efforts to share both knowledge and best public health practices across national boundaries. For example, the World Health Organization (WHO) has developed a program for ensuring global health security by strengthening country capacity in microbiology and epidemiology to improve national preparedness (see Box 4-1). Financial and technical assistance to international agencies, governments, and nongovernmental organizations has already proven to be an effective means of addressing global disease threats. The Centers for Disease Control and Prevention (CDC) continues to support reference laboratories and provide technical assistance for disease outbreaks. Likewise, the National Institutes of Health (NIH) has expanded the number of international research and treatment centers. Financial and technical support has also come from private foundations and other U.S. agencies and organizations, and has been particularly effective in supporting efforts to combat HIV, tuberculosis, malaria, and polio.

The United States should seek to enhance the global capacity for response to infectious disease threats, focusing in particular on threats in the developing world. *Efforts to improve the global capacity to address microbial threats should be coordinated with key international agencies such as the World Health Organization (WHO) and based in the appropriate U.S. federal agencies (e.g., the Centers for Disease Control and Prevention [CDC], the Department of Defense [DOD], the National Institutes of Health [NIH], the Agency for International Development [USAID], the Department of Agriculture [USDA]), with active communication and coordination among these agencies and in collaboration with private organizations and foundations. Investments should take the form of financial and technical assistance, operational research, enhanced surveillance, and efforts to share both knowledge and best public health practices across national boundaries.*

BOX 4-1
The World Health Organization Office in Lyon

Epidemics and emerging infections continue to threaten human health worldwide, and many developing countries lack the capacity and expertise necessary to address these threats effectively. The World Health Organization (WHO), headquartered in Geneva, Switzerland, is working to ensure global health security.

In 2001, WHO's Department of Communicable Diseases, Surveillance, and Response opened an office in Lyon, France. To strengthen country capacity in microbiology and epidemiology, this new office provides a training program focused on enhancing the capacity of national public health laboratories, supporting field epidemiology training programs, and improving the capacity to detect and respond to disease outbreaks. The overall objective of the program is to strengthen diagnostic and surveillance capabilities at all levels. This goal can be achieved through an increase in reference diagnostic capabilities for communicable diseases; the development of appropriate core public health administrative practices; the development of rapid, sustainable national and international laboratory communications networks; the development of rapid, efficient, and safe means for shipment of diagnostic materials and laboratory specimens; and the establishment of appropriate quality control principles and practices.

The 2-year training program is designed for senior laboratory staff. Throughout the course of the program, participants receive training in essential laboratory diagnostic practices and techniques, biosafety, data collection and management, statistical analysis, basic disease epidemiology, and personnel management and administration. Following an initial 8-week session in Lyon, the trainees return to their home organizations. Over the course of the next 2 years, they are followed up in their home countries and return to Lyon for two shorter visits. Upon completion of the program, participants should be able to contribute effectively to the rapid detection of epidemic and emerging diseases in their countries.

Each year the program enrolls 15 participants for two sessions. It is estimated that after 5 years, the program will have trained 150 specialists from 45 countries. The first training cohort consisted of participants from 7 African countries who were selected for their senior roles in the management of their country's national public health reference laboratory. The first training session consisted of three modules: laboratory, surveillance, and information technology; laboratory response; and laboratory management. The second group of trainees was selected from Middle Eastern and North African countries and began training in 2002.

SOURCE: World Health Organization, 2001h.

Improving the global capacity to respond to microbial threats will require sustained efforts over time. Given the imminent nature of many infectious disease threats, however, it is critical that immediate action be taken toward achieving this capacity. Mobilization of young graduates in the health sciences has proven to be a successful strategy for meeting the goals identified by government agencies responsible for improving health domestically. For example, the National Health Service Corps, administered by the Health Resources and Services Administration (HRSA), has created a mechanism for dedicated health professionals to work in underserved communities where they are most needed nationwide. A similar mechanism could be used to established a Global Health Services Corps, offering loan forgiveness in exchange for service in areas of global public health need. Such a program could provide the stimulus for an immediate U.S. workforce to serve as a means of increasing global response capacity by assisting developing countries in creating the infrastructure, knowledge, and skills necessary to sustain long-term independent success. In addition to building developing-country capacity to respond, the program could enable U.S. public health agencies (e.g., CDC, NIH) to maintain expertise in epidemiology and laboratory issues related to diseases no longer endemic in the United States through training of U.S. scientists within countries where these diseases remain endemic. The same is true for diseases that are potential bioterrorist agents, particularly since the cadre of U.S. experts in rare diseases has declined (see the later discussion of educating and training the microbial threats workforce).

Expansion of programs in infectious disease research and training for health professionals from other countries is also needed. Notable successes in this area include the NIH Fogarty International Center for Advanced Study in the Health Sciences (FIC) that sponsors U.S. schools of medicine and public health in providing training for foreign scientists from developing countries through its AIDS International Training and Research Program (NIH, 1999). Since the center's inception, more than 2,000 scientists from more than 100 countries and territories have received training. In addition, over 46,000 students and health professionals have been provided short-term training through courses conducted in 65 countries. FIC also supplies funding for competitive supplemental awards under the Tuberculosis International Training and Research Program, a collaborative program with the National Institute of Allergy and Infectious Diseases (NIAID), CDC, and USAID. An aim of this funding is to foster global health research efforts and public health capacity to better respond to the threat posed by tuberculosis and multidrug-resistant tuberculosis. In yet another collaborative program, FIC and NIAID provide awards to U.S. universities under the International Training and Research Program in Emerging Infectious Diseases, which expands NIH research training efforts in the study of microbial threats. The long-term objective is to train teams of scientists in regions of the world that offer unique opportunities to understand the fundamental biology, epidemiology, and control of emerging microbial diseases.

IMPROVING GLOBAL INFECTIOUS DISEASE SURVEILLANCE

The need to strengthen global infectious disease surveillance is vital. As noted earlier, in addition to the United States' humanitarian objective of aiding countries in crisis, it is critical to U.S. national security that quality population-based data on disease burden and trends in the developing world be obtained through global surveillance (Hyder and Morrow, 2000). Yet disease burden estimates and projections are often based on only fragmentary data (Murray and Lopez, 1997). The reality in many developing societies is that deaths and births are not recorded, and a formal system of medical care is unavailable to most of the population (Cooper et al., 1998). Health care infrastructures that lack simple diagnostic tests for diseases such as tuberculosis or that have insufficient resources to perform diagnostic tests add to the lack of knowledge of disease burden. Developing countries in which high proportions of the population experience morbidity and/or mortality from infectious diseases may be the least likely to be encompassed by official statistics because of this lack of resources. Basic health indices, such as death rates or causes of death, are unknown in such contexts. Health ministries may generate health reports, but the data are generally unreliable. Such numbers have been used as the basis for broad policy recommendations; if the numbers are incorrect, however, the resulting policies can be damaging.

In addition to monitoring disease burden, surveillance efforts should be expanded and diversified to include the capacity to recognize previously unknown illnesses or unusual outbreaks of disease that may have global significance. With today's rapid and often mass global movements of people, animals, and goods, the transnational spread of infectious diseases can occur quickly and easily. Global surveillance, especially for newly recognized infectious diseases, is therefore crucial in responding to and containing microbial threats before isolated outbreaks develop into regional or worldwide epidemics.

U.S. agencies have been working with WHO and other partners to achieve the goal of a comprehensive global surveillance system, and efforts to date are aptly described as creating a "network of networks" (see Figure 4-1). In Europe, countries have made significant progress through the development of networks such as those for travel-related Legionnaires' disease, enteric organisms (Enter-net), and drug resistance. The United States has also supported efforts to establish regional networks. An example is DOD's support for laboratory-based surveillance in the 21 countries of the Caribbean Epidemiology Center, in collaboration with the Pan American Health Organization and CDC. Likewise, CDC and others have worked in many areas to assist regional surveillance networks. Examples include the Amazon and Southern Cone networks, which encompass eight laboratories

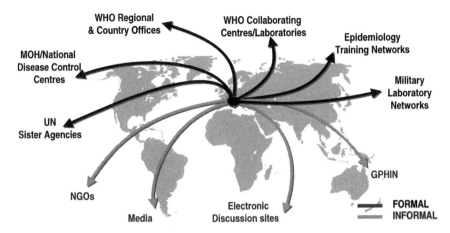

FIGURE 4-1 Global surveillance of communicable diseases: a network of networks.
SOURCE: WHO, Communicable Diseases.

in six countries of South America (CDC, 2002r), and the MeKong Delta
Surveillance Network, which includes five countries of Asia, as well as the
province of Yunan in China.

In 1996, DOD was mandated to use its long-standing and well-re-
spected overseas research laboratories in Egypt, Indonesia, Kenya, Peru,
and Thailand to establish the Global Emerging Infections Surveillance
(GEIS) program. GEIS is a critical and unique resource for the United States
in the context of global infectious disease surveillance; it is the only U.S.
entity with broad-based laboratory capacity in overseas settings. GEIS has
already demonstrated its excellent potential to detect the emergence of
disease in those and surrounding countries (IOM, 2001e). CDC has assigned several epidemiologists to GEIS to provide increased epidemiologic
capacity at these overseas sites. CDC plans to establish multiple international programs to address emerging infections, the first of which was
established in Thailand in 2001 (CDC, 2002r). As more DOD overseas
laboratories and CDC Emerging Infections Programs are established, increased collaboration between the two agencies will be beneficial, and serious consideration must be given to which geographic sites will fill the most
critical gaps in surveillance worldwide.

Also important for global surveillance are novel training programs
initiated by NIAID that provide the opportunity for field training in Asia,
Africa, and South America, along with laboratory-based training in the
United States, with incentives to return trainees to their home countries.
Such programs require expansion in particular in the "hot zones" of Africa
and Asia that are recognized as epicenters for the emergence of such agents

as Ebola, HIV, Nipah, and influenza. NIAID initiatives on pandemic preparedness for influenza in Asia, which promote zoonotic surveillance and preparation of the necessary reagents, are prototypes for the programs necessary for global surveillance.

The WHO Global Influenza Surveillance Program, now 50 years old, was responsible for the early identification of the H5N1 influenza A virus, as well as the H9N2 virus that occurred later—viruses that had previously been detected only in birds. The reagents necessary for identification of these viruses were developed by NIAID and were made available to the WHO program. Because WHO must issue recommendations for the composition of influenza vaccines twice a year—once for the Northern Hemisphere in February and once for the Southern Hemisphere in September—data must be gathered throughout the year. The infrastructure in place allows the identification of new variants, whether they are new epidemic variants or new variants with pandemic potential. The infrastructure rests on a number of national influenza centers that serve as the key laboratories for the isolation and identification of influenza viruses, using a kit of reagents produced by CDC and distributed globally. The laboratories also collect epidemiological information for transmittal to WHO headquarters in Geneva. International collaborating centers, including CDC, conduct comparative analyses of influenza viruses from around the world. Collaboration with industry is essential because the strains that are identified as vaccine candidates are provided free of charge to the pharmaceutical industry for vaccine production.

Globally, advances in information technology have also allowed novel uses of the Internet in disease surveillance. The Program for Monitoring Infectious Diseases (Pro-Med) uses electronic communications to provide up-to-date news on disease outbreaks and is open to all users. A team of experts in human, animal, and plant diseases screens, reviews, and investigates reports before posting notices. The system was designed to promote communication among the international infectious disease community, and to provide for the exchange of information about outbreaks and other matters of interest regarding emerging infectious diseases (International Society for Infectious Diseases, 2001). PacNet, an Asian network of health professionals on 20 Pacific Islands, is another such network, established to allow the exchange of information among health professionals regarding epidemics in that region. An even more innovative system, established by Health Canada in collaboration with WHO, is the Global Public Health Intelligence Network (GPHIN), an Internet-based application that continuously scans global electronic media (news wires, websites) for information on global public health risks, including infectious disease outbreaks (WHO, 1998b) (see Box 4-2). In line with the growth of electronic media, approximately 65 percent of the world's first news about infectious disease events

BOX 4-2
Global Outbreak Alert and Response Network

The Global Outbreak Alert and Response Network enables WHO to monitor disease outbreaks continuously. This network was formally launched in 2000 and links over 72 existing networks around the world, some of which are able to diagnose and detect unusual agents and handle dangerous pathogens. The four critical tasks of the network are epidemic intelligence and detection, verification of rumors and reports, immediate alert, and rapid response.

The Global Outbreak Alert and Response Network gathers global disease intelligence using a number of sources, such as ministries of health, WHO country offices and collaborating centers, laboratories, academic institutes, and nongovernment organizations. The Global Public Health Intelligence Network (GPHIN), an electronic system that constantly performs surveillance of worldwide communications for disease events, is one of the most important informal sources from which the network gathers data. GPHIN was developed for WHO through a collaboration with Health Canada in 1996.

The intelligence gathered is converted by the WHO Outbreak Alert and Response team, which then determines whether a reported disease event constitutes cause for international concern. The team meets each morning to review reports and rumors, assess their epidemiological significance, and determine actions needed. The team creates a detailed report that is distributed electronically each day to specific WHO staff around the world. From 1998 to 2001, WHO verified 578 outbreaks in 132 countries.

The network electronically connects WHO member countries, disease experts, institutions, agencies, and laboratories to keep them constantly informed of outbreak events, rumored and confirmed. The network also provides real-time alerts through an outbreak verification list, offering detailed information on current outbreaks that is regularly updated and maintained. In addition, WHO posts information on outbreaks on its Disease Outbreak News website.

Rapid response is a critical task of the Global Outbreak Alert and Response Network. Once an outbreak has been verified, the Outbreak Alert and Response team determines whether an international response is needed to contain it. When an international response is necessary, partners in the global health network are called upon to provide specific support, from investigations and patient management to logistics, including the provision of necessary staff and supplies. WHO and the Nuclear Threat Initiative recently partnered to create an Emergency Outbreak Response Fund to ensure that the rapid response teams can be at a designated site within 24 hours of a detected outbreak. Since 2000, WHO and the network have launched effective international responses to outbreaks in Afghanistan, Cote d'Ivoire, Egypt, Ethiopia, and other countries.

SOURCE: World Health Organization, 2003b.

during the past 4 years has come not from official country notifications, but from informal sources, including press reports and the Internet (Heymann, 2001). Recent efforts to increase capacity for translation to the six official United Nations languages will further enhance the GPHIN system.

As described earlier, surveillance of and response to emerging infectious disease threats in other parts of the world can directly benefit the United States as well as the country in which an occurrence is detected. For example, the investigation of hantavirus in Korea in the 1970s and the development of a diagnostic test were useful in the identification of and response to the epidemic of hantavirus infection in the southwestern United States in 1993. Similarly, the investigation of the H5N1 influenza virus in Hong Kong in 1997 alerted the United States and the world to the threat posed by influenza viruses in avian species as sources of pandemic influenza viruses in humans, and highlighted the urgency of influenza pandemic planning globally. The rapid measures taken to control H5N1 influenza in Hong Kong exemplify increasing global cooperation in disease surveillance. WHO, together with experts from the United States, Europe, and the Pacific region, provided information to the Hong Kong authorities on the virological and epidemiological properties of the H5N1 threat, and as a consequence, the local authorities decided to slaughter all poultry in Hong Kong. This decision resulted in a dramatic cessation of human cases of H5N1, providing a direct benefit to Hong Kong, China, and the global community. Similar steps to stamp out the epidemic of Nipah viruses among livestock and humans in Malaysia provide yet another example of the importance of global disease surveillance and the benefits to global health. Likewise, liaisons between the U.S. and European sentinel surveillance networks have led to the identification and removal of products being marketed in numerous countries, including the United States, that were contaminated with bacterial pathogens.

Several national and international groups, including the National Science and Technology Council (1995) and the Denver Summit of the Eight (1997), have echoed the 1992 IOM recommendation to establish a global disease and outbreak surveillance system. Significant efforts have been made to enhance global surveillance, but the system remains skeletal and is inadequate to monitor disease incidence and prevalence in most parts of the world.

The United States should take a leadership role in promoting the implementation of a comprehensive system of surveillance for global infectious diseases that builds on the current global capacity of infectious disease monitoring. *This effort, of necessity, will be multinational and will require regional and global coordination, advice, and resources from participating nations. A comprehensive* *system is needed to accurately assess the burden of infectious diseases in developing countries, detect the emergence of new microbial threats, and direct prevention and control efforts. To this end, CDC should enhance its regional infectious disease surveillance; DOD should expand and increase in number its Global Emerging Infections Surveillance (GEIS) overseas program sites; and NIH should increase its global surveillance research. In addition, CDC, DOD, and NIH should increase efforts to develop and arrange for the distribution of laboratory diagnostic reagents needed for global surveillance, transferring technology to other nations where feasible to ensure self-sufficiency and sustainable surveillance capacity. The overseas disease surveillance activities of the relevant U.S. agencies (e.g., CDC, DOD, NIH, USAID, USDA) should be coordinated by a single federal agency, such as CDC. Sustainable progress and ultimate success in these efforts will require health agencies to broaden partnerships to include nonhealth agencies and institutions, such as the World Bank.*

REBUILDING DOMESTIC PUBLIC HEALTH CAPACITY

The U.S. capacity to respond to microbial threats to health is contingent on a public health infrastructure that has suffered years of neglect. Upgrading current public health capacities will require considerably increased investments across differing levels of government. Most important, this support will have to be sustained over time. Such an investment will have lasting and measurable benefits for all humankind. With recent increased funding for bioterrorism preparedness, the United States has an opportunity to develop programs and policies that will both protect against acts of bioterrorism and improve the U.S. public health response to all microbial threats. However, it is alarming that some of these funds have been diverted from multipurpose infrastructure building to single-agent preparedness.

The threat of bioterrorism is intimately related to that of naturally occurring infectious diseases. The response to bioterrorism is much like the response to any microbial threat to health, and the necessary resources for building the public health infrastructure are, in essence, the same as those needed to respond to bioterrorism. It would be counterproductive to develop an ancillary system for bioterrorist threats. Rather, such efforts must be integrated with those addressing the continuum of infectious disease concerns and potential disasters to which public health agencies are already charged to respond. While preparedness for bioterrorist-inflicted outbreaks will require certain specialized program elements and policies (related, e.g., to law enforcement, evidence collection), the human health aspects of this new challenge mirror many of the requirements for preventing and responding to a range of naturally occurring infectious disease threats. Wherever possible, therefore, effective strategies should build on existing systems that are used routinely and can be useful for both purposes. In short, the objectives of the funding that has been allocated for bioterrorism will be met only if the public health infrastructure is enhanced first and foremost. Otherwise, preparedness programs will be inadequate, and critical opportunities to protect both human populations and agriculture (food animals and plants) from a range of disease threats, both naturally occurring and maliciously caused, may be missed.

Strong and well-functioning local, state, and federal public health agencies working together represent the backbone of effective response to a major outbreak of infectious disease, including a bioterrorist attack. How quickly public health agencies can recognize and respond to an emerging threat dramatically influences the ability to reduce casualties, control contagion, and minimize panic and disruption. Unfortunately, an overall shortage of qualified public health workers makes it difficult to meet this demand. Following the events of 2001, public health agencies were asked to develop new programs and add new staff despite the lack of available candidates. An estimated 3,200 to 4,000 new positions were requested in the bioterrorism cooperative agreements submitted to CDC. In addition, an estimated 13,000 to 15,000 persons are needed to provide 24-hour emergency coverage at the local level (Center for Infectious Disease Research and Policy, 2002). Yet a wide range of administrative barriers prevent public health agencies from obtaining qualified staff. These include noncompetitive pay scales, cumbersome hiring procedures, lack of system flexibility, and inadequate incentives for retaining qualified personnel. Local health departments range in coverage from small areas served by part-time staff with little or no formal public health training to large urban health districts with inadequate resources to support the continuing education and training of their workforce. Some of the smaller local health departments could be consolidated and strengthened to ensure needed professional expertise and coverage on a more regional basis. To strengthen the public health infrastructure for infectious disease detection and response, it will be necessary to train, equip, and expand the workforce to provide both on-the-ground epidemiologic expertise and laboratory capability.

Communication, including computer connectivity, must also be strengthened to efficiently collect, analyze, and share information among public health and other officials at the local, state, and federal levels. Enabling public health agencies to obtain fast and secure Internet access is key in facilitating linkages between health departments and health care providers. For example, the Health Alert Network (HAN) is being developed by

CDC as a nationwide, integrated, secure, electronic communications system that will provide high-speed Internet connections, enabling public health officials to engage in distance learning and share laboratory findings, health advisories, and other information relevant to disease outbreaks. The network's primary goal is to improve the information technology infrastructure of local and state health departments. The Health Alert Network is designed to be the nation's rapid online system for health communication and will serve as the electronic platform for the National Electronic Disease Surveillance System (NEDSS) (discussed later), Epi-X (see Box 4-3), and

---

BOX 4-3
Epidemic Information Exchange

The Epidemic Information Exchange (Epi-X) is a secure, web-based communications network for public health officials. Developed by CDC in 2001, it enables health officials to rapidly report and discuss public health information on disease outbreaks and other health events as they are identified and investigated.

Since its launch, Epi-X has provided health officials throughout the United States with up-to-the-minute information, reports, alerts, and discussions about terrorist events, disease outbreaks, and other events of public health significance. Public health officials and other designated users can use Epi-X to post reports, notify colleagues, and receive feedback on ongoing epidemiological investigations, as well as research current and past outbreaks.

Epi-X will strengthen bioterrorism preparedness efforts by supporting information sharing about disease outbreaks and other health events over a secure communications system. The network includes a Forum area in which state epidemiologists can post information on surveillance and response activities for approximately 500 public health officials in the United States, including those in the U.S. military.

As of 2002, Epi-X had posted over 1000 reports of disease outbreaks, other public health activities, and requests for epidemiologic assistance from CDC. Over 1,000 public health officials at the federal, state, and local levels had used Epi-X to communicate with colleagues and experts across a secure, encrypted web-based network; track information for outbreak investigations and response; conduct online conferences to discuss such topics as West Nile virus and anthrax investigations; alert health officials by pager, phone, and e-mail to urgent events; request CDC assistance in investigations; and communicate with bioterrorism preparedness programs.

Plans to expand Epi-X are under way and include increasing its user base and expanding secure communications for public health and safety officials, as well as expanding the network to provide information on international outbreaks that might affect public health in the United States.

SOURCE: Center for Disease Control and Prevention, 2002s.

other applications. HAN can assist health agencies in assessing their technology needs, acquiring equipment to help meet these needs, establishing Internet connection and e-mail capabilities, and developing training programs. The network was activated on September 11, 2001, and within 4 hours of the terrorist attacks in New York and Washington, D.C., was transmitting health messages to 250 top health officials in the United States. The network has continued to transmit health alerts, advisories, and updates, and has been expanded to reach an estimated 1 million recipients, including public health officials, physicians, nurses, laboratory staff, and other health professionals.

To rebuild the public health workforce needed to respond to microbial threats, health profession students (especially those in the medical, nursing, veterinary, and laboratory sciences) must be educated in public health as a science and as a career. Even for students within schools of public health, education has traditionally focused on academic research training, not public health practice. A 1988 IOM report notes that "many observers feel that some [public health] schools have become somewhat isolated from public health practice and therefore no longer place a sufficiently high value on the training of professionals to work in health agencies" (IOM, 1988:15). A more recent IOM report states that in 1998, only 56 of 125 medical schools required courses on such topics as public health, epidemiology, or biostatistics (IOM, 2002e). The report recommends that *all* medical students receive basic public health training. It also concludes that all nurses should have at least an introductory grasp of their role in public health, and that all undergraduates should have access to education in public health. Educational strategies in which applied epidemiology programs provide exposure to state and local health departments may help increase awareness of the role of public health in population-based infectious disease control and prevention, and provide for exposure to public health as a potential career choice (see the later discussion on educating and training the microbial threats workforce).

Managing and controlling epidemic diseases requires deep engagement and coordination on the part of both the public health and the medical communities. Recent experiences with both anthrax (intentionally caused) and West Nile virus (naturally occurring) reinforced the importance of links between educated, alert medical providers and a responsive public health system. Rapid recognition of an event requires that health care providers be trained to recognize unusual symptoms of disease that may reflect an emerging health problem, whatever the source. The experience with anthrax and West Nile virus demonstrated the potential difficulties involved in distinguishing naturally occurring from intentionally caused disease outbreaks early on. In fact, in some instances, the source of an outbreak and whether the infectious agent was intentionally introduced may never be known.

A strengthened relationship between public health and clinical medicine is also vitally important to the development of plans for a surge of patients in the nation's health care system, whose facilities routinely operate at or near capacity. The need to have such plans in place is just as important for preparedness for a severe flu season as for preparedness for a bioterrorist attack. To control most infectious disease epidemics, public health agencies must be closely linked with those who can deliver medical care to persons in need and provide prophylactic treatment or vaccines that may be required for disease control.

Looking to the future, the nation's public health system will continue to be challenged to combat both routine and unexpected outbreaks of disease. In fact, we may anticipate discoveries of an increasing array of previously unknown infectious disease threats, including newly bioengineered microbial agents for which we may have no effective control or treatment strategies. A successful response to these new threats will require that the nation make a renewed and much-needed commitment to public health and address the threat of bioterrorism in the broader context of infectious disease. We must recognize and act on the understanding that public health is an essential aspect of public safety and a critical pillar in our national security framework. Our programs and policies must reflect this recognition; adequate public health and infectious disease expertise must be present at the table when critical decisions are made; and public health professionals must be part of our national security team.

U.S. federal, state, and local governments should direct the appropriate resources to rebuild and sustain the public health capacity necessary to respond to microbial threats to health, both naturally occurring and intentional. *The public health capacity in the United States must be sufficient to respond quickly to emerging microbial threats and monitor infectious disease trends. Prevention and control measures in response to microbial threats must be expanded at the local, state, and national levels and be executed by an adequately trained and competent workforce. Examples of such measures include surveillance (medical, veterinary, and entomological); laboratory facilities and capacity; epidemiological, statistical, and communication skills; and systems to ensure the rapid utility and sharing of information.*

IMPROVING DOMESTIC SURVEILLANCE THROUGH BETTER DISEASE REPORTING

Surveillance is the foundation for infectious disease prevention and control. Surveillance provides information crucial to monitoring the health of the public, identifying public health problems and priorities, taking public health actions to prevent further illness, and evaluating the effectiveness of these actions. Surveillance of infectious diseases is dependent largely on timely and accurate diagnosis by health care providers and prompt reporting of disease to relevant public health authorities. Open lines of communication and good working relationships between health care providers and public health authorities are essential to a robust system of surveillance and effective implementation of disease investigation and response activities.

No single surveillance system captures all the information required to monitor the health of the public. Such a capability is impossible given the existence of multiple data sources, differing information requirements, multiple distinct users, and different partners with which CDC collaborates to obtain data for specific programs areas (CDC, 2000f). To better manage and enhance the large number of current surveillance systems and allow the public health community to respond more quickly to public health threats, CDC has developed the National Electronic Disease Surveillance System (NEDSS). NEDSS is an initiative designed to promote the use of data and information system standards to advance the development of efficient, integrated, and interoperable surveillance systems at the federal, state, and local levels (CDC, 2002t). The vision of NEDSS is to have integrated surveillance systems that can transfer appropriate public health, laboratory, and clinical data efficiently and securely over the Internet. Gathering and analyzing information quickly and accurately will help improve the nation's ability to identify and track emerging infectious diseases and potential bioterrorism attacks, as well as to investigate outbreaks and monitor disease trends.

The long-term vision for NEDSS is that of complementary electronic information systems that automatically gather health data from a variety of sources on a real-time basis; facilitate monitoring of the health of communities; assist in the ongoing analysis of trends and detection of emerging public health problems; and provide information for setting public health policy. CDC is focusing on the development, testing, and implementation of standards to serve as the framework that will support more complete and comprehensive integration of systems in the future. While the various systems developed by CDC and state and local health departments will remain distinct from one another, the use of standards will ensure that surveillance data can readily be shared, that users familiar with one system can easily use another, and that software can be shared across programs.

Largely in response to recommendations in *Emerging Infections: Microbial Threats to Health in the United States* (IOM, 1992), CDC initiated several new surveillance programs, including the Emerging Infections Program for population-based surveillance and research (see Box 4-4). In addition, several sentinel surveillance systems were established for various infectious diseases or conditions in emergency departments, in travelers' clinics, and through a network of infectious disease clinicians (see Table 4-1). These systems have been extremely useful in improving surveillance, particularly for invasive bacterial diseases, including foodborne illnesses, and in several other specific areas of infectious disease control.

Notification of public health officials of the occurrence of an unusual illness has been, and will continue to be, vital to the detection of emerging microbial threats. Health care providers are an essential component of surveillance programs. Astute clinicians are the first line of defense for the identification of most emerging microbial threats. Health care providers are critical in recognizing unusual presentations of illness or clusters of unusual illnesses, and report their observations to local or state health officials. Reports are likely to be generated because of close clustering, unusual morbidity and mortality, novel clinical features, or the availability of medical expertise. Recent diseases identified as initial clusters of unusual illness include Legionnaires' disease, Lyme disease, hantavirus pulmonary syndrome, and West Nile encephalitis in North America. At the same time, other medical personnel, such as infection control professionals, could play an enhanced role in detecting outbreaks and increases in emergency department visits or hospital admissions for diagnoses that may be of public health importance; some played this role effectively during the anthrax events of 2001. Infection control professionals are well situated to detect unusual disease clusters throughout a hospital, including the emergency department and the intensive care unit; they have a close collaboration with both the infectious disease specialists and the microbiologists within a health system. This potentially critical link with local and state public health agencies must be supported within the health care environment. Unfortunately, the ranks of these professionals are thinning.

CDC monitors disease burden in the United States through the National Notifiable Diseases Surveillance System (NNDSS), implemented in 1961. The list of nationally notifiable diseases is maintained and revised as needed by the Council of State and Territorial Epidemiologists (CSTE) in collaboration with CDC (see Box 4-5). Regulatory authority for disease surveillance in the United States is provided through state legislation; health officials in every state report voluntarily to CDC. All states generally report the internationally quarantinable diseases (yellow fever, cholera, and plague) in compliance with WHO's International Health Regulations (CDC, 2002t). Most states include within their disease reporting requirements a provision for the reporting of any unusual presentation of illness or death (in an individual or cluster of individuals), especially those for which a cause cannot be identified. In addition, states can elect to add other diseases to their list that may be relevant for their geographic area. Some states include conditions other than infectious diseases. Current data on nationally re-

---

BOX 4-4
Emerging Infections Program

In 1994, CDC developed a new proposal to improve and strengthen infectious disease surveillance. This initiative, outlined and expanded in CDC's 1998 publication *Preventing Emerging Infectious Diseases: A Strategy for the 21st Century*, has been implemented in collaboration with many public health partners (CDC, 1998c).

CDC implemented the Emerging Infections Program (EIP) as a result of this strategic initiative. The EIP is a collaboration among CDC, state health departments, and other public health partners for the purpose of conducting population-based surveillance and research on infectious diseases. The EIP network comprises nine EIP sites: California (San Francisco Bay area), Colorado, Connecticut, Georgia, Maryland, Minnesota, New York, Oregon, and Tennessee. These sites conduct population-based surveillance and research that go beyond the routine functions of local health departments to address important issues in infectious diseases and public health.

The primary objective of the EIP is to act as a national resource for the surveillance, prevention, and control of emerging infectious diseases (CDC, 2002u). The EIP network is able to achieve this objective by addressing important issues in infectious diseases, participating in emergency responses to outbreaks, providing public health agencies with new information, recognizing the importance of training in all EIP activities, and making prevention of infectious diseases a priority (Schuchat et al., 2001). The EIP sites have performed investigations of meningococcal and streptococcal disease, and have also established surveillance for unexplained deaths and severe illness in an attempt to identify diseases and infectious agents, known and unknown, that can lead to severe illness or death (CDC, 1998c).

Two projects are conducted through the entire EIP network: Active Bacterial Core surveillance (ABCs) and Foodborne Diseases Active Surveillance Network (FoodNet). ABCs is a population-based surveillance system that conducts active surveillance for

---

portable diseases are available in CDC's *Morbidity and Mortality Weekly Report*.

Efforts to educate physicians and other health care professionals are critical to improving national surveillance through disease reporting. As noted earlier, practicing health care providers have detected and reported many recent emerging threats, including inhalational anthrax in Florida. In addition, it is essential that strong links be established between animal care providers (e.g., veterinarians, wildlife officials) and public health officials to enhance reporting of animal infections of relevance to human health; the emergence of West Nile virus has clearly demonstrated this need.

Many health care providers do not fully understand their role in infectious disease surveillance, including their role as a source of data (IOM, 2000). Health care providers receive little formal education in infectious disease surveillance: few medical or other health science schools include the

invasive disease caused by *Streptococcus pneumoniae*, group A streptococcus, group B streptococcus, *Neisseria meningitidis*, and *Haemophilus influenzae*. A population of 17 to 30 million is actively surveyed for the presence of these bacterial pathogens which were the cause of 10,000 deaths in the United States in 1998 (Schuchat et al., 2001). In 1999, the most recent complete year of surveillance, 7,632 cases of invasive disease due to the five pathogens were reported (7,067 isolates collected). Other ABCs accomplishments include a study of the risk of invasive group A streptococcal (GAS) infections among household contacts of index patients, analysis of a population-based case-control study of other risk factors for invasive GAS, and the development of a procedures manual and database for use in a post-licensure efficacy study of a pneumococcal conjugate vaccine.

FoodNet is a collaboration among the CDC EIP sites, the U.S. Food and Drug Administration, and the U.S. Department of Agriculture, created in 1996 to conduct population-based, active surveillance for foodborne infections. The primary objectives of FoodNet are to (1) determine the epidemiology of bacterial, parasitic, and viral foodborne diseases; (2) determine the prevalence of foodborne diseases in the United States; and (3) investigate the link between certain foods and the proportion of foodborne disease caused by their ingestion (Yang, 1998). FoodNet conducts surveillance for *E. coli* O157:H7, *Campylobacter*, *Listeria*, *Salmonella*, *Shigella*, *Yersinia*, *Vibrio*, *Cryptosporidium*, and *Cyclospora*.

The EIP network has scored several accomplishments. From 1993 to 1998, ABCs detected a decline in the incidence of group B streptococcal disease in newborns in the monitored population. The results of this surveillance provided the basis for guidelines for the prevention of mother-to-child transmission of group B streptococcus through the use of intrapartum antibiotics (Schrag et al., 2000). FoodNet has been successful in monitoring, tracking trends, and defining risk factors for causes of foodborne illnesses, and in estimating the burden of foodborne illnesses in the United States (CDC, 2002u).

importance of and requirements for reporting diseases of public health significance to public health authorities in their curricula; residency programs seldom address the need for provider participation in public health surveillance; and little, if any, continuing medical education exists on the topic, nor is it widely integrated into board certification exams.

CDC should take the necessary actions to enhance infectious disease reporting by medical health care and veterinary health care providers. *Innovative strategies to improve communication between health care providers and public health authorities should be developed by working with other public health agencies (e.g., the Food and Drug Administration [FDA], the Health Resources and Services Administration [HRSA], USDA, the Department of Veterans Affairs [VA], state and local health departments), health*

TABLE 4-1 Selected Sentinel Surveillance Systems for Monitoring Infectious Diseases

EMERGEncy ID NET	EMERGEncy ID NET is an interdisciplinary, multicenter, emergency department-based network based at 11 university-affiliated, urban hospital emergency departments with more than 900,000 combined annual patient visits. Research projects include investigation of bloody diarrhea; prevalence of *Shiga toxin-producing Escherichia coli*; rabies postexposure prophylaxis practices, and nosocomial emergency department *M. tuberculosis* transmission.
Foodborne Diseases Active Surveillance Network (FoodNet)	FoodNet is a collaborative project among the CDC, the 9 Emerging Infections Program sites (EIPs), the U.S. Department of Agriculture (USDA), and the U.S. Food and Drug Administration (FDA). FoodNet consists of active surveillance of laboratories, physicians, and the general population for foodborne diseases and related epidemiologic studies designed to help public health officials better understand the epidemiology of foodborne diseases in the United States.
Gonococcal Isolate Surveillance Project (GISP)	GISP is a collaborative project to monitor antimicrobial resistance in *Neisseria gonorrhoeae* in the United States. Participants of GISP include the CDC, five regional laboratories, and selected local STD clinics.
National Molecular Subtyping Network for Foodborne Disease Surveillance (PulseNet)	PulseNet is a national network of local public health laboratories that performs DNA "fingerprinting" on pathogens that may be foodborne. The network permits rapid comparison of these "fingerprint" patterns through an electronic database at the CDC.
National Nosocomial Infections Surveillance (NNIS) System	The NNIS system is conducted by the Hospital Infections Program to collect high-quality nosocomial infection surveillance data that can be aggregated into a national database. NNIS is a cooperative effort between the CDC and acute care general hospitals that volunteer to participate in this surveillance system.
Unexplained Deaths and Critical Illnesses Surveillance System	Active population-based surveillance through coroners and medical examiners is conducted in 4 Emerging Infections Program sites (EIPs) with a total population of 7.7 million 1- to 49-year-olds. Surveillance is passive for clusters of unexplained deaths and illnesses.
United States Influenza Sentinel Physicians Surveillance Network	Approximately 260 physicians around the country report each week to the CDC the total number of patients seen and the number of those patients with influenza-like illness by age group.

SOURCE: CDC.

BOX 4-5
Nationally Notifiable Infectious Diseases
in the United States, 2003

Acquired immunodeficiency syndrome (AIDS)
Anthrax
Botulism
   Botulism, foodborne
   Botulism, infant
   Botulism, other (wound and unspecified)
Brucellosis
Chancroid
Chlamydia trachomatis, genital infections
Cholera
Coccidioidomycosis
Cryptosporidiosis
Cyclosporiasis
Diphtheria
Ehrlichiosis
   Ehrlichiosis, human granulocytic
   Ehrlichiosis, human monocytic
   Ehrlichiosis, human, other or unspecified agent
Encephalitis/meningitis, Arboviral
   Encephalitis/meningitis, California serogroup viral
   Encephalitis/meningitis, eastern equine
   Encephalitis/meningitis, Powassan
   Encephalitis/meningitis, St. Louis
   Encephalitis/meningitis, western equine
   Encephalitis/meningitis, West Nile
Enterohemorrhagic *Escherichia coli*
   Enterohemorrhagic *Escherichia coli*, O157:H7
   Enterohemorrhagic *Escherichia coli*, shiga toxin positive, serogroup non-O157
   Enterohemorrhagic *Escherichia coli* shiga toxin+ (not serogrouped)
Giardiasis
Gonorrhea
Haemophilus influenzae, invasive disease
Hansen disease (leprosy)
Hantavirus pulmonary syndrome
Hemolytic uremic syndrome, post-diarrheal
Hepatitis, viral, acute
   Hepatitis A, acute
   Hepatitis B, acute
   Hepatitis B virus, perinatal infection
   Hepatitis C, acute

Hepatitis, viral, chronic
   Chronic hepatitis B
   Hepatitis C virus infection (past or present)
HIV infection
   HIV infection, adult(≥13 years)
   HIV infection, pediatric (<13 years)
Legionellosis
Listeriosis
Lyme disease
Malaria
Measles
Meningococcal disease
Mumps
Pertussis
Plague
Poliomyelitis, paralytic
Psittacosis
Q fever
Rabies
   Rabies, animal
   Rabies, human
Rocky Mountain spotted fever
Rubella
Rubella, congenital syndrome
Salmonellosis
Shigellosis
Streptococcal disease, invasive, Group A
Streptococcal toxic-shock syndrome
Streptococcus pneumoniae, drug resistant, invasive disease
Streptococcus pneumoniae, invasive in children <5 years
Syphilis
   Syphilis, primary
   Syphilis, secondary
   Syphilis, latent
   Syphilis, early latent
   Syphilis, late latent
   Syphilis, latent unknown duration
   Neurosyphilis
   Syphilis, late, non-neurological
Syphilis, congenital
   Syphilitic stillbirth
Tetanus
Toxic-shock syndrome
Trichinosis
Tuberculosis
Tularemia
Typhoid fever
Varicella (morbidity)
Varicella (deaths only)
Yellow fever

SOURCE: CDC.

sciences educational programs, and professional medical organiza-
tions (e.g., the American Medical Association, the American Soci-
ety for Microbiology, the American Nurses Association, the Amer-
ican Veterinary Medical Association, the Association for
Professionals in Infection Control and Epidemiology, the Associa-
tion of Teachers of Preventive Medicine).

In addition to improving disease reporting by health care providers, efforts are needed to expand disease reporting from clinical laboratories. Automated laboratory reporting of notifiable infectious diseases from private clinical laboratories has been shown to improve dramatically the timeliness and quality of disease reporting for many notifiable infectious diseases, such as foodborne bacterial diseases (Effler et al., 1999; Overhage et al., 1997; Panackal et al., 2002). CDC has developed the standards and security measures needed for automated reporting of notifiable infectious diseases, having achieved consensus on critical issues. As of June 2002, however, relatively few states had implemented automated reporting of infectious diseases from major clinical laboratories using these standards.

CDC should expeditiously implement automated electronic laboratory reporting of notifiable infectious diseases from all relevant major clinical laboratories (e.g., microbiology, pathology) to their respective state health departments as part of a national electronic infectious disease reporting system. *The inclusion of antimicrobial resistance patterns of pathogens in the application of automated electronic laboratory reporting would assist in the surveillance and control of antimicrobial resistance.*

EXPLORING INNOVATIVE SYSTEMS OF SURVEILLANCE

Advances in information technology that allow automated reporting from laboratories may also be helpful in the development of other new systems, such as those incorporating remote sensing, as well as automated systems of syndromic surveillance.[1] In some sites, data describing patient illnesses before definitive diagnosis (e.g., fever, cough) are being transmitted electronically by health care providers and monitored centrally by those responsible for disease surveillance.

Syndromic surveillance is not new, although advances in information technology may improve its potential usefulness (see Appendix B for a more detailed discussion of syndromic surveillance). Historically, syndromic sur-

---

[1]For the purposes of this discussion, syndromic surveillance is defined as the surveillance of disease syndromes (groups of signs and symptoms), rather than specific clinical or laboratory-defined diseases.

veillance has proven quite useful in limited circumstances. For example, cruise ships that dock in U.S. ports are required to notify the U.S. Public Health Service when the number of visits to the ship's clinic reaches a threshold; public health investigation of and response to these threshold events has led to a marked reduction in the frequency of bacterial food- and waterborne illnesses among passengers in the past two decades.

It has been argued that surveillance of presenting symptoms of illness in emergency departments or clinics could be used to detect a mass release of a biological agent earlier than would be possible through more traditional surveillance. The influx of resources for enhancing recognition of bioterrorism events has resulted in numerous attempts to automate potentially relevant data and provide these data to a central entity responsible for epidemic detection. However, reporting of data from many clinics and hospitals is currently difficult to accomplish in real time in much of the civilian sector because of the number of incompatible systems in operation.

One of the more advanced and efficient systems of encounter-level data is the Electronic Surveillance for Early Notification of Community-based Epidemics (ESSENCE), developed by DOD, which provides syndromic surveillance in military treatment facilities using a grouping of International Classification of Disease (ICD) codes. Evaluation of the usefulness of this system for the timely detection of epidemics is ongoing (see Box 4-6).

In 2001, the Department of Health and Mental Hygiene in New York City established a surveillance system for detection of bioterrorism events. The technical setup and daily statistical analyses, as well as any disease investigations, if needed, occur at the Department of Health. The system was labor-intensive in its first few weeks, in the immediate aftermath of September 11, 2001, when staff were placed at every participating hospital to ensure that the medical providers completed daily forms and to conduct real-time data entry. Beginning in October 2001, the system was transitioned to a completely electronic system for data transfer so that staff on site were no longer required, and existing data systems were used so as not to require additional work by the hospital staff. The system was the first to detect the start of widespread influenza activity in the New York City, as well as the first indicator of norovirus activity in the area—well before the increased reports of institutional and cruise ship outbreaks. As one of the major purposes of this system is to ensure rapid detection of disease syndromes that might indicate the prodrome of a bioterrorist event, the analysts err on the side of increased sensitivity and are required to investigate several false alarms in the process.

Another approach is reflected in the Rapid Syndrome Validation System, developed by Sandia National Laboratories. This system enables health care providers in emergency departments to enter clinical and demographic

BOX 4-6
The Electronic Surveillance System for Early Notification of Community-Based Epidemics

The Electronic Surveillance System for Early Notification of Community-Based Epidemics (ESSENCE) is a syndromic surveillance system for the detection of infectious disease outbreaks at military treatment facilities worldwide. ESSENCE was initially developed by DOD's Global Emerging Infections System (GEIS) to serve 104 primary and emergency care clinics in the National Capital Region. Since the September 11, 2001, terrorist attack, it has been expanded to include the entire Military Health System (121 Army, 110 Navy, 80 Air Force, and 2 Coast Guard installations worldwide).

ESSENCE uses data from the Ambulatory Data System, which contains diagnoses of DOD health care beneficiaries and is located at all military treatment facilities. The data are captured at the military treatment facilities and are then sent to a centralized server in Denver, which feeds information directly into the secure server located at the Walter Reed Army Institute of Research, the Central Hub of GEIS. Data are captured daily; however, there is a lag time in the transfer of data of 1 to 4 days from the time of the initial patient visit.

Data are classified according to seven syndrome groups that have been identified based on International Classification of Diseases, 9th Revision (ICD-9) codes. These groups are as follows:

1. Respiratory (common cold, sinus infection)
2. Fever/malaise/sepsis
3. Gastrointestinal (vomiting, diarrhea, abdominal pain)
4. Neurological (headache, meningitis)

data on patients with infectious disease syndromes and to report directly to the health department (Sandia National Laboratories, 2002).

The resource requirements for automated reporting of syndromic data from most hospitals, clinics, or emergency departments are currently high, but these costs may be reduced over time with standardization of software. The resources required may also be reduced if the surveillance system uses data that are already being collected, and data transfer can occur automatically without requiring staff resources on either end. The primary resource requirements for such systems are analytic staff to evaluate the data and disease investigators to respond to any potential outbreaks detected. The most critical need for these systems is to ensure effective links to local and state public health agencies that would need to respond in the event of an alarm. The central role of public health agencies in the effectiveness of any such system is crucial, since they have both the authority and the expertise for investigations needed to respond should an attack be detected.

The use of other existing health databases, including 911 calls and pharmacy records, is also being explored. A clinical validation study of the

5. Dermatological-infectious (vesicular rash)
6. Dermatological-hemorrhagic (bruising, petechiae)
7. Coma/sudden death

Graphs are created and historical data are used in baseline comparisons of the data to monitor the defined syndromes for trends that could signify an event due to an emerging infectious disease. A geographic information system (GIS) is used to perform data visualization, as well as to determine the geographic component of an outbreak. The central hub of ESSENCE can provide data in terms of syndrome, age, gender, clinic, location, and health care provider. The graphs are made available daily to public health officials on a secure website so they can review and analyze any potential emerging infection outbreak scenarios.

GEIS was recently awarded a 4-year, $12 million grant from the Defense Advanced Research Projects Agency (DARPA) for the creation of ESSENCE II. This effort involves collaboration with the Johns Hopkins School of Public Health, the George Washington University School of Public Health, Carnegie Mellon University, IBM, and Cycorp. These partners will work together to create a surveillance system for detecting a potential biological attack on the U.S. military. Plans are for the system to actively obtain data on the following: health maintenance organization (HMO) billing, over-the-counter drug sales, school absenteeism, and military pharmacy, laboratory, and radiology orders. ESSENCE II will track these data continually to detect abnormalities, and will transmit alerts and notifications when an abnormal situation appears. In addition to the partners listed above, a team of epidemiologists and computer researchers will be involved in the development of ESSENCE II.

SOURCE: Department of Defense–Global Emerging Infections System, 2002.

Emergency Management Services 911 syndromic surveillance system showed sensitivity in detecting illness suggestive of influenza, although the system had poor specificity (Greenko et al., 2002). Surveillance of antimicrobial and over-the-counter drugs is being explored for its usefulness in early detection of an epidemic in a community.

Some evidence indicates that these systems may be used to detect epidemics of influenza and some gastrointestinal illnesses earlier than would otherwise be the case (J. Duchin, Public Health, Seattle and King county, personal communication, January 30, 2002; J. Pavlin, GEIS, personal communication, January 28, 2002). Data from these systems have also been used in tabletop exercises for a bioterrorism event and have filled a critical need for rapid and continuous assessment of health care utilization for particular problems; this is likely to be the case as well for naturally occurring epidemics, such as influenza pandemics and other crises.

The potential usefulness of these systems for early detection of individual class A biological agent infections is unclear. The assumptions on which these systems are based require closer examination with regard to their usefulness in the early detection of bioterrorism. A key issue for syndromic surveillance systems is determining statistical thresholds for response that are sufficiently sensitive and specific to detect severe illnesses (such as anthrax) earlier than would be possible through traditional methods without overtaxing the public health system with false alarms. This determination is difficult for a rare event or an event causing severe illness or death. Numerous false signals from these systems have to date resulted in the diversion of limited public health resources, and some areas are raising the threshold for which they may investigate a "signal" at the expense of loss of sensitivity and timeliness. Geospatial coding may be useful in this regard.

In summary, syndromic surveillance is likely to be increasingly helpful in the detection and monitoring of epidemics, as well as the evaluation of health care utilization for infectious diseases. At the same time, the potential exists for syndromic surveillance to draw resources away from other systems that have proven to be robust in the detection of microbial threats. Although novel approaches utilizing nonspecific data may prove useful, particularly for conditions for which empirical diagnosis and treatment represent the standard of care, a balance should be sought between strengthening what is known to be helpful (e.g., diagnosis of patients with infectious illness, strengthening of the liaison between clinical care providers and health departments) and the exploration and evaluation of new approaches.

Research on innovative systems of surveillance that capitalize on advances in information technology should be supported. *Before widespread implementation, these systems should be carefully evaluated for their usefulness in detection of infectious disease epidemics, including their potential for detection of the major biothreat agents, their ability to monitor the spread of epidemics, and their cost-effectiveness. Research on syndromic surveillance systems should continue to assess such factors as the capacity to transmit existing data electronically, to standardize chief complaint or other coded data, and to explore the usefulness of geospatial coding; CDC should provide leadership in such evaluations. In addition, promising approaches will need to be coordinated nationally so that data can be shared and analyzed across jurisdictions.*

DEVELOPING AND USING DIAGNOSTICS

Etiologic diagnosis—identifying the microbial cause of an infectious disease—is the cornerstone of effective disease control and prevention efforts, including surveillance. The first recognized case of inhalational anthrax in the 2001 bioterrorist attack was diagnosed by examination of a

Gram stain of the patient's cerebrospinal fluid. Yet for various reasons, including restrictions imposed by managed care, laboratory regulations (e.g., CLIA[2]), and the increasing use of empirical therapy, etiologic diagnosis has declined significantly over the past decade; as a result, the quality of clinical care, surveillance, and training has been compromised. In addition, a dangerous consequence of decreased etiologic diagnosis has been an increase in the inappropriate use of broad-spectrum antibiotics and the emergence of antimicrobial resistance. A specific diagnosis, including results of antimicrobial resistance testing, allows for more appropriate treatment, avoids the inappropriate use of antibiotics, and also informs public health actions.

The dramatic rise in the number of unexplained causes of community acquired pneumonia in adults is testament to the current crisis in etiologic diagnosis. For example, prospective studies evaluating the causes of community acquired pneumonia in adults have failed to identify the cause in 40 to 60 percent of cases (Bartlett et al., 2000). In virtually all studies of community acquired pneumonia when diagnoses have been made, *Streptococcus pneumoniae* has accounted for two-thirds of all bacteremic cases. It has been suggested that sputum cultures in the large percentage of undiagnosed cases have failed to yield *S. pneumoniae* mainly because of inadequate specimen collection; delays in seeding cultures; use of less sensitive techniques for recovering the organism (Bartlett et al., 1998); and barriers imposed by meeting requirements of individual health care plans, such as the requirement to send specimens to a specified laboratory regardless of geographic location or availability of tests of highest quality. Permitting these unacceptable practices to persist is causing problems for the U.S. capacity to respond to microbial threats.

Current diagnostic approaches for collection of environmental samples or clinical specimens involve primarily hands-on, ad hoc procedures using a variety of devices and instruments. In the clinical arena, these procedures result in specimens of variable quantity and quality. The process is relatively laborious and nonstandardized. A few common methods for specimen disruption are applied to each specimen type without particular regard for the possible diversity of pathogens and their requirements, nor are special precautions taken in a uniform manner to minimize degradation of pathogens. Recovery of fastidious microbes from clinical specimens has almost certainly suffered as a result of the time demands and resource

---

[2]Congress passed the Clinical Laboratory Improvement Amendments (CLIA) in 1988, establishing quality standards for all laboratory testing to ensure the accuracy, reliability, and timeliness of patient test results regardless of where the test is performed.

constraints typical of today's clinical workplaces, as well as recent laboratory downsizing (Bartlett et al., 1998). Technology developments, such as the use of microsonicators for efficient rapid microbial lysis (Belgrader et al., 1999a; Taylor et al., 2001b), are likely to improve the current situation. Problems with lack of standardization and nonuniformity of procedures are even more prevalent in environmental microbial detection; air and water are among the environmental specimen types that are collected and processed most frequently.

Disincentives to conduct careful laboratory diagnoses include the costs of additional tests, particularly comprehensive ones, and claims that the test results return too late to be of use in clinical management. However, a precise diagnosis obtained from skilled laboratory analysis can be invaluable and cost-effective, even if specific therapy is not available for the condition diagnosed, and is important for public health surveillance. This is particularly true for acute respiratory infections such as bronchitis and pharyngitis, illnesses with a low percentage of bacterial infection that are nonetheless often treated with antibiotics (Gonzales et al., 2001). Treating such illnesses with antibiotics is costly and represents the type of inappropriate antibiotic use that fosters drug resistance and exposes patients to the risks associated with antibacterial drug consumption (see the discussion later in this chapter). Progress has been made in etiologic diagnosis of pediatric patients in some communities. In Finland, for example, etiologic diagnosis is made in 90 percent of cases of severe respiratory disease in children (Nohynek et al., 1991). This success rate is attributed to an emphasis on etiologic diagnosis, coupled with a situation in which highly skilled microbiologists work within the relatively compact health care system that characterizes the Scandinavian medical community. In the United States, however, the underuse of etiologic diagnosis and the overuse of antibiotics remain significant health care problems.

Clinical microbiology continues to rely heavily upon cultivation-based methods and should continue to do so. Cultivation methods have improved considerably over the past several decades, with advances being made in the scope and diversity of media components, control of environmental conditions, use of heterologous host cells, and use of growth-promoting factors (Mukamolova et al., 1998). A number of recently recognized and newly described microbial pathogens, including spirochetes, rickettsia, actinomycetes, and a variety of viruses, have been cultivated successfully in the laboratory. Cultivation is the most widely used approach in laboratories, clinics, and health care facilities throughout the world, especially in developing countries, and hence is currently the most common microbial detection platform for international surveillance. It is important to note that cultivation, despite being slow, limited in sensitivity for some clinically relevant microbes, and the least technologically sophisticated approach, nevertheless provides the most ready assessment of complex microbial phenotypes (behaviors), such as drug resistance. Cultivation allows for the "fingerprinting" of an organism, important for the understanding of microbes and how they spread.

Diagnostic Pathology

The ability of diagnostic pathology to help in recognizing and understanding diseases—both old and emerging, both in humans and in animals—is often overlooked. Basic anatomic pathology involves analyzing tissues from dead specimens, making observations, interpreting the findings, and following up with histopathology studies of samples under a microscope. In recent years, the advent of molecular pathology has heightened the power of diagnostic pathology. With such tools as immunohistochemistry, in situ hybridization, and polymerase chain reaction (PCR) assays, pathologists can now identify etiology more rapidly than ever before and, in many cases, where doing so would previously have been impossible (see Appendix C for a more detailed discussion of advanced diagnostic methods). Diagnostic immunohistochemistry was key to confirming both the West Nile virus and the anthrax outbreaks. However, current disease surveillance systems, for human diseases and zoonoses alike, fail to make adequate use of diagnostic pathology. No infectious disease pathology program is currently supported, in contrast with other specialty pathology training programs, such as those in cardiovascular disease. In the medical community today, many unexplained deaths evade rigorous pathological studies. Overall, the number of autopsies being performed has declined, and the system is highly capricious as to the determination of when an autopsy is necessary. In addition, there is overarching concern about training and skill levels with respect to ensuring that the latest technologies in diagnostic pathology are being applied (see Box 4-7).

The availability of archived biological samples can facilitate the understanding of new pathogens and the response to outbreaks. More countries should be encouraged to maintain (publicly aknowledged) registries of blood and tissue specimens, whether from zoonotic or human events, to make it feasible to search for specific susceptibility factors. For example, in 1998 an outbreak of viral encephalitis occurred in Malaysia. Analysis of archival collections of 1995 serum samples from pigs showed that some of those samples contained antibodies to the previously unrecognized Nipah virus. This finding allowed investigators to conclude that the virus had been circulating in the population for some time. A large and invaluable resource of archived samples is DOD's Triservice Serum Repository, begun in 1985, which contains 25 million specimens collected from military personnel. This resource serves many research needs; it provided important informa-

---

BOX 4-7
The Value of Autopsies

The records of medical examiners and coroners provide vital information about patterns and trends of mortality in the United States and are excellent sources of data for public health studies and surveillance. For example, during the outbreak of West Nile encephalitis in New York, autopsies were performed under the jurisdiction of New York City's Office of the Chief Medical Examiner because of the obvious public health implications (Shieh et al., 2000). Other notable cases in which autopsies contributed to the discovery or increased understanding of emerging infectious diseases include investigations of hantavirus pulmonary syndrome, Ebola hemorrhagic fever, leptospirosis associated with pulmonary hemorrhage, new variant Creutzfeldt-Jakob disease, and Nipah virus encephalitis.

Autopsy rates are decreasing in the United States (Shieh et al., 2000; Sinard, 2001). National statistics reveal that the performance of autopsies declined from 41 percent of hospital deaths in 1961 to 5 to 10 percent in the mid-1990s (CDC, 2001n; Hasson and Schneiderman, 1995; Burton and Nemetz, 2000). A survey of 244 hospitals conducted by the College of American Pathologists in 1994 showed that half of U.S. hospitals had autopsy rates at or below 8.5 percent, and three-quarters had autopsy rates below 13.5 percent. Accreditation programs in internal medicine recommend maintaining an autopsy rate of at least 15 percent (CDC, 2001n).

Autopsy rates have fallen for a variety of reasons. First is a lack of insurance reimbursement, so that hospital financial managers and pathology departments must absorb the autopsy costs. Second is lack of incentive. Managed care has resulted in fewer pathologists who have to work longer and harder, imposing workforce burdens with little incentive to take on the added workload imposed by increasing the rate of autopsies. Third is a decreased emphasis on pathology in medical schools. Many medical students graduate with no training in autopsy procedure or little opportunity to view an autopsy in progress. Fourth is the misconception that other diagnostic modalities, such as computed tomography and magnetic resonance imaging, have replaced the need for autopsies. And finally, some pathologists have become concerned about the increased risk of occupational exposure to potentially fatal pathogens (Hanzlick and Baker, 1998).

---

tion on hantavirus from samples that had been obtained from military recruits from the southwestern United States.

Microbiological Diagnosis and Development of New Diagnostic Tools

At the same time that traditional, available diagnostic tools are not being utilized, newer, improved etiologic diagnostic tools are needed. The capability for etiologic diagnosis could be significantly improved if inexpensive, rapid, sensitive, and specific tests were available to differentiate not only between viruses and bacteria, but also among different types of viruses and bacteria. The sensitivity of detection methods for cultivation-amenable microorganisms is currently suboptimal. When traditional diagnostic methods are rigorously applied to syndromes of suspected infectious etiology, such as pneumonia, encephalitis, lymphocyte-predominant meningitis, pericarditis, acute diarrhea, and sepsis, only a minority of cases can be explained microbiologically. In addition, a long list of chronic inflammatory diseases with features of infection remain poorly understood and inadequately explained from a microbiological perspective.

Newer technologies can succeed where methods for pathogen identification through serology or cultivation have failed in the past because of the absence of specific reagents or fastidious requirements for agent replication. The newly available technologies include methods based on the analysis of microbial nucleic acid sequences (e.g., DNA microarrays, PCR), analysis of microbial protein sequences (e.g., mass spectrophotometry), immunological systems for microbe detection (e.g., expression libraries), and host response profiling. Over the past decade, the use of molecular pathogen discovery methods has resulted in the identification of several novel agents, including Borna disease virus, hepatitis C virus, Sin Nombre virus, HHV-6, HHV-8, *Bartonella henselae*, and *Tropheryma whippelii*. The advent of molecular pathology has heightened the power of diagnostic pathology. Despite these achievements, however, sensitive and specific rapid diagnostic tools that can be used to diagnose common diseases in the office, clinic, and emergency room simply are not being used or are unavailable.

For example, although many different microbe-specific PCR assays have been described, only a small proportion has actually entered into routine clinical practice. Examples include assays for *N. gonorrheae*, *C. trachomatis*, herpes simplex virus, and HIV. A modest number of recent studies have confirmed that the use of these molecular diagnostic tests can reduce patient-care costs and favorably impact patient management (Dumler and Valsamakis, 1999; Ramers et al., 2000). In particular, the development of rapid, real-time (semiquantitative) PCR with point-of-care microbial detection within 30 minutes (Belgrader et al., 1998, 1999b) could potentially alter the use of antibiotics on a widespread scale and reduce antibiotic resistance (Bergeron and Ouellette, 1998). Some of the factors that may have limited more widespread use of these theoretically appealing molecular approaches include difficulty in obtaining specimens and transporting them to the laboratory, a paucity of studies that address clinical validation, and the need for specialized expertise.

CDC and NIH should work with FDA, other government agencies (e.g., DOD, USDA, the national laboratories), and industry on the development, assessment, and validation of rapid, inexpensive and cost-effective, sensitive, and specific etiologic diagnostic tests for microbial threats of public health importance.

Strategies for developing and deploying inexpensive, sensitive, and specific rapid diagnostics will need to be developed for several different scenarios, including ambulatory and bedside, as well as use in developing countries. Ambulatory diagnostics should target primarily childhood respiratory diseases; these tests need to be as inexpensive as possible and widely available for use in both offices and clinics to ensure timely results. For hospitalized patients or those with more serious conditions, a single platform for diagnosis of multiple agents is needed. For example, if pneumonia is the issue, a single PCR assay that can detect common bacterial and viral pathogens should be able to provide an etiologic diagnosis and allow specific therapy. Hospitals could adopt a single platform as an interim standard that would allow tests to be developed at multiple sites with some assurance that they could be implemented at most sites. Using the same platform for bioterrorist threats would stimulate the more rapid availability of local testing for bioterrorist agents and would not preclude competing test platforms or research on better approaches. Overseas diagnostics should be rugged, simple, inexpensive, and tailored to diseases and zoonotic agents of local importance.

Public health agencies and professional organizations (e.g., those concerned with patient care, health education, and microbiological issues) should promulgate and publicize guidelines that call for the intensive application of existing diagnostic modalities and new modalities as they are established. *Such guidelines should be incorporated into continuing education programs, board examinations, and accreditation practices. Payers for health care should cover diagnostic tests for infectious diseases to increase specific diagnoses and thereby inform both public health and medical care, including monitoring of inappropriate use of antimicrobials.*

As diagnostic tests become more sensitive and increasingly capable of detecting the presence of and differentiating among various types of microorganisms, it is imperative that health care practitioners be able to make clinical sense of the results. Again, a renewed emphasis on laboratory and etiologic diagnostic training should be a regular part of medical education. A positive laboratory test, coupled with corresponding clinical signs and symptoms of disease, can assist decision-making regarding appropriate therapy; treatment decisions should not rest purely on diagnostic test results, however, regardless of their sensitivity and specificity. As necessary as improved diagnostic tests are, enthusiasm for them must not override their meaning in the clinical presentation of illness.

EDUCATING AND TRAINING
THE MICROBIAL THREAT WORKFORCE

The number of qualified individuals in the workforce required for microbial threat preparedness is dangerously low. For example, in 2001 the need for at least 600 new epidemiologists in public health departments across the United States was identified because of the requirements for bioterrorism preparedness alone. Yet only 1,076 students graduated with a degree in epidemiology in the year 2000 and are potentially seeking employment in government, academia, or private industry, and the largest percentage are trained in chronic disease, not infectious disease epidemiology. According to the National Association of City and County Health Officers, the most needed occupations between 1999 and 2000 were public health nurses, environmental scientists and specialists, epidemiologists, health educators, and administrative staff.

The real-world information and skills needed for confronting microbial threats must be better integrated into the training of *all* health care professionals to ensure a prompt and effective response to any and all infectious disease threats, whether naturally occurring or maliciously introduced. It is vital that on-the-job training opportunities, especially for students and new health professionals, be further developed to ensure that professionals responsible for infectious disease control are well trained in real-life situations, and to expose health professions students to career paths in infectious disease prevention and control. Academic health centers are the intellectual hub of these types of professional training programs, and as such serve as the ideal recipients for increased investment in microbial threat education and outreach. Training programs are also urgently needed for health care workers who are currently in mid- and upper-level management positions.

Training programs in applied epidemiology are critical for the development of a strong microbial threat workforce. Currently, some applied epidemiology training programs are in place both domestically and internationally. These programs may provide a solid foundation on which present programs can be expanded and future epidemiology training programs modeled. One example of such a program is the Epidemic Intelligence Service (EIS), a 2-year postgraduate program at CDC that currently enrolls about 70 new officers each year. A typical class comprises primarily medical doctors, but also includes nurses, veterinarians, dentists, and doctoral graduates in epidemiology and the social and behavioral sciences. The majority of EIS officers (also known as "disease detectives") train at CDC headquarters, and the remainder go to either a state or a large local health department. The latter officers are trained in broad, front-line public health experience; officers deal with surveillance using this information to focus investigations and to implement policy. The officers at CDC headquarters are trained in specialized, disease- or problem-specific areas.

The initial EIS program, which started over 50 years ago, was focused on communicable disease, but over the years has expanded to include officers trained in environmental health, chronic disease, injuries, and maternal and child health. EIS officers provide international outbreak assistance through investigations in all regions of the world. The success of the program has led to the development of similar training offices in 20 countries worldwide.

EIS officers have played a pivotal role in the success of many investigations, including polio eradication in Africa and Asia, hantavirus outbreak in the southwestern United States, West Nile virus outbreak in the northeastern and southeastern United States, Ebola outbreaks in Uganda and Zaire, and bioterrorism preparedness. Still, there is room for improvement. In particular, EIS needs to be expanded to include more officers who spend full- or part-time assignments in infectious disease control programs at state and local public health departments. In addition, it should be recognized that this is a training program. Thus, while EIS officers often provide an invaluable service during their training, their true value lies in their development as a much-needed cadre of professionals for the future.

For more than 20 years, CDC has collaborated with ministries of health around the world to help establish field epidemiology training programs (FETPs). The goal of these programs is to provide service to the sponsoring government or agency while also training public health workers in epidemiology and outbreak investigation. During training, staff members, trainers, and trainees (or fellows) work with ministries of health and national governments to provide and enhance core public health functions, including disease prevention and control, surveillance, and the supplying of information needed to support informed policy and legislation. In most countries, applied training programs also serve as the backbone for the development and implementation of health information and surveillance systems, bulletins that give program managers and decision makers timely information, and supervision and training of other health workers in the health care system.

The FETPs have trained more than 900 international public health leaders in epidemiology and outbreak investigation, and approximately 420 more are currently in training (CDC, 2002r). Many of these programs have contributed to efforts in infectious disease control and prevention. The FETPs would be enhanced if all programs were assured of laboratory support in the diagnosis of infectious diseases, as is the case with the Thailand FETP.

The Association of Public Health Laboratories' Emerging Infectious Diseases Laboratory Fellowship Program trains qualified bachelor's and

BOX 4-8
Training in Foreign Animal Disease Control

Plum Island (located 1 1/2 miles off the northeastern end of Long Island, New York) under the administration of the U.S. Department of Agriculture's Agricultural Research Service (ARS) and the Animal and Plant Health Inspection Source (APHIS) is one of the principal locations in the United States where infectious foreign animal disease agents are studied.

Scientists on Plum Island have the laboratory capability to diagnose more than 35 exotic animal diseases, and they perform thousands of diagnostic tests each year to detect the presence of foreign animal disease agents. The tissue and blood samples that are tested are submitted by veterinarians suspecting an exotic disease in domestic livestock or by animal import centers testing quarantined animals for foreign diseases. Samples are also submitted by animal health professionals in other countries who need help with a diagnosis.

An integral part of the laboratory's mission is training animal health professionals in the recognition of foreign animal diseases. Staff present several courses each year at Plum Island to give veterinarians, scientists, professors, and veterinary students the opportunity to study the clinical signs and pathological changes caused by foreign animal diseases.

SOURCE: Animal and Plant Health Inspection Service, 1992.

master's candidates in laboratory science so they can understand the role and importance of public health laboratory services, and it trains doctoral candidates (microbiologists in particular) to conduct high-priority infectious disease research in public health laboratories. The program is highly competitive and limited to a small number of trainees each year. This program should be evaluated to assess how well it is meeting the purpose for which it was initiated and to provide recommendations for further expansion and enhancement. Increased training in the recognition and diagnosis of animal diseases that can indirectly affect human health is also needed (see Box 4-8).

CDC, DOD, and NIH should develop new and expand upon current intramural and extramural programs that train health professionals in applied epidemiology and field-based research and training in the United States and abroad. *Research and training should combine field and laboratory approaches to infectious disease prevention and control. Federal agencies should develop these programs in close collaboration with academic centers or other potential training sites. Domestic training programs should include an*

educational, hands-on experience at state and local public health
departments to expose future and current health professionals to
new career options, such as public health.

VACCINE DEVELOPMENT AND PRODUCTION

Vaccines are an essential element in the success of modern medical science. Vaccines have played a central role in providing people around the world with longer and better lives. Indeed, it is difficult to exaggerate the impact of vaccination on the health of the world's population. With the exception of safe water, no other modality, not even antibiotics, has had such a large effect on mortality reduction and population growth (Plotkin and Mortimer, 1994; Szucs, 2000). As we enter the twenty-first century, however, vaccine development and production are dependent on a complex set of issues, including the translation of basic research into the development of effective vaccines, regulatory requirements, liability concerns, market forces, and competing priorities that have led to periodic shortages of routine vaccines, as well as a lack of vaccines for diseases that affect predominantly developing regions of the world. Added to this complex situation is the need for vaccines to protect against microbial agents that could be used in a bioterrorist attack.

Despite these challenges, opportunities for major breakthroughs in vaccine development are more promising than ever before as the front across which the basic sciences are advancing broadens. In the past decade, scientists have made great strides forward in biotechnology, genomics, and understanding of the molecular basis of pathogenesis. Advances in immunology include the development of tetramer technology that permits functional analysis of T cells (Klenerman et al., 2002); understanding of the role of dendritic cells in antigen processing and presentation (Guermonprez et al., 2002), of antigen-receptor signaling (Myung et al., 2000), and of the role of heat-shock proteins in antigen presentations (Srivastava, 2002); and demonstration of the induction of both antibody-mediated and cell-mediated immune responses to a wide range of infectious disease agents. Success in using virus-like particles may soon lead to the development of vectors that simultaneously carry several different antigens (Moss, 1996).

The development of new delivery systems is likely to continue to be an important area of innovation in vaccines. The improved fundamental knowledge of helper T cells offers opportunities to create new means of encouraging cell-mediated immunity. Mucosal immunity is being studied extensively, as are new types of adjuvants. Opportunities also exist to follow up the success with hepatitis B vaccine by developing other recombinant vaccines (IOM, 2001d). Advances in viral pathogenesis reveal that disease agents such as vaccinia have multiple strategies to circumvent both antibody- and cell-mediated responses (Moss and Shisler, 2001). New knowledge about the role of cytokines in immune responsiveness and function (Hunter and Reiner, 2000) offers hope for adjuvants for immune responses. Characterization of the antigenic domains on multiple organisms and the ability to express them on a single organism provides the opportunity to vaccinate against multiple disease agents (Henderson and Moss, 1999). And recent advances in reverse genetics for negative-stranded RNA viruses now permit influenza virus to be made to order, permitting rapid development of new vaccine strains (Neumann and Kawaoka, 2001). On all of these fronts, additional, well-funded basic research is likely to have significant social benefits (Kurstak, 1993).

Meeting the Need for Translating Basic Research

Despite the remarkable advances in basic knowledge of immunology and microbiology, proportional translation of these findings to new vaccine development has not occurred. Reflecting on the HIV pandemic and the terrible toll it has taken throughout both the developed and, in particular, the developing world, no clearer need for an effective vaccine exists. After two decades of substantial progress in the field of HIV/AIDS, however, we are still short of the target of having a vaccine to prevent the spread of infection.

An increased commitment to research is necessary to ensure the development of vaccines for the numerous infectious diseases that threaten the world's human population. Vaccines against acute respiratory infections, diarrheal diseases, malaria, tuberculosis, STDs, and dengue are desperately needed. Vaccines are in the pipeline for many diseases that burden the developing world—Chagas' disease, onchocerciasis and lymphatic filariasis, leishmaniasis, schistosomiasis, and malaria—but they are in the predevelopment stage and are still far from ready for use in humans (WHO, 1999a). Efficacious vaccines for malaria and dengue, arguably two of the most important arthropod-borne diseases, are not available despite extensive developmental efforts. The problems associated with the development of malaria vaccines have been the subject of many scientific and lay publications, and an efficacious vaccine is not likely to be available soon. Development of a dengue vaccine has been complicated by the issue of the potential for immune enhancement. Four serotypes of dengue virus exist; infection with one serotype typically provides lifelong immunity against reinfection with the homologous serotype, but does not provide immunity against infection with a heterologous serotype. Such secondary heterologous infections are an important risk factor for dengue hemorrhagic fever and shock syndrome (Beaty, 2000). Thus, development of a vaccine strategy that will result in balanced immunity to all four serotypes is a necessity;

however, achieving this has proven to be very difficult, and a number of new strategies are now undergoing investigation.

Responding to Marketplace and Policy Issues

Numerous economic and public health policy issues complicate efforts in vaccine development, production, and deployment. In the last 40 years, few pharmaceutical manufacturers have considered vaccines an attractive business opportunity because of the low return on investment and the exposure to legal liability (Rappuoli et al., 2002). Companies perceive little market incentive to develop vaccines for diseases that occur sporadically and affect the poorest populations—vaccines that may also have little chance of being employed effectively. This has certainly been seen in the area of tropical diseases, especially arthropod- and rodent-borne diseases. Even if inexpensive and efficacious vaccines or drugs are developed, their use by those most in need may be hampered by a lack of public health infrastructure. For example, a safe and effective vaccine for yellow fever has existed for decades. Yet this disease continues to be a pathogen of significant importance in humans in Africa and South America, and its emergence remains a constant threat in urban areas of the tropics and potentially even in Asia, where it would represent a public health catastrophe (Monath, 2001).

The infrastructure for the manufacture of vaccines is steadily deteriorating, and shortages currently exist even in the availability of certain routine vaccines. For example, the difficulty of producing sufficient influenza vaccine in extremely mild interpandemic years, such as 2000 and 2001, signals a potential disaster during a pandemic year. In 2000, supplies of the tetanus and diptheria booster fell short. By the fall of 2001, CDC was reporting shortages of five vaccines, some of which are combination vaccines that protect against eight childhood diseases. Of the eight recommended routine childhood vaccines, five are produced by a single major manufacturer; consequently, if supply is interrupted or a manufacturer ceases production, there may be few or no alternative sources of vaccine (GAO, 2002). The reality is that the infrastructure does not exist to produce even a sufficient supply of currently licensed vaccines, let alone to develop new vaccines against emerging microbial threats. Thus in the event of an outbreak—whether naturally occurring or an act of bioterrorism—the United States will not have the capacity to produce sufficient vaccines to safeguard the population.

The anthrax attacks of 2001 in the United States generated widespread public awareness of infectious agents that had previously not been regarded as worthy of much public attention or substantial federal research funding. Before September 2001, several infectious agents had been identified as being of concern for possible use in a biological attack. As a result, early efforts were undertaken to explore new avenues for the development of needed vaccines. For example, DOD proposed that government-owned, contractor-operated (GOCO) facilities investigate, develop, and produce vaccines against potential biological agents such as tularemia, plague, and anthrax. Recognizing that neither the government nor private industry alone could develop protection against these threats, DOD initiated a set of new partnerships and contracting strategies to prevent a national catastrophe.

To reap the advantages of scientific advances, private, industrial sources of innovation in vaccines must be strengthened and protected. Here the base is clearly too narrow. In contrast to the vast complex of institutions and individuals involved in basic medical research, only four leading companies worldwide have been responsible for developing new vaccines during the past two decades. It was not mergers and acquisitions that concentrated responsibility for vaccine innovation in the hands of four multinational firms; rather, the economic forces that drove firms out of the industry were the rising costs of innovation, production, and distribution and the shrinking margins allowed by monopsony, or the concentration of buying power in the hands of a relatively small number of public agencies. In the United States, several large companies ceased vaccine production because the total world market for vaccines was so much smaller than that for pharmaceuticals, government purchases allowed only narrow profit margins, and liability continued to be an issue (Galambos and Sewell, 1995; IOM, 2001d).

The current economic situation surrounding vaccine innovation has not improved, and thus will not encourage the entry or reentry of large pharmaceutical companies with extensive resources that could be dedicated to vaccine innovation. If anything, the economic situation has deteriorated further. The increasing costs associated with discovery have become a major barrier. In 1976, it cost an estimated $54 million to develop a new chemical entity (Hansen, 1979). By 1987 that figure had increased to $231 million (DiMasi et al., 1991). Today it costs an estimated $500 million to devise a new drug or vaccine, and that figure includes only the cost of discovery. If one adds the charges for development and clinical evaluation, the total cost increases to $800 million to $1 billion. Moreover, before any of that investment can be recovered, a new vaccine must pass through a complex and lengthy regulatory process. Without lowering standards, the United States has made progress in streamlining the regulatory process, yet cooperative improvements in regulatory systems must continue to be examined and addressed.

Incremental changes along these lines will be important, but improvements with global—not national or even regional—distribution will also be essential. A major development that could have a significant impact on the economic problems outlined above would be international harmonization of the industry's technical requirements and regulatory processes. The European Union (EU) has demonstrated how to change on a regional basis; now the move must be made to an international level of standardization and regulation. Cooperative measures short of thoroughgoing harmonization would help. Clinical trials and designs could be standardized, and testing authorities could begin to accept lot release test results without major structural changes on a national basis. By working with increased vigor toward the development of international standards and an international compact that would finally eliminate redundancy in a costly and time-consuming process, it may be possible to improve substantially the economic conditions that have in the past sharply reduced the number of firms contributing to vaccine innovation.

The pricing problem with vaccines is a critical issue. To prevent further defections from the industry and encourage healthy entry into the market, this problem must be addressed head-on. To some extent, a price-controlled market for vaccines exists in the United States, and to a greater extent, price control through government purchasing exists in much of the developed and developing worlds. Half of the vaccines in the United States are purchased by the Vaccines for Children Fund and other government-controlled programs. The creation of these funds was a major step forward. So, too, was the development of vaccine production capabilities in the developing world, where 75 percent of the world's supply of vaccines is now manufactured. India, China, Pakistan, Egypt, Nigeria, Brazil, and other developing nations produce diphtheria, tetanus, and pertussis (DTP) vaccine for use in their countries. In Europe and Japan, government-controlled markets have long prevailed. Under political pressures to hold down costs, many government agencies place downward pressure on margins, which makes it difficult to sustain the needed level of innovation and production.

Only the developed nations can afford a pricing system that favors innovation. The manner in which vaccines are priced in the U.S. market cannot be applied to markets in Africa, Latin America, and Southeast Asia. The European market is also likely to have a different level of pricing, although that situation should change as the EU makes further progress toward consolidation and growth. With a consolidated market comparable to that of the United States, the EU should, at some point, be able to make a contribution to sustaining innovation similar to that of the United States. This development would have the enormous advantage of alleviating some of the political pressures that are mounting in the United States against differential pricing.

With the necessary political will and effective leadership from the developed world, a new economic environment for vaccine innovation can be created. By developing and deploying new vaccines, it will be possible to build on the tremendous accomplishments of the WHO campaigns; deal effectively with the massive problems created by rotavirus, malaria, dengue, tuberculosis, and reemerging organisms; and perhaps even cope with the threat of biological terrorism. Without changes in the economics of vaccine innovation, however, significant progress on these fronts cannot be expected.

A State of Crisis

Our nation—and the world—faces a serious crisis with respect to vaccine development, production, and deployment. Concern has increased over the inadequacy of vaccine research and development efforts, periodic shortages of existing vaccines, and the lack of vaccines to prevent diseases that affect persons in developing countries disproportionately. Yet, too little has been done to resolve these issues. The evolving threat of intentional biological attacks makes the need for focused attention and action even more critical.

The challenges associated with vaccine innovation, production, and deployment are many and complex. Solutions will require a novel, coordinated approach among government agencies, academia, and industry. Issues that must be examined and addressed in a more meaningful and systematic fashion include the identification of priorities for research, the determination of effective incentive strategies for developers and manufacturers, liability concerns, and streamlining of the regulatory process. Currently, the federal government is neither addressing all of these challenges at a sufficiently high level nor providing adequate resources. Leadership, empowerment, and accountability are urgently needed at the cabinet level to ensure a comprehensive, integrated vaccine strategy that will address the following critical elements:

The U.S. Secretary of Health and Human Services should ensure the formulation and implementation of a national vaccine strategy for protecting the U.S. population from endemic and emerging microbial threats. *Only by focusing leadership, authority, and accountability at the cabinet level can the federal government meet its national responsibility for ensuring an innovative and adequately funded research base for existing and emerging infectious diseases and the development of an ample supply of routinely recommended vaccines. The U.S. Secretary of Health and Human Services should work closely with other relevant federal agencies (e.g., DOD, the Department of Homeland Security, VA), Congress, industry, academia, and the public health community to carry out this responsibility.*

The U.S. Secretary of Defense, the U.S. Secretary of Health and Human Services, and the U.S. Secretary of Homeland Security should work closely with industry and academia to ensure the rapid development and deployment of vaccines for naturally occurring or intentionally introduced microbial threats to national security. *The federal government should explore innovative mechanisms, such as cooperative agreements between government and industry or consortia of government, industry, and academia, to accelerate these efforts.*

The Administrator of USAID, the U.S. Secretary of Health and Human Services, and the U.S. Secretary of State should work in cooperation with public and private partners (e.g., leaders of foundations and other donor agencies, industry, WHO, UNICEF, the Global Alliance for Vaccines and Immunization) to ensure the development and distribution of vaccines for diseases that affect populations in developing countries disproportionately.

NEED FOR NEW ANTIMICROBIAL DRUGS

Antibiotics

Unfortunately, complacency toward infectious diseases in the 1960s, overconfidence in existing antibiotics, and competition from highly profitable opportunities for pharmaceutical development and sale in other fields of medicine resulted in a lag in the production of new classes of antibiotics. This occurred despite significant advances in the fundamental science that has fueled pharmaceutical innovation in many other areas.

As a result of the looming crisis previously discussed, public pressure, and apparent scientific opportunities, many companies intensified their efforts in antibiotic drug discovery in the early 1990s. The complete sequencing of all major bacterial pathogens affecting humans, development of high-throughput screening, combinatorial chemistry, and microarray assays promised a golden age of antibiotic drug discovery. Indeed, at first glance, the situation with respect to antibiotics currently in clinical development looks encouraging. Several new antibiotic variations are in the first three phases of clinical development, with billions of dollars having been invested in their development (see Table 4-2). Not one new class of antibiotics, however, is in development. Rather, these "new" antibiotics belong to existing classes, including macrolides and quinolones, that have been used to treat humans for years. The absence of new classes in the pipeline and the fact that, even for compounds in Phase I, an additional 8 years is required on average before launch, is alarming when one considers the ever-increasing number of antibiotic-resistant organisms.

It has become apparent that the discovery of new antibiotics is not as easy as was once believed. Despite a plethora of highly validated targets, these targets are not feasible unless a chemical entity can be found that penetrates the cell wall and inhibits growth. In addition, the chemical compound must not be highly toxic and preferably should have good oral bioavailability. These technical hurdles, coupled with competition for resources within pharmaceutical companies from other significant medical needs with larger market opportunities, have led to reduced investment in or, in the case of most companies, elimination of antibiotic drug discovery programs. In fact, today there is only one large pharmaceutical company with a robust antibiotic research program.

Recent discoveries have linked many chronic diseases to infectious etiologies, and it remains to be seen whether this will inspire a renewed interest in antibiotic development for these conditions. Nevertheless, the development of an antibiotic is an expensive and risky process; no guarantee can be made that the antibiotic will remain effective and the investment will be regained before the patent period has ended. Bacterial threats associated with bioterrorism raise additional concerns. In an initial bacterial bioterrorist attack, the level of antibiotic susceptibility will not be known. More than one bacterial agent may be released simultaneously, and bacterial weapons resistant to even the newest antibiotics (e.g., quinolones) can be generated. Thus, new classes of broad-spectrum antibiotics are urgently needed.

Antivirals

Expanding knowledge in the fields of genomics, cell biology, structural biology, and combinatorial chemistry has resulted in the rapid development of some new antivirals. This is exemplified by the dramatic increase in antiviral drugs targeting HIV and, to a much lesser extent, influenza viruses. Yet only a few broad-spectrum antiviral agents are on the market, and the availability of specific antivirals to the majority of RNA and DNA viruses is largely lacking. This situation is exacerbated by the fact that many viruses evolve to circumvent the action of antivirals and the immune response through the development of resistance.

Despite the rapid advances in technology, antivirals for only HIV, hepatitis B and C, herpes viruses, and influenza have been targeted for development. As with vaccines, this situation is due, in large part, to marketing considerations, the absence of a profit margin large enough to repay the costs of development, and the limited potential for sufficient net profit. The problem is well illustrated by the case of influenza. Four companies were

TABLE 4-2 Antibiotics and Antivirals in Development

Product Name	Company	Indication	Development Status
Antibiotics			
antibiotic (topical)	Antex Biologics *Gaithersburg, MD*	skin and soft tissue infections	Phase I
Augmentin SR beta lactam antibiotic (modified release formulation)	GlaxoSmithKline *Philadelphia, PA* *Rsch. Triangle Park, NC*	respiratory tract infections, including penicillin-resistant *Streptococcus pneumoniae*	application submitted
Cidecin© daptomycin for injection	Cubist Pharmaceuticals *Lexington, MA*	complicated skin and soft tissue infections, community-acquired pneumonia and certain resistant infections	Phase III
Cleocin© clindamycin XR	Pharmacia *Peapack, NJ*	acute bacterial sinusitis, dental infections, streptococcal pharyngitis/tonsillitis, uncomplicated skin and skin structure infections	Phase I
dalbavancin	Versicor *Fremont, CA*	skin and soft tissue infections	Phase II
daptomycin	Cubist Pharmaceuticals *Lexington, MA*	complicated skin and soft tissue infections	Phase III completed
		bacteremia in endocarditis, community-acquired pneumonia requiring hospitalization, VRE infections	Phase III
		complicated urinary tract infections	Phase II completed

Product	Company	Indication	Status
E1010 (carbapanem antibiotic)	Elsai, Teaneck, NJ	broad spectrum antibiotic	Phase I
Factive broad-spectrum fluoroquinolone antibiotic (IV formulation)	GlaxoSmithKline, Philadelphia, PA, Rsch. Triangle Park, NC	respiratory tract infections	Phase III
Factive broad-spectrum fluoroquinolone antibiotic (oral formulation)	GlaxoSmithKline, Philadelphia, PA, Rsch. Triangle Park, NC	respiratory and urinary tract infections	application submitted
Helicide© bismuth subutrate, tetracycline and metronidazole	Axcan Pharma, Mont St.-Hiliare, Quebec	eradication of *Helicobacter pylori*	application submitted
Iseganan HCl oral solution	IntraBiotics Pharmaceuticals, Mountain View, CA	prevention of oral mucositis caused by radiotherapy and chemotherapy	Phase III
Iseganan HCl solution for inhalation	IntraBiotics Pharmaceuticals, Mountain View, CA	prevention of ventilator-associated pneumonia	Phase II
		treatment of respiratory infections in cystic fibrosis patients	Phase I/II
ISV-401	InSite Vision, Alameda, CA	bacterial conjunctival infections	Phase II

continues

TABLE 4-2 Continued

Product Name	Company	Indication	Development Status
Ketek© ketolide	Aventis Pharmaceuticals *Bridgewater, NJ*	first-line therapy for respiratory tract infections in adults first-line therapy for respiratory tract infections in children	application submitted Phase I/II
Levaquin™ levofloxacin	Janssen Research Foundation *Titusville, NJ* R.W. Johnson P.R.I. *Raritan, NJ*	nosocomial pneumonia community-acquired pneumonia (short-course therapy), prostatitis	application submitted Phase III
Lumenax™ rifaximin	Salix Pharmaceuticals *Raleigh, NC*	traveler's diarrhea	application submitted
MB1 594AN	Micrologix Biotech *Vancouver, British Columbia*	*Propionibacterium* acnes	Phase II
MB1 594AN	Micrologix Biotech *Vancouver, British Columbia*	*Propionibacterium* acnes	Phase II
oritavancin	InterMune Pharmaceuticals *Brisbane, CA*	treatment of gram-positive bacterial infections	Phase III
ramoplanin	Genome Therapeutics *Waltham, MA*	prevention of bloodstream infections caused by the gram-positive bacteria vancomycin resistant enterococci (VRE)	Phase III

Drug	Company	Indication	Phase
Tequin™ gatifloxacin	Bristol-Myers Squibb *Princeton, NJ*	prostatitis otitis media, pediatric meningitis	Phase III Phase II
Ligecycline	Wyeth Pharmaceuticals *Philadelphia, PA*	infection caused by antibiotic-resistant bacteria	Phase III
ABT-492 (quinolone)	Abbott Laboratories *Abbott Park, IL*	respiratory and urinary tract infections	Phase II
ABT-773	Abbott Laboratories *Abbott Park, IL*	respiratory infections; ketolide	Phase III
Antivirals			
ACH-126,443 (beta-L-Fd4C)	Achillion Pharmaceuticals *New Haven, CT*	chronic hepatitis B	Phase II
ACH-126,445 (L-Oddu)	Achillion Pharmaceuticals *New Haven, CT*	Epstein-Barr virus	Preclinical
adefovir dipivoxil	Gilead Sciences *Foster City, CA*	chronic hepatitis B	Phase III
adenovirus antiviral	Barr Laboratories *Pomona, NY*	undetermined	Phase I
amdoxovir (DAPD)	Triangle Pharmaceuticals *Durham, NC*	chronic hepatitis B	Phase II
clevudine (L-FMAU)	Triangle Pharmaceuticals *Durham, NC*	chronic hepatitis B	Phase II

continues

TABLE 4-2 Continued

Product Name	Company	Indication	Development Status
Coviracil© emtricitabine	Triangle Pharmaceuticals *Durham, NC*	chronic hepatitis B	Phase II
EHT899	Enzo Biochem *Farmingdale, NY*	chronic active hepatitis associated with hepatitis B	Phase II
MIV-210	Medivir *Huddinge, Sweden*	hepatitis B	Phase I
MIV-606	Medivir *Huddinge, Sweden* Reliant Pharmaceuticals *Liberty Corner, NJ*	herpes zoster	Phase II
Picovir™ pleconaril	Aventis Pharmaceuticals *Bridgewater, NJ* ViroPharma *Exton, PA*	viral respiratory infection (adult)	application submitted disapproved by FDA, terminated
PNU-243672	Pharmacia *Peapack, NJ*	prevention and treatment of infections caused by herpes viruses in immunocompromised patients	Phase I
relbivudine (LdT)	Novirio Pharmaceuticals *Cambridge, MA*	treatment of chronic hepatitis B	Phase II

torcitabine (LdC)	Novirio Pharmaceuticals *Cambridge, MA*	treatment of chronic hepatitis B	Phase II
Valtrex© valacyclovir	GlaxoSmithKline *Philadelphia, PA* *Rsch. Triangle Park, NC*	cold sores, HSV suppression in immunocompromised patients, prevention of HSV transmission	Phase III
XTL-001 in combination with lamivudine	XTL Biopharmaceuticals *Rehovot, Israel* *New Ipswich, NH*	treatment of chronic hepatitis B	Phase II
XTL-002	XTL Biopharmaceuticals *Rehovot, Israel* *New Ipswich, NH*	treatment of hepatitis C	Phase I

NOTE: The content of this survey was obtained through government and industry sources based on the latest information. Survey current as of March 1, 2002 (http://www.phrma.org). A list of medicines approved and in development for HIV infection and AIDS can be found in PhRMA's report, *New Medicines in Development for AIDS.*
SOURCE: Adapted from PhRMA, 2002.

initially developing antineuraminidase inhibitors. After two consecutive years of mild influenza, two of the companies ceased their development of the drugs, and the fact that only two remaining companies were producing them raised concern regarding the market's capacity to support continued production. This situation could have catastrophic results during the next emergence of pandemic influenza. Stockpiling of these drugs is critical, and strategies that have been proven effective in maintaining an adequate supply of them must be implemented.

The development of new, improved therapies for influenza and other viruses is essential. However, incentives may be necessary to foster the development of antivirals for those viruses that do not represent large market opportunities but have high morbidity and mortality. The threat of certain viruses being used as agents of biological terrorism emphasizes the increased need for the development of new antivirals, as well as broad-spectrum antivirals and immunomodulators, especially for those agents for which there are no vaccines, such as Ebola and Marburg. The possible targets for antiviral development include each step in the replication cycle, from virus attachment to release (see Table 4-3).

Antivirals to Human Immunodeficiency Virus (HIV)

An effective vaccine to prevent HIV infection has not yet been developed. The remarkable advances in the treatment of HIV have resulted largely from advances in antiviral chemotherapy. Combination chemotherapy that suppresses the replication of HIV results in a pronounced reduction in illness and death. Multidrug treatment of patients with indinavir, zidovudine, and lamivudine can reduce the serum levels of HIV to less than 50 copies per ml (see Figure 4-2). Although these treatments reduce replication, however, they do not completely suppress viral replication, and it is probable that a smoldering virus replication is present and difficult to detect. Nonetheless, the immune function of both CD4 and CD8 cells is regenerated, and persistent opportunistic infections are often resolved. It is this restoration of the immune function that has transformed the natural history of AIDS (Richman, 2001). The dramatic restoration of immune function comes at a cost, however—the expense, inconvenience, and toxicity of antiretroviral therapy.

Approximately 10 billion (10^{10}) HIV virus particles are generated daily in an infected host (Perelson et al., 1996). With a mutation rate of about 10^{-5} nucleotides per replication cycle and no proofreading mechanism for reverse transcription, approximately one mutation is generated for each new genome of 92,000 nucleotides (Mansky and Temin, 1995). Thus, genomes with a mutation in any gene, as well as many with double mutations, could be generated daily. As a result, drug-resistant mutants can develop

TABLE 4-3 Stages of Virus Replication and Possible Targets of Action of Antiviral Agents

Stage of Replication	Classes of Selective Inhibitors	Viruses
Cell Entry		
Attachment	Soluble receptor decoys, antireceptor antibodies, fusion protein inhibitors	General[A] Retroviruses (HIV)[R]
Penetration	Soluble ICAM,[B] anti ICAM	Picornaviruses[R]
Uncoating	Ion channel blockers, capsid stablizers	Influenza A[R]
Release of viral genome		Picornaviruses[R]
Transcription of viral genome*	Inhibitors of viral DNA polymerase, RNA polymerase, reverse transcriptase, helicase, primase, or integrase	Retroviruses (HIV)[R], Herpesviruses[R], Hepatitis B[R], Hepatitis C[R]
Transcription of viral Messenger RNA		
Replication of viral genome	Ribavirin	Respiratory Syncitical Virus (RSV), Arenaviruses (Lassa), Hanta viruses
Translation of viral proteins	Interferons, antisense oligonucleotides, Ribozymes	General[A] Papillomaviruses
Regulatory proteins (early)		
Structural proteins (late)	Inhibitors of regulatory proteins	General[R]
Posttranslational modifications		
Proteolytic cleavage	Protease inhibitors	Retroviruses (HIV)[R] Picornaviruses[R]
Myristoylation, glycosylation		
Assembly of virion components	Interferons, assembly protein inhibitors	General[A]
Release	Neuraminidase inhibitors, antiviral antibodies, cytotoxic lymphocytes	Influenza A[R], B[R]
Budding, cell lysis		General[A]

*Depends on specific replication strategy of virus, but virus-specified enzyme required for part of process
AGeneral, potentially applicable to all viruses.
BIntercellular adhesion molecule.
REmergence of resistance.
SOURCE: Modified from Hayden, 2001.

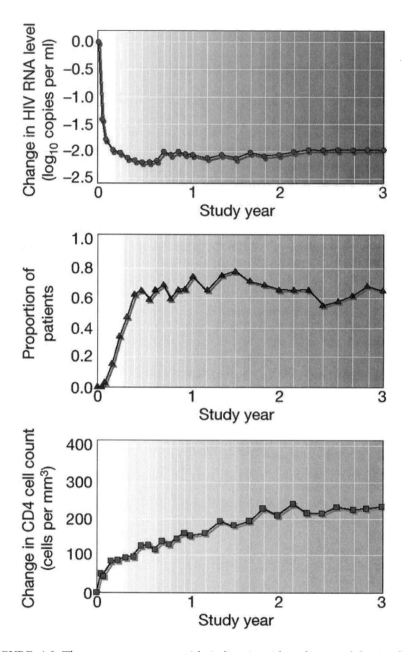

FIGURE 4-2 Three-year treatment with indinavir, zidovudine, and lamivudine. Reprinted with permission from Richman (2001). Copyright 2001 by Nature Publishing Group.

TABLE 4-4 Approved Antiretroviral Drugs

Nucleoside reverse-transcriptase inhibitors	
Abacavir (ABC)	Stavudine (d4T)
Didanosine (ddI)	Zalcitabine (ddC)
Lamivudine (3TC)	Zidovudine (AZT)
Non-nucleoside reverse-transcriptase inhibitors	
Efavirenz	Nevirapine
Delavirdine	
Protease inhibitors	
Amprenavir*	Nelfinavir
Indinavir*	Ritonavir
Lopinavir*	Saquinavir*

*Often or usually used with low-dose ritonavir for pharmacological enhancement.
Reprinted with permission from *Nature* (Richman, 2001) copyright (2001) Macmillan Publishers Ltd.

rapidly and are highly transmissible, leading to treatment failure. The emergence of multidrug-resistant HIV means that new drugs are needed, and drugs against additional targets are in fact under development (see Table 4-4). Yet new drugs will face problems of bioavailability and the inevitable emergence of resistance. The other difficulty is the high cost of the drugs, making optimal chemotherapy for HIV available only to persons in the upper socioeconomic groups, even in the developed world.

Two approaches to augmenting HIV-specific immunity are under investigation: therapeutic vaccination and strategic treatment interruption (STI). Therapeutic vaccination may induce new cellular and humoral immune responses in HIV-infected persons. STI is based on the hypothesis that after the arrest of progressive disease and the partial recovery of the immune system through potent antiretroviral therapy, the temporary interruption of therapy will release HIV antigen. This "autoimmunization," followed by reprotection of the immune system with reintroduced chemotherapy, can be performed in cycles until augmented immunity can change the natural history of infection. The combined use of chemotherapy and immunological approaches is in its infancy and is an important topic for further research. Insight gained into combination chemo- and immunotherapy will also be used in addressing the extensive viral epidemics of chronic hepatitis B and C.

Antivirals to Influenza Viruses

The first option for the control of influenza is efficacious, economically beneficial vaccines. However, it takes at least 6 months to prepare a new influenza virus vaccine. In the face of an emerging pandemic strain, a specific vaccine would not be immediately available, and less-specific antivirals would be the only option. Two families of antivirals are available for influenza viruses: (1) two derivatives of adamantine—amantadine (Symmetrel) and rimantadine (Flumadine), and (2) two neuraminidase inhibitors—zanamivir (Relenza) and oseltamivir (Tamiflu). Amantadine and rimantadine target primarily the M2 ion channel, with the hemagglutinin as a secondary target; they are efficacious for influenza A viruses but do not inhibit influenza B viruses (Hay et al., 1985). The two neuraminidase inhibitors block the enzymatic site on both influenza A and B viruses and are efficacious on all subtypes of the viruses, including the H5N1 and H9N2 viruses that were transmitted to humans in Hong Kong (Gubareva et al., 2000). Therapeutic benefits from each of these antineuraminidase influenza drugs are dependent on early initiation of therapy; they include shortening of the infection by 1.5 days and reduction in the sequelae of influenza, such as middle-ear infection (Gubareva et al., 2000; Hayden et al., 1999; Walker et al., 1997).

Both families of anti-influenza drugs are approved for prophylaxis, and the degree of protection provided is essentially complete. Unfortunately, therapeutic use of amantadine and rimantadine results in the rapid emergence of resistant strains, which are shed and transmitted to treated patients (Hayden and Hay, 1992). However, resistant strains are rarely detected in naturally circulating influenza A viruses. Resistance to the neuraminidase inhibitors has also been recognized, but is much more difficult to achieve either experimentally or in the field. Mutations are usually detected first in the hemagglutinin near the receptor binding sites, resulting in a reduction in the affinity of binding and easier release of virus by the enzyme activity of the neuraminidase. Under continued drug pressure from neuraminidase inhibitors, mutations occur in the neuraminidase enzyme active center, leading to resistance. This resistance comes at a price to the virus, including compromised enzyme stability, a change in optimal pH (McKimm-Breschkin et al., 1996; Gubareva et al., 1997), and reduced transmissibility of the resistant virus in animals (Herlocher et al., 2002). The importance of immune surveillance in combination with chemotherapy became apparent for immunocompromised patients when prolonged use of antineuraminidase inhibitors in an influenza-infected transplant patient resulted in selection of drug-resistant mutants (Gubareva et al., 1998). Thus, future developments in antiviral research must address the emergence of resistant mutants and include strategies that incorporate immunostimulation with vaccines and/ or cytokines.

Other Antiviral Agents

Approved efficacious antiviral agents for herpes simplex virus (HSV) and varicella virus, including a number of nucleoside analogues (e.g., adenine arabinoside [Ara-A], acyclovir [Zovirax], valacyclovir [Valtrex]; see Field and Laughlin, 1999), are widely used for therapy and prophylaxis. If patients have normal immune response to HSV, the development of resistance to nucleoside analogues is not a significant problem, but the current antivirals are not curative. Antiviral agents for hepatitis B and C (interferons plus antivirals) are approved or in development. Ribavirin, a triazole nucleoside analogue, inhibits RNA polymerases and transcription and is broadly reactive against respiratory syncitial virus, papillomaviruses, and arenaviruses (see Table 4-3).

As a result of increasing antibiotic resistance, drug options for treatment of some bacterial infections (e.g., vancomycin-resistant enterococci and vancomycin-resistant staphylococci) are increasingly limited. Although defining the precise public health risk of emergent antibiotic resistance is not simple, the problem is global in scope and very serious. Many generic but essential antibiotics are in short supply (Strausbaugh, 2001), and the development of new antibiotics has been severely curtailed. Antivirals are available for only a limited number of viruses, and few are in development. When one considers the bacterial and viral threats of bioterrorism and the ability to generate antibiotic-resistant bacterial weapons, the urgent need for new antimicrobials becomes clear. Thus, many of the issues raised regarding vaccine production apply also to antibiotics and antivirals.

The U.S. Secretary of Health and Human Services should ensure the formulation and implementation of a national strategy for developing new antimicrobials, as well as producing an adequate supply of approved antimicrobials. *The U.S. Secretary of Health and Human Services should work closely with other relevant federal agencies (e.g., DOD, the Department of Homeland Security), Congress, industry, academia, and the public health community to carry out this responsibility.*

Need for Stockpiling

The 2001 anthrax outbreak clearly demonstrated the need to have access to a stockpile of effective antimicrobial agents for immediate use during the aftermath of a bioterrorist attack. In the absence of vaccines, antimicrobials are the only effective population-based preventive measure for use against a bioterrorist attack once exposure has occurred, provided, of course, that an effective drug exists. Fortunately, ciprofloxacin was determined to be the appropriate drug in this situation, and an ample supply was readily available. The same may not be true when the next influenza pandemic eventually occurs, likely resulting in tens of thousands of deaths. Although stockpiling of antiviral drugs for influenza is a component of the pandemic plan developed by the United States and WHO (WHO, 1999e), we have yet to begin stockpiling antivirals effective against influenza. The time has come to move forward with this plan and determine which drugs are needed; the quantity required; the costs of production, storage, and distribution; and the authority under which the drugs will be used.

The U.S. Secretary of Health and Human Services and the U.S. Secretary of Homeland Security should protect our national security by ensuring the stockpiling and distribution of antibiotics, antivirals (e.g., for influenza), and antitoxins for naturally occurring or intentionally introduced microbial threats. *The federal government should explore innovative mechanisms, such as cooperative agreements between government and industry or consortia of government, industry, and academia, to accelerate these efforts.*

INAPPROPRIATE USE OF ANTIMICROBIALS

For a variety of reasons previously discussed, the pharmaceutical industry is developing fewer new antimicrobials than in previous years. Whereas it appeared at one time that an endless supply of effective new drugs to treat resistant infections would exist, such is no longer the case. Therefore, immediate action must be taken to preserve the effectiveness of available drugs.

Factors leading to the increasing problem of antimicrobial resistance are well known and understood. Many genes for resistance occur on cassettes that can move between organisms, across species boundaries (Leverstein-van Hall et al., 2002), and between chromosomes and plasmids. Resistance genes in bacteria are commonly grouped together on the same mobile genetic elements, with the crucial practical consequence that the use of any single drug may select for resistance to a wide group of drugs. Thus, an antimicrobial employed in food and animal production that has never before been used to treat infection in humans can select for resistance to other drugs used to treat humans.

Resistant bacteria often persist in vivo even in the absence of continued selection by antibiotics, although in some cases resistance gradually diminishes once antibiotic pressures have been reduced. One explanation for continued resistance involves the lethal effect of the loss of certain plasmids when bacteria divide. Some resistant microbes are less fit, but resistant strains arising in a clinical context are generally virulent and can often persist for extended periods of time once established. Therefore, it is imperative to actively pursue and address the problem; it will be too late to effect useful change once most microbes have become resistant to the available drugs.

Antibiotic resistance resulting from the inappropriate overuse of antibiotics is not a new problem. A number of expert committees and professional organizations have studied the problem, issued reports, and made recommendations (Alliance for the Prudent Use of Antibiotics, 2001; CDC, 2001o; FDA, 2000; GAO, 1999; Center for Science in the Public Interest, 1998; NRC, 1999). Unfortunately, little has been done to change the situation, especially in the United States. Resistance due to the inappropriate use of antibiotics compromises the efficacy of many classic and highly effective antibiotics, such as penicillin for pneumococci and vancomycin for enterococci, as well as that of some newer antibiotics, such as ciprofloxacin and other types of fluorinated quinolones for gonococci, *Salmonella*, and *Campylobacter*. The recent discovery of an enterococcal gene for vancomycin resistance in *S. aureus* was alarming even though it had been predicted on the basis of the ability of the genes to transfer across species boundaries during mixed culture (CDC, 2002d). In the case of enterococcal and staphylococcal infection, alternative therapies have been introduced, but resistance to these new drugs has already been documented (Tsiodras et al., 2001; Herrero et al., 2002). The specter of untreatable infections—a regression to the pre-antibiotic era—is looming just around the corner.

Preventing the overuse of antimicrobials is not an easy task because of the revolutionary effects the drugs have had on human and animal health. Because antimicrobials are highly effective, there is an understandable tendency to use them in any situation in which they might be helpful. These effective drugs are relatively inexpensive compared with other medical interventions. Patients demand the drugs when they have an illness they imagine to be treatable with antibiotics. Doctors prescribe antibiotics for that same reason, often in the absence of diagnostic tests to determine the etiology of infection, and also because patients want and expect to be treated with them. In many areas of the world where little money is available for health care, antimicrobials are readily available without a doctor's prescription, and as a result are often taken unnecessarily or inadequately. Many problems associated with antimicrobial resistance have arisen in poor and developing areas of the world, and have subsequently spread globally.

In addition to avoiding the inappropriate use of antibiotics to treat viral disease, prudence dictates use of the appropriate antimicrobial when an etiologic diagnosis is made. For example, the rapid rise in drug-resistant malaria has led to the development of newer, generally more expensive therapies for the disease. This in turn has resulted in an increase in the prescribing of these newer drugs, even in areas where there is no demon-strated resistance to first-line therapies. The use of first-line therapies must be continued in areas where resistance has not been documented, and newer therapies should be used only when first-line therapies are ineffective or in areas of resistance. To this end, it is essential to monitor resistance patterns around the world.

Decreasing Inappropriate Use of Antimicrobials in Human Medicine

Decreasing the inappropriate use of antimicrobials in human medicine is a complex task that requires a multipronged effort fueled by a sense of urgency. The inappropriate use of antibiotics for treatment of viral diseases can be averted by the increased use of available diagnostic tests and the development of better point-of-care, inexpensive, rapid, sensitive, and spe-cific diagnostic tests, which would enable the rational use of new antivirals as they become available (see the earlier discussion of the development of diagnostics). The decreased use of antibacterials for viral respiratory infec-tions and other syndromes should lessen selective pressures for the emer-gence of resistant bacteria. FDA has recently included this message on label inserts of antibiotics.

If this important objective is to be achieved, the general public and health care providers must be better educated and informed about the importance of administering antimicrobial therapy properly. The need is urgent to both educate and monitor all categories of practitioners and drug dispensers in developing countries where medicines are sold directly to the public over the counter and dispensed by private practitioners in an ad hoc manner. More attention needs to be given to improving practitioner educa-tion and compliance. Patient care would be improved by the development and dissemination of better evidence-based treatment guidelines. More re-search is needed on methods for treating infections to minimize the emer-gence of resistance without a loss of efficacy. Infection control programs must be supported in hospitals in an effort to decrease the transmission of resistance both within the hospitals and in the community. Surveillance for patterns of resistance in hospitals and in the community must be continued and expanded; this will require a coordinated effort among public health organizations, private medicine, and industry. Because resistant microbes arise throughout the world and travel broadly to all regions, the needs and problems of the economically and health care disadvantaged regions of the world must be considered.

The world is facing an imminent crisis in the control of infectious diseases as the result of a gradual but steady increase in the resistance of a number of microbial agents to available therapeutic drugs. Although defin-ing the precise public health risk of emergent antimicrobial resistance is not a simple task, there is no doubt that the problem is of global concern and is creating dilemmas for the treatment of infections in both hospitals and community health care settings.

CDC, FDA, professional health organizations, academia, health care delivery systems, and industry should expand efforts to decrease the inappropriate use of antimicrobials in human medicine through (1) expanded outreach and better education of health care providers, drug dispensers, and the general public on the inherent dangers associated with the inappropriate use of antimicrobials, and (2) the increased use of diagnostic tests, as well as the development and use of rapid diagnostic tests, to determine the etiology of infection and thereby ensure the more appropriate use of antimicrobials.

Decreasing Inappropriate Overuse of Antimicrobials in Animal Husbandry and Agriculture

Clearly, a decrease in the inappropriate use of antimicrobials in human medicine alone is not enough. Substantial efforts must be made to decrease inappropriate overuse of antimicrobials in animals and agriculture as well.

Although estimates vary widely, the total amount of antimicrobials used in Europe and the United States in animal husbandry and agriculture far outweighs the total used in humans (McEwen and Fedorka-Cray, 2002). The majority of this use is for growth promotion or preventive therapy in healthy animals. Mounting evidence suggests a relationship between antimicrobial use in animal husbandry and an increase in bacterial resistance in humans (Alliance for the Prudent Use of Antibiotics, 2002), a view supported by an IOM committee that reviewed the use of drugs in food animals (IOM, 1999b). The use of antimicrobials in food animals leads to antibiotic resistance, which can then be transmitted to humans through the food supply (Swartz, 2002; Fey et al., 2000; Smith et al., 2002; White et al., 2001).

A study published in 2001 found that 20 percent of ground meat samples obtained from supermarkets in the Washington, D.C., metropolitan area were contaminated with *Salmonella*. Of these bacteria, 84 percent were resistant to at least one antibiotic and 53 percent to at least three antibiotics (White et al., 2001). This study supports previous findings that foods of animal origin are potential sources of ceftriaxone-resistant *Salmonella* infections in humans. Similarly, researchers found that between 17 and 87 percent of chickens obtained in supermarkets in four states contained strains of *Enterococcus faecium* that were resistant to quinupristin–

dalfopristin, an approved antimicrobial for use in humans (McDonald et al., 2001). The researchers believed that the use of virginiamycin, an antibiotic of the streptogramin group, in farm animals had created a reservoir of streptogramin–resistant *E. faecium* in the food supply, which could contribute to foodborne dissemination of resistance as the clinical use of quinupristin–dalfopristin increases.

Substantial evidence supports that certain types of resistant organisms, such as vancomycin-resistant enterococci, emerged initially in animals because of the use of similar drugs for growth promotion or prophylaxis (O'Brien, 2002). Consideration of this association led to a ban on the use of avoparacin, a vancomycin analogue, in Europe (Wegener et al., 1999). The decreased use of antimicrobials for growth promotion or prophylaxis in many European countries has been associated with a subsequent stabilization in resistance or a gradually decreasing resistance in animal flora (Aarestrup et al., 2001). WHO has called for all antimicrobials used for disease control in food animals to be prescribed by veterinary health care providers, and for termination or rapid phase-out of antimicrobials used for growth promotion if they are used for human treatment (WHO, 2000f). Various other groups have suggested that because of the increasing risk of antimicrobial resistance, the subtherapeutic use of antibiotics for growth promotion should be banned (some would include use for prophylaxis in the ban as well) if they are also used in humans (Union of Concerned Scientists, 2002; Alliance for the Prudent Use of Antimicrobials, 2002).

The main argument against a ban is the potential economic hardships to livestock and poultry producers, which would result in higher costs for consumers. According to the IOM Committee on the Use of Drugs in Food Animals, such a ban would increase the price of meat by an estimated 0.013 to 0.06 cents per pound; this translates to $4.84 to $9.72 per person each year, depending on the meat and the cut (IOM, 1999b). Yet, evidence suggests that animals can be raised efficiently without the use of growth-promoting antimicrobials (Emborg et al., 2001; Wierup, 2001).

Critics of the ban also argue that it would result in poorer production efficiency and an increased incidence of infectious disease in animals. However, it has been noted that subtherapeutic antibiotics are most effective in animals under the stress of inadequate nutrition and suboptimal sanitary conditions (Braude et al., 1953); therefore, improved hygiene and changes in animal husbandry practices to control disease could potentially eliminate the need for growth promoters (Emborg et al., 2001). In Denmark, the elimination of antimicrobial growth promoters from broiler chicken feed did not result in a change in death rates or a decrease in kilograms of broilers produced per square meter. Danish scientists also reported that the decreased use of virginiamycin and avilamycin in animals was followed by decreases in resistance to these drugs (Aarestrup et al., 2001).

FDA should ban the use of antimicrobials for growth promotion in animals if those classes of antimicrobials are also used in humans.

The committee endorses the Public Health Action Plan to Combat Antimicrobial Resistance developed by the Interagency Task Force on Antimicrobial Resistance and the recommendations of the WHO Global Strategy for the Containment of Antimicrobial Resistance (see Boxes 4-9 and 4-10). Although the broad scope of these recommendations defies easy implementation, we must seize the opportunity immediately to do as much as we can while organizing the resources and plans needed to carry out other initiatives. To do nothing is, in effect, to allow the continued evolution of antimicrobial-resistant microbes, which poses serious near- and long-term threats to global health. The total burden of human illness due to resistant bacteria that have been transferred from animals to humans is unknown, but the guiding principle should be that we must do what the available evidence suggests will help stem the tide of increasing resistance before it is too late. By endorsing these recommendations, we will join belatedly much of the rest of the developed world, which already has made similar recommendations and, in many cases, implemented them. These changes should be accompanied by substantial outcomes research on the effects on animal health, resistance prevalence in animals and humans, and the economics of food production.

VECTOR-BORNE AND ZOONOTIC DISEASE CONTROL

The majority of emerging infectious diseases are zoonoses (i.e., diseases transmitted from animals to humans under natural conditions). Vector-borne and rodent-borne diseases are especially notable in this regard, remaining major causes of morbidity and mortality in humans in the tropical world and representing a large proportion of newly emerged diseases (see the discussion in Chapter 3). Exacerbating the situation is the potential for many of these agents to be weaponized and used by bioterrorists. Because of their resurging public health importance and their exceptional ability to cause epidemics, vector-borne and zoonotic diseases will undoubtedly continue to pose significant risks to human health in the future.

Unfortunately, the national and international capacity to address these diseases is limited. The many reasons for this include (1) the lack of efficacious vaccines for many of these pathogens; (2) decreased support for and deterioration of the public health surveillance and control infrastructure for vector-borne and zoonotic diseases; (3) erosion in the numbers of scientists trained in relevant fields, including medical entomology, vector ecology, zoonoses, and tropical medicine; (4) the development of resistance to drugs

BOX 4-9
WHO Global Strategy for Antimicrobial Resistance

In response to the growing problem of antibiotic resistance, WHO has worked with many partners, including the American Society for Microbiology and the Alliance for the Prudent Use of Antibiotic (APUA), to develop the WHO Global Strategy for Containment for Antimicrobial Resistance. The seven key recommendations emanating from the 25 expert reports used to formulate the strategy are summarized below.

Increase Awareness of the Antibiotic Resistance Problem
International organizations:
  Obtain worldwide commitments to establish prudent antibiotic use policies
National and municipal organizations:
  Publicize the outcomes of programs from other countries
  Educate the general public
  Promote communication
  Evaluate the curricula of universities
Health care institutions:
  Use effective teaching methods for education prescribers
Health care workers:
  Educate the general public

Improve Surveillance of Antibiotic Resistance
National and municipal organizations:
  Coordinate local surveillance networks
  Recruit leaders for surveillance networks
  Support a reference laboratory
  Share results of surveillance with international organizations
  Monitor resistance in food animals
  Monitor sentinel human populations
Health care institutions:
  Develop local surveillance network
  Maintain a laboratory with adequate quality assurance and trained technicians

Health care workers:
  Initiate a local surveillance network
Pharmaceutical companies:
  Undertake postmarking surveillance to detect the emergence of resistance to new antibiotics
  Support surveillance networks

Improve Antibiotic Use in People
National and municipal organizations:
  Enforce the prudent use of antibiotics
  Create national and regional guidelines
  Update guidelines based on surveillance data
  Eliminate financial incentives that promote the misuse of antibiotics
  Monitor advertising
  Consider the impact of new drugs on resistance during the drug approval process
  Limit general access to new drugs
  Establish postmarking surveillance accords
Health care institutions:
  Establish an Infection Control Committee
  Establish a Drugs and Therapeutics Committee
  Establish guidelines for appropriate antibiotic use
  Appoint an antimicrobial resistance monitor
  Reduce the spread of infection
  Create pharmacy reports

Establish and disseminate list of essential drugs
Educate employees
Maintain a laboratory
Health care workers:
Prescribe antibiotics prudently
Improve hygiene

Improve Antibiotic Use in Animals
National and municipal organizations:
Increase awareness of the antibiotic resistance problem
Regulate antibiotic prescriptions for animals
Restrict growth promoter use in animals
Regulate antibiotic use in animals
Set a risk standard for resistance
Consider human and nonhuman uses simultaneously
Monitor advertising
Veterinarians:
Promote a prudent use of antibiotics in animals
Develop local guidelines for antibiotic use
Food animal producers:
Improve farm hygiene
Reduce the use of antibiotics as growth promoters
Improve animal husbandry
Researchers:
Perform risk–benefit analysis of growth promoter use
Assess environmental impact
Examine food processing and distribution methods

Encourage New Product Development
National and municipal organizations:
Provide incentives to industry
Protect intellectual property rights
Facilitate networking
Pharmaceutical companies:
Increase research and development in several areas

Increase Resources to Curb Antibiotic Resistance in the Developing World
International organizations:
Share results of surveillance internationally
Secure technical and financial support for developing countries
Invest in a worldwide vaccine strategy to reduce antibiotics
Ensure the availability of vaccines and quality drugs
Facilitate communication among the countries of the world
Safeguard privacy and human rights
Promote appropriate international laws
National and municipal organizations:
Decrease the risk of infectious disease
Ensure antibiotic availability
Share resources with other countries

Increase Funding for Surveillance, Research, and Education
National and municipal organizations:
Increase funding for a surveillance network
Increase funding for research
Increase funding for education

SOURCE: World Health Organization, 2001i.

BOX 4-10
Public Health Action Plan to Combat Antimicrobial Resistance

A Public Health Action Plan to Combat Antimicrobial Resistance was developed by an Interagency Task Force on Antimicrobial Resistance that was created in 1999. This plan reflects a broad-based consensus of federal agencies on actions needed to address antimicrobial resistance. Part I focuses on domestic issues, Part II, yet to be developed, will identify actions that address international concerns more specifically. The following is a summary of the Task Force's recommendations on the four domestic focus areas.

1. Surveillance
Develop and implement a coordinated national plan for antimicrobial resistance
Ensure the availability of reliable drug susceptibility data for surveillance
Monitor patterns of antimicrobial drug use
Monitor antimicrobial resistance in agricultural settings to protect the public's
    health by ensuring a safe food supply, as well as animal and plant health

2. Prevention and Control
Extend the useful life of antimicrobial drugs through appropriate use policies that
    discourage overuse and misuse
Improve diagnostic testing practices
Prevent infection transmission through improved infection control methods and
    use of vaccines
Prevent and control emerging antimicrobial resistance problems in agriculture and
    human and veterinary medicine
Ensure that comprehensive programs to prevent and control antimicrobial resistance
    tance involve a wide variety of nonfederal partners and the public so these programs
    grams become a part of routine practice nationwide

3. Research
Increase understanding of microbial physiology, ecology, genetics, and mechanisms
    nisms of resistance
Augment the existing research infrastructure to support a critical mass of researchers
    ers in antimicrobial resistance and related fields
Translate research findings into clinically useful products, such as novel approaches
    es to detecting, preventing, and treating antimicrobial-resistant infections.

4. Product Development
Ensure that researchers and drug manufacturers are informed of current and projected
    jected gaps in the arsenal of antimicrobial drugs, vaccines, and diagnostics and
    of potential markets for these products
Stimulate the development of priority antimicrobial products for which market incentives
    centives are inadequate while fostering their appropriate use
Optimize the development and use of veterinary drugs and related agricultural
    products that reduce the transfer of resistance to pathogens that can infect humans
    mans

SOURCE: CDC, 2001o.

in pathogens and to chemical pesticides in arthropods; (5) population growth associated with rampant and unplanned urbanization in the tropics and increased juxtapositions of humans, animal reservoirs, and vectors; (6) increased trafficking of pathogens, vectors, and animal reservoirs; and (7) societal and behavioral changes and practices that contribute to greatly increased disease incidence.

To deal with the many needs and issues involving vector-borne and zoonotic diseases is an overwhelming task. Nonetheless, a number of key issues must be addressed promptly to provide the expertise, infrastructure, resources, and tools required to develop the capacity to respond to the threats posed by vector-borne and zoonotic diseases.

Human Resource Capacity

The critical national needs for specialists in vector-borne and zoonotic diseases (e.g., medical entomologists, vector biologists, vector ecologists, mammologists, ornithologists) were illustrated dramatically by the recent emergences of Sin Nombre virus and West Nile virus in the United States. The loss of medical entomologists, for example, was recognized as a national problem in the 1980s (NRC, 1983). However, attitudes changed little in academic departments across the nation as a result. Medical entomology positions were invariably lost when occupants retired or moved. This situation resulted in a dramatic reduction overall in the number of medical entomologists/vector biologists. For example, the United States is facing a critical shortage of morphological systematists who are also field biologists capable of collecting arthropod vectors within the context of their specific environments. As newer molecular taxonomic approaches become more established in monitoring vectors, traditional systematists are needed to guide and verify the application of such approaches. Specialists in vector ecology are also increasingly in short supply, as are academic institutions capable of the relevant training (Spielman, 1994). Experts in the ecology of both vectors and reservoirs are needed to monitor the distribution, abundance, composition, and density of species, and the prevalence of infections that are relevant to human health.

With the emergence of Lyme disease, human erlichiosis, and West Nile encephalitis in the United States and the resurgence of vector-borne diseases throughout the world (Gratz, 1999; Gubler, 1998), some progress has been made as organizations such as CDC, NIH, WHO, and foundations have begun to promote research in molecular vector biology. Increased funding and program development opportunities, especially in molecular vector biology, have led to greater numbers of scientists entering the field, many of whom are now assuming faculty positions in universities. Perhaps as the public health importance of vector-borne and zoonotic disease control is better recognized, student demand will grow, and previously lost positions in much-needed related areas of science will be regained. The end result would be a renewed stream of students to replenish the depleted ranks of medical entomologists, ecologists, and vector biologists at all levels.

The momentum to address national and international needs in medical entomology/vector biology could be leveraged in numerous ways. For example, CDC could establish a medical entomology/vector biology Epidemic Intelligence Service (EIS) program, and its entomologic EIS officers could provide support to national and international jurisdictions requesting entomologic expertise. In addition, regional centers of excellence in medical entomology/vector biology could be established to provide needed services, training, and research. These centers would preferably be incorporated into larger interdisciplinary infectious disease centers (see the later discussion), which would serve as resources to regions and nations in addressing issues involving vector-borne and other emerging diseases and bioterrorism.

Efficient training strategies are necessary to address the human resource needs at all levels, from understanding disturbances in the enviroment that impact on the abundance and distribution of vectors and animal reservoirs, to identification and processing of species, to gene identification and characterization, to development of geographic information systems (GIS) and other approaches for control of vector-borne and zoonotic diseases. The emergence of West Nile virus resulted in an intensive effort by CDC to train individuals in mosquito identification, processing, and control, and the emergence of Sin Nombre virus led to similar efforts by CDC to train individuals in rodent identification, surveillance, and control. WHO provides workshops devoted to specific important issues concerning vector-borne diseases in disease-endemic areas. Web-based training programs, courses, and texts might be used to address critical short term-needs. However, alternative approaches will be necessary to develop a new generation of leaders and trainers in the field.

The Biology of Disease Vectors course is notable in this regard. This intensive 2-week course, which is supported by the MacArthur Foundation, the WHO Special Program for Research and Training in Tropical Diseases, and the Howard Hughes Medical Institute, provides learning and networking opportunities for vector biologists. The course alternates annually between the United States and a disease-endemic country. Students participating in the course come from both developed and developing countries, and internationally recognized faculty provide invaluable networking and career opportunities. Such courses, strategically targeted to an area of national need, not only expedite the development of new leaders, but can also advance fields scientifically.

In efforts to rebuild the human resource capacity needed to address vector-borne and zoonotic diseases, it will be critical to increase training and research opportunities in applied, field-oriented vector biology and zoonotic disease research. CDC, DOD, NIH, and other federal agencies should continue to encourage research projects and programs that investigate the biological, behavioral, entomological, and environmental determinants of pathogen emergence, and that incorporate modern and robust molecular and quantitative tools into these investigations. Notable successes in this area include CDC's partnering with state and university scientists to address newly emergent vector-borne and rodent-borne diseases, such as Lyme disease, West Nile fever, and hantavirus pulmonary syndrome. These efforts leveraged CDC funds and talents to address emerging disease issues, supported applied epidemiological research and training in disease-endemic sites, and enhanced communication and partnering between CDC and state and local institutions.

The continued presence of long-term, sustainable laboratories in selected disease-endemic countries is critical. Such laboratories are invaluable for research, training, and surveillance for tropical and emerging infectious diseases. Historically, Naval Medical Research Units, United States Army, and WHO laboratories have provided opportunities for trainees to obtain tropical disease research experience. More recent programs, such the NIH International Collaborations in Infectious Disease Research (ICIDR) and Tropical Disease Research Units, provide training and research opportunities in field-oriented vector biology and control. The NIH ICIDR grants, together with the companion Actions for Building Capacity Program at the Fogarty Center, emphasize epidemiological research and training in disease-endemic areas in the context of NIH-funded research. Such programs also initiate interactions with collaborators in tropical regions, and yield long-term benefits in terms of establishing public health infrastructure, training and research opportunities, and listening posts in areas of the world where many pathogens emerge.

CDC, DOD, NIH, and USDA should work with academia, private organizations, and foundations to support efforts at rebuilding the human resource capacity at both academic centers and public health agencies in the relevant sciences—such as medical entomology, vector and reservoir biology, vector and reservoir ecology, and zoonoses—necessary to control vector-borne and zoonotic diseases.

Need to Increase the Armamentarium for Vector Control

Expanded research into the biological and ecological determinants of vector maintenance and transmission of pathogens, together with the explosion of information that will occur in the mosquito post-genomics era (Holt et al., 2002) are likely to result in new and unforeseen approaches and targets to control vector-borne diseases. Examples of research areas with the potential to increase the armamentarium for control of vector-borne diseases and to augment currently available control approaches are described below.

For the foreseeable future, traditional approaches to reducing vector populations or repelling vectors will remain the first lines of defense against emerging and resurging vector-borne diseases. Clearly, the development of new, environmentally acceptable pesticides will be critical to mitigate the potential for dramatic increases in such diseases (Sina and Aultman, 2001).

Improved Pesticides

Discontinuance of DDT usage has exacerbated the burden of vector-borne diseases in many parts of the world (Attaran et al., 2000). The resurgence of vector-borne diseases and resistance to alternative pesticides, therefore, has forced some countries to resume DDT usage. Since domicile treatment with DDT has not been associated with major adverse environmental consequences, this practice should be allowed for vector control in public health emergencies until equally effective and inexpensive substitutes for DDT are developed. DDT may help control vector-borne diseases, such as dengue and malaria, not only by killing vectors, but also by repelling them (Roberts et al., 2000). Residual DDT in homes may repel mosquitoes, thereby disrupting the close association between the human host and anthropophilic and endophilic vectors and dramatically reducing opportunities for pathogen transmission. At the same time, care will be needed to ensure that the availability of DDT for public health uses does not result in its use in agricultural applications. The development of efficacious and environmentally sensitive alternatives to DDT needs to become a major research objective.

Novel Strategies to Prolong Pesticide Usage

Pesticide usage in integrated pest management programs, which incorporate established agricultural practices for mitigating the evolution of resistance (e.g., rotation of pesticides used, inclusion of refugia with no pesticide applications), would extend the useful life of existing pesticides. Incorporating new molecular tools for diagnosing pesticide resistance into control programs could also result in more effective and efficient pesticide usage. Moreover, the development of novel strategies for prolonging pesticide efficacy, such as negative cross-resistance, should be possible in this era of high-throughput screening (Pittendrigh and Gaffney, 2001). More information on the effect of the prevalence of resistance to pesticides on the control of vector-borne diseases would be of great value for risk assessment.

New Repellents

As noted, repellents remain a first line of defense against emerging or resurging vector-borne diseases. DEET is the most efficacious repellent currently available commercially; however, its relicensing has been problematic because of adverse effects associated with its overuse in children, presumably due to its lipophilic nature (Qiu et al., 1998). Modern high-throughput and genomic approaches may permit the identification of new molecules with repellent activity similar to that of DEET (and DDT), but without adverse effects. Understanding of the molecular basis of vector olfaction and host seeking (Hill et al., 2002) could lead to the development of new repellents and attractants to control vectors (Day et al., 2001).

New Biopesticides and Biocontrol Agents to Augment Chemical Pesticides

The increase in pesticide resistance necessitates new investigations into biocontrol agents, such as viruses and bacteria, that could be incorporated into integrated pest management approaches for vector control. New formulations of *Bacillus thruringiensis* and *Bacillus sphaericus* show promise for control of vectors, even in tropical regions (Thiery et al., 1997; Regis et al., 2001). Baculoviruses from mosquitoes may be useful for vector control (Afonso et al., 2001). Other biopesticide agents could be improved using molecular genetic approaches to make them more efficacious control agents. For example, viruses could be used to transduce effector molecules in order to enhance vector knockdown or manipulate vector phenotypes.

Novel Strategies to Interrupt Pathogen Transmission

Strategies for vector-borne disease control remain focused on approaches that involve immunizing humans, using pesticides to reduce vector populations, or repellents to reduce contact with vectors. If pesticide resistance and parasite resistance to drugs continue to increase, if public health infrastructure cannot be rebuilt, and if mortality rates from vector-borne diseases persist or increase, novel approaches now emerging from investigations of vector molecular biology and pathogen–vector–host interactions may be necessary to control these diseases.

Insights into the molecular basis of pathogen–vector–host interactions suggest new strategies for controlling vector-borne diseases (Foy et al., in press; Willadsen, 2001). Immunizing hosts to vector-specific determinants of pathogen transmission (e.g., salivary effector proteins that enhance pathogen infection; see Titus and Ribeiro, 1988) could provide broad-spectrum protection against multiple pathogens or strains (Kamhawi et al., 2000, Valenzuela et al., 2001). Other critical determinants of pathogen infection of and transmission by vectors (e.g., vector proteolytic enzymes, which process arbovirus proteins and condition vector infection) could be targeted for transmission-blocking vaccines (Carter, 2001). Immunizing vertebrate hosts to immunologically privileged antigens of vectors could kill or impair blood-feeding mosquitoes, a strategy that works for ticks (Willadsen and Billingsley, 1996) and may also be useful against mosquito vectors, which frequently feed on humans (Foy et al., in press). Theoretically, these vectors would feed on other hosts (zooprophylaxis), thereby reducing pathogen transmission.

Genetic approaches in which vector populations are manipulated to become incompetent vectors are being investigated for their potential to interrupt pathogen transmission. Such approaches could minimize potential environmental issues associated with pesticide usage and prevent an ecological vacuum that other vectors could occupy. The vector population could theoretically be genetically immunized to make it nonpermissive to pathogen transmission. The "immunogens" could be driven into vector populations by harnessing naturally occurring arthropod systems, such as transposable elements, symbionts, or transducing viruses, which would be vector-specific (Beaty, 2000). RNAi, which was recently documented in vectors (Adelman et al., 2001), could be exploited in such programs. Proof of principle has been provided that vectors can be molecularly manipulated to make them refractory to arboviruses and trypanosome and malaria parasites (Beard et al., 2002; Olson et al., 1996, Ito et al., 2002). Recent progress in vector molecular biology suggests that continued research in these areas may provide new approaches for the control of vector-borne diseases, although the success of genetic manipulation in control programs is by no means certain (Boete and Koella, 2003). Research utilizing genetically manipulated vectors would require ecological studies (Scott et al., 2002) to determine the feasibility of such an approach to vector control and would require addressing the benefits, risks, and social and political issues associated with such a control strategy (Alphey et al., 2002).

DOD and NIH should develop new and expand upon current research efforts to enhance the armamentarium for vector control. *The development of safe and effective pesticides and repellents, as well as novel strategies for prolonging the use of existing pesticides by mitigating the evolution of resistance, is paramount in the absence of vaccines to prevent most vector-borne diseases. In addition, newer methods of vector control—such as biopesticides and biocontrol agents to augment chemical pesticides, and novel strategies for interrupting vector-borne pathogen transmission to humans—should be developed and evaluated for effectiveness.*

Geographic Information Systems and Robust Models for Predicting and Preventing Vector-borne and Zoonotic Diseases

Also complicating the control of vector-borne and zoonotic diseases has been a lack of knowledge of fundamental epidemiologic, genetic, biologic, and environmental determinants that condition potential increased transmission to humans by the respective nonhuman vectors or reservoirs. Because biological and ecological factors condition the transmission of pathogens by vectors and from animal reservoirs to humans, GIS and robust models (see Appendix E for a discussion of modeling) offer the potential to provide predictive capability for the emergence of vector-borne and zoonotic diseases. The ecological and quantitative capabilities of GIS make it possible to identify some of the determinants of endemicity and emergence. The developing hantavirus GIS models are promising in this regard (Boone et al., 1998; Glass et al., 2000; Hjelle and Glass, 2000; Yates et al., 2002b). The inclusion of genetic information concerning vector competence and rodent permissiveness, as well as other epidemiologically important information, such as gene flow in vector and reservoir populations (e.g., Black et al., 2001; Gorrochotequi-Escalante et al., 2002), may improve surveillance and risk assessment strategies for zoonoses and enhance the predictive capability of GIS and model systems. New GIS and robust models could revolutionize surveillance, risk assessment, and prevention strategies for zoonoses and permit the focusing of resources and talent on prevention efforts in areas of greatest risk, an especially important capability in resource-limited environments.

CDC, DOD, and NIH should work with state and local public health agencies and academia to expand efforts to exploit geographic information systems (GIS) and robust models for predicting and preventing the emergence of vector-borne and zoonotic diseases.

COMPREHENSIVE INFECTIOUS DISEASE RESEARCH AGENDA

Research remains an essential underpinning of the capacity to prevent and control infectious diseases. Despite recommendations made in the 1992 IOM report *Emerging Infections: Microbial Threats to Health in the United States*, calling for increased research on factors underlying the emergence of infectious diseases and an extramural grant program for research on surveillance and applied control methods, significant gaps remain in the overall infectious disease research agenda of the United States. To ensure that the nation is strategically poised to protect itself against the threat of infectious diseases and to maximize its assistance to developing countries in their efforts to combat these diseases, further investments must be made to support a diverse array of multidisciplinary research domains. These new investments must be part of an overall strategy for improved public health preparedness and protection against infectious disease threats, and a comprehensive system of accountability must be in place to ensure that no critical areas are neglected.

The considerable amount of new resources now becoming available for biodefense research makes this a critical time to develop a comprehensive research agenda. The most effective use of these new funds will involve integration of the evolving threat posed by the intentional use of biological agents as weapons into the broader context of infectious disease research. As previously noted, bioterrorism represents but the extreme end of a continuum of serious infectious disease threats, including the emergence of new infectious diseases, the resurgence of old ones, the appearance of new antimicrobial-resistant forms of old diseases, recognition of the infectious etiology of chronic diseases, and the creation of bioengineered organisms that produce disease in unforeseen ways. For such an integrated agenda to be effective, it must address both long- and short-term needs, involve both basic science and applied public health research, be multidisciplinary in nature, and utilize modern and robust molecular and quantitative tools.

Scientific research can yield a greater understanding of the biology and pathogenesis of organisms that cause disease, the biology of disease-spreading vectors, and the ways in which the human immune system responds to infection and disease. Several factors beyond these traditional foci of infectious disease research, however, play significant roles in the emergence of infectious disease threats (see Chapter 3). For example, malnutrition has long been known to play a role in susceptibility to death from diarrhea, respiratory infection, and malaria. Not as well understood are the roles of famine, war, crowding, urbanization, and population growth. Risky behaviors, such as illicit drug use and unprotected sex, are closely linked to several emerging infectious diseases. Ecological factors surrounding a lack of clean water and poor sanitation have also been linked to diseases such as cholera and plague. Additional ecological factors (e.g., deforestation or other forms of land use change) are associated with many emerging vector-borne and zoonotic diseases, such as dengue, malaria, yellow fever, Lassa fever, Lyme disease, and West Nile encephalitis, but remain poorly understood. New grounds for mosquito breeding have developed in waste dumps, threatening vector control efforts that have traditionally focused on vector breeding in swamps and marshes. As previously noted, agricultural practices have been closely linked to the spread of antibiotic resistance, influenza outbreaks, and diseases of food crops and animals. Migration, travel, and commerce have been associated with several microbial threats to health.

Human development and large-scale social phenomena are closely connected to infectious disease threats at a global level. National security and an enlightened self-interest require that countries recognize the direct impact of social, economic, political, and ecological factors, especially in developing countries. In additional to technical and financial support, a research program focused on the global social and ecological factors affecting infectious disease emergence should be established. Only recently have studies been conducted within the traditional biomedical, social epidemiology, and medical anthropology research arenas to begin to address these factors and the interventions necessary to combat them.

Inferences about the etiology of disease are typically drawn through statistical association of natural observations or experiments. Recognizing, however, that the emergence of infectious disease is usually not attributable to any single factor, but the result of complex interactions among numerous and often unknown physical, biological, ecological, and socioeconomic variables, it is clear that multidisciplinary studies, including dynamic analyses of such interactions, are needed.

NIH should develop a comprehensive research agenda for infectious disease prevention and control in collaboration with other federal research institutions and laboratories (e.g., CDC, DOD, the U.S. Department of Energy, the National Science Foundation), academia, and industry. *This agenda should be designed to investigate the role of genetic, biological, social, economic, political, ecological, and physical environmental factors in the emergence of infectious diseases in the United States and worldwide. This agenda should also include the development and assessment of public health measures to address microbial threats. A sustained commitment to a robust research agenda must be a high priority if the United States is to dramatically reduce the threat of naturally occurring infectious diseases and intentional uses of biological agents. The research agenda should be flexible to permit rapid assessment of new and emerging threats, and should be rigorously reevaluated* *on a 5-year basis to ensure that it is addressing areas of highest priority.*

Successfully carrying out such an integrated, comprehensive research agenda will entail collaboration among multiple government agencies, academia, and the private sector. Collaborations between the academic research and public health communities are essential to ensure that priority research areas are addressed in a timely manner and that findings can be readily applied. Research driven by grants in the infectious disease arena rarely includes the kind of practical research, such as evaluations of programs and interventions, that is of value to public health workers in the field. Even within schools of public health, applied public health research has not been a priority. This problem can be addressed, in part, by creating faculty positions that are accountable to both academic centers and health departments. A coordinated approach must extend from fundamental laboratory science through operation, evaluation, and intervention research. In addition, the full support and engagement of a range of professional disciplines, including such often-overlooked fields as entomology, ecology, and anthropology, are needed.

INTERDISCIPLINARY INFECTIOUS DISEASE CENTERS

As previously noted, addressing the highly complex nature of infectious disease emergence requires the involvement of experts from a broad range of disciplines and health sectors. Collaborative links within and between universities and among international, federal, and state governments currently exist. The present structure of academic and public health institutions, however, requires that most of these arenas operate independently of each other. Opportunities for convergence and synergism are often lost unless experts convene under the same roof (or on the same campus) to discuss a problem. Not only are opportunities lost for collaboration, but there are often unnecessary redundancies of effort and expense. Furthermore, the absence of an interdisciplinary collaborative approach results in failure to adequately train the workforce needed to address the emerging microbial threats facing the world today. While federally proposed Research Centers of Excellence in Biodefense and Emerging Infections may provide some of the infrastructure needed to address specific emerging disease threats (e.g., basic research, vaccine and antimicrobial drug development), they do not meet the need for such an approach.

Many types of infectious disease problems—including the search for infectious triggers of chronic disease, the emergence of antibiotic resistance, nosocomial infections, and zoonotic infections—could be addressed through an interdisciplinary approach. The majority of emerging diseases that threaten humans are of zoonotic origin. In the past 10 years, the world has had to respond to Sin Nombre virus and other hantaviruses from rodents, Nipah virus from bats via pigs, influenza viruses from aquatic birds, and West Nile virus from birds via mosquitoes. Zoonotic diseases have also emerged when domestic animals have served as reservoirs. As discussed earlier, antimicrobial-resistant organisms have emerged in part as a result of the agricultural use of antimicrobials for disease prevention and growth promotion in chickens, pigs, cattle, and even fish and shellfish. Indeed anthrax, used as an agent of bioterrorism in 2001, is a naturally occurring zoonotic disease. The vulnerability of the United States and the developed world to agroterrorism attack using agents such as foot and mouth disease virus and the high socioeconomic cost of diseases of livestock could be better addressed through an interdisciplinary approach to microbial threats. It is imperative that those in the human, animal, agricultural, and environmental sciences come together to examine such threats.

Our understanding of many recent emerging disease threats has come mostly from a cadre of scientists who are at home in the laboratory, in the clinic, or in the field. These scientists have usually been formally trained in one medical/biomedical/veterinary discipline, but have gained additional training and experience in other disciplines pertinent to disease prevention and control. The disciplinary base of this cadre of scientists has been remarkably diverse, including clinical medicine, veterinary medicine, microbiology, virology, molecular biology, pathology, immunology, toxicology, epidemiology, public health, mammalogy, wildlife biology, medical entomology, and ecology. Some of these scientists have had valuable tertiary expertise as well, in such areas as epidemiologic modeling, GIS and remote sensing technologies, health education, administration and management, and public policy. Other relevant disciplines include economics, anthropology, and ethics.

This cadre of scientists has provided invaluable knowledge and skills to address the multidisciplinary nature of infectious disease control. Younger counterparts rely increasingly on molecular approaches and computer-based tools, and often lack training and experience in the basic disciplines most pertinent to infectious disease prevention and control, such as epidemiologic field observations and investigations. Unfortunately, today there are too few scientists who can bring to bear all the various tools and approaches that may be of use in the detection, diagnosis, investigation, prevention, and control of emerging infectious diseases.

These problems are not unique to infectious diseases. In the past, one solution has been to create centers of interdisciplinary excellence, perhaps best exemplified by the cancer research centers that have proven invaluable to advances in cancer prevention and treatment. Denmark has met the need for an interdisciplinary perspective in addressing emerging infectious diseases by developing a zoonosis center as an element of its national public health institution, the Statens Serum Institut, uniting veterinary and human health professionals. The committee believes much could be gained if the United States were to create similar interdisciplinary infectious disease centers for research, education, training, and public service. Given the nation's lack of infrastructure in this area, such centers would have to be established with bricks and mortar, not as completely virtual centers.

Interdisciplinary infectious disease centers should be developed to promote a multidisciplinary approach to addressing microbial threats to health. *These centers should be based within academic institutions and link (both physically and virtually) the relevant disciplines necessary to support such an approach. They would collaborate with the larger network of public agencies addressing emerging infectious diseases (e.g., local and state health agencies, CDC, DOD, the U.S. Department of Energy, FDA, the Food Safety and Inspection Service, NIH, the National Science Foundation, USAID, USDA), interested foundations, private organizations, and industry. The training, education, and research that these centers would provide are a much-needed resource not only for the United States, but also for the entire world.*

The proposed centers would provide space to bring people together so that their proximity would generate work across intellectual discipline–driven boundaries on a research agenda that requires a cross-disciplinary approach. This is exactly what comprehensive cancer centers have done so well, bringing together clinicians (pediatricians, internists, oncologists, radiologists, and surgeons), basic scientists, epidemiologists, pharmacologists, immunologists, virologists, cell biologists, structural biologists, radiation biologists, and radiation therapists. Interdisciplinary work requires that those involved have not only good will toward and awareness of each other, but also a means of actually talking to each other frequently, often casually—contacts that in time lead to new kinds of work that bridge multiple disciplines. Seminars on various arenas of work given regularly in a center help bring people and ideas together. Economists, sociologists, medical anthropologists, epidemiologists, medical geographers, and others might need to pool their talents with those of immunologists, vaccine developers, and infectious disease clinicians and health care workers to solve persistent problems of community- or regionally-based outbreaks of infection. A center would help unite faculty of schools of public health, medical school basic and clinical faculty, and local and state public health officials.

Nowhere is the opportunity for interdisciplinary work greater than in the global infectious diseases arena. To make such work a reality, we need to create space and support for people from multiple disciplines to work

---

A Vision for Interdisciplinary Infectious Disease Centers

Interdisciplinary, multidisciplinary research projects. The centers would foster interactions among university faculty in public health, clinical medicine, veterinary medicine, and the relevant basic and social sciences, as well as among those working in local, state, and national public health systems. The centers would focus on high-priority public health problems and leverage expertise across multiple organizations.

A training venue. The aim would be to develop future scientists and leaders with the kind of broad perspective needed to work across boundaries in their efforts to control new and reemerging microbial threats to health. A venue providing a point of entry or primary exposure for young scientists might take the form of summer fellowship programs, internships, and other training opportunities.

A link to primary and reference laboratory diagnostic systems. No common ground for developing a proper national reference diagnostic system and communal repository of infectious agent stocks and other diagnostic reagents currently exists. The centers would also provide an ideal venue for creating such a system and for training in laboratory technologies.

Information/database systems. Databases would provide pertinent epidemiological, diagnostic, and other important information for all members of the scientific community. Some aspects of this information/database system might be made available via the Internet, and an e-mail network (perhaps as a subunit of the highly successful Pro-Med system) might also be provided.

---

together. Emerging infectious diseases and persistent infections create an urgent need for such centers. In addition to helping to meet national and even international needs in addressing emerging infectious diseases, the proposed centers would play a critical role in improving our national capacity to deal with nosocomial infections, drug resistance, socioeconomic issues in the emergence and transmission of infection, and the infectious etiologies of cancer and chronic inflammatory and degenerative diseases. Individual centers would be expected to have different foci of interest, so as to provide the nation with a broad-based ability to deal with infections of all kinds.

A case in point to suggest the value of such centers is the importance of addressing the zoonotic aspects of influenza. While WHO oversees global surveillance of human influenza through centers in London, Atlanta, Tokyo, and Melbourne, there is little interaction between this program and animal influenza surveillance programs. Influenza viruses that have been transmitted from wild aquatic bird reservoirs through domestic poultry and pigs and then on to humans represent the most significant threat of influenza to humans. Although the Office International des Epizooties (OIE) deals with the reportable diseases of animals, only certain influenza virus types that are highly pathogenic for poultry are of concern—those viruses that are found to be rather nonpathogenic in poultry, but for which a potential threat to humans exists, are ignored. Given the remarkable mutability of influenza viruses, it might be expected that there would be strong links between WHO and its human influenza tracking system and OIE and its still-primitive animal influenza tracking system. It can be argued that such linkage will be effected only through the development of several interdisciplinary infectious disease centers focused on zoonoses.

Epilogue

As the work of this committee draws to an end, none of its members are sanguine about what the future may hold with respect to microbial threats to health. Certainly, it is clear many forces in our complex global village converge to make us more vulnerable to these threats. At the same time, however, this study has identified many opportunities to make a real and enduring difference in preventing disease and improving health.

Today's outlook with regard to microbial threats to health is bleak on a number of fronts. AIDS is out of control in much of sub-Saharan Africa, India, China, and elsewhere; bioterrorism has become a reality; the relentless rise of antimicrobial resistance continues; we have no viable strategy or acceptance of responsibility for the replacement of obsolescing antibiotics; many disappointments surround efforts to develop vaccines for diseases such as malaria and HIV, as well as the range of new vaccines that may be needed for natural and manmade threats; in some countries a poorly informed popular movement against vaccination has led to a resurgence of common childhood infections; and cholera, drug-resistant malaria, and dengue fever continue to spread to new areas. Moreover, microbial threats present us with new surprises every year.

Yet bright spots on the global scene have also occurred, including the gratifying model of the utility and availability of ivermectin for onchocerciasis in Africa; the containment of H5N1 flu in Hong Kong in 1997, along with ongoing surveillance; and the reduced mortality from HIV/AIDS in the United States, attributable to a combination of behavioral change and the availability of protease inhibitors and combination antiretroviral therapy.

227

Many developments hold promise for achieving further progress. These include signs of public, philanthropic, and political awareness of the significance of global infectious diseases; a new recognition of the importance of a strong and vital public health infrastructure; the extraordinary advances made in microbial genomics offering enormous potential for new technologies to prevent and cope with infection; the emergence of broad ecological and evolutionary perspectives on the biology of host–microparasite symbiotic interrelationships; and a greater appreciation of the socioeconomic settings of disease emergence.

At the same time, it is essential to recognize that infectious diseases have always been closely interwoven with world history, and the present situation is no exception. The world is changing and in many respects is quite unstable, as evidenced by the realignment of powers with the end of the cold war; the eruption of interethnic hostility in the Balkans and Central Africa, the political and religious conflicts raging in many areas of the world, and the escalation of international terrorism. Such political turbulence is paralleled by the state of the global economy, including the massive burden of third-world debt, currency and banking crises, and the cycling of economic bubbles and collapses—all of which have eroded the resources available for public health and for entrepreneurial investment in antimicrobials and vaccines to counter the microbial threats identified in this report. Not surprisingly, the interdependence of health status and economic and social development is also interwoven with issues of leadership, whether at critical health institutions or in various national regimes.

The developed world has financial and technological resources that should enable the successful application of old and new methods to contain infection. Nevertheless, we live in a society where many competing factors—including market forces, regulatory pressures, and environmental and ethical concerns, to name but a few—influence research and development priorities and portfolios. Inevitably, tensions arise that may override or diminish the potential community health benefits of such measures as the development of pesticides or vaccines adapted to the needs of the developing world.

Thus while dramatic advances in science and medicine have enabled us to make great strides in our struggle to prevent and control infectious diseases, we cannot fall prey to an illusory complacency. We must understand that pathogens—old and new—have ingenious ways of adapting to and breaching our armamentarium of defenses. We must also understand that factors in society, the environment, and our global interconnectedness actually increase the likelihood of the ongoing emergence and spread of infectious diseases. It is a sad irony that today we must also grapple with the intentional use of biological agents to do harm, human against human.

No responsible assessment of microbial threats to health in the twenty-first century, then, could end without a call to action. The magnitude and urgency of the problem demand renewed concern and commitment. We have not done enough—in our own defense or in the defense of others. As we take stock of our prospects with respect to microbial threats in the years ahead, we must recognize the need for a new level of attention, dedication, and sustained resources to ensure the health and safety of the United States—and of the world.

Glossary

Agent any power, principle, or substance capable of producing an effect, whether chemical, physical, or biological.

AIDS acquired immunodeficiency syndrome, the end stage of HIV disease.

Airborne the dissemination of microbial agents through a suitable portal of entry, usually the respiratory tract. Microbial aerosols are suspensions of particles in the air consisting partially or wholly of microorganisms.

Allograft a homograft between allogeneic individuals.

Anthropophilic attracted to humans especially as a source of food (*anthropophilic* mosquitoes); indicating relative attraction to humans.

Antibiotic chemical substance produced by a microorganism that has the capacity to inhibit the growth of or to kill other microorganisms; antibiotics that are nontoxic to the host are used as chemotherapeutic agents in the treatment of infectious diseases.

Antibody a protein produced by the immune system in response to the introduction of a substance (an antigen) recognized as foreign by the body's immune system. Antibody interacts with the other components of the immune system and can render the antigen harmless, although for various reasons this may not always occur.

Antigen a molecule capable of eliciting a specific antibody or T-cell response; a molecule specifically reacting with an antibody.

Antigenic having the properties of an antigen.

231

Antimalarial   a chemotherapeutic agent that inhibits or destroys malarial parasites.

Antimicrobial   a drug for killing microorganisms or suppressing their multiplication or growth. For the purposes of this report, antimicrobials include antibiotics and antivirals.

Antiretroviral   substance that stops or suppresses the activity of a retrovirus such as HIV.

Antiviral   drugs, including interferon, that stimulate cellular defenses against viruses, reducing cell DNA synthesis and making cells more resistant to viral genes, enhancing cellular immune responses or suppressing their replication.

Arbovirus   shortened form of arthropod-borne virus. Any of a group of viruses that are transmitted to humans and animals by mosquitoes, ticks, and sand flies; they include such agents as yellow fever and eastern, western, and Venezuelan equine encephalitis virus.

Arenavirus   any group of viruses composed of pleomorphic virions of varying size, one large and one small segment of single-stranded RNA, and ribosomes within the virions that cause the virus to have a sandy appearance. Examples are Junin, Machupo, and Lassa fever viruses. Rodents are common reservoirs of the arenaviruses.

Arthropod   as used in this report, refers to insects and ticks, many of which are medically important as vectors of infectious diseases.

Arthropod-borne   capable of being transmitted by insect and tick (arthropod) vectors.

B cell   one of two general categories of lymphocytes (white blood cells) involved in the humoral immune response. When help is provided by T lymphocytes, B lymphocytes produce antibodies against specific antigens.

Bacillus   rod-shaped bacterium.

Bacteremia   refers to the presence of bacteria in the blood.

Bacteria   one of the two major classes of prokaryotic organism.

Beta-lactam   an active portion of an antibiotic (e.g., penicillin or cephalosporin) that is part of the chemical structure of the antibiotic and that can be neutralized by a beta-lactamase produced by certain microorganisms (e.g., some staphylococci).

Beta-lactamase   an enzyme that neutralizes the effect of an antibiotic containing beta-lactam.

Bioterrorism   terrorism using biological agents. Biological diseases and the agents that might be used for terrorism have been labeled by the CDC and comprise viruses, bacteria, rickettsiae, fungi, and biological toxins. These agents have been classified according to the degree of danger each agent is felt to pose into one of three categories.

BL-4   level of containment required for safe handling of the most contagious pathogenic microbes.

Case-fatality rate   usually expressed as the percentage of persons diagnosed as having a specified disease who die as a result of that illness within a given period.

Category A   high-priority agents include organisms that pose a risk to national security because they can be easily disseminated or transmitted person-to-person, cause high mortality, with potential for major public health impact, might cause public panic and social disruption, and require special action for public health preparedness. These diseases include anthrax, botulism, plague, smallpox, tularemia, and viral hemorrhagic fevers.

Category B   second-highest priority agents include those that are moderately easy to disseminate, cause moderate morbidity and low mortality, and require specific diagnostic capacity and enhanced disease surveillance. These agents/diseases include Q fever brucellosis, glanders, ricin toxin, epsilon toxin, and staph toxin.

Category C   third-highest priority agents include emerging pathogens that could be engineered for mass dissemination in the future because of availability, ease of production and dissemination, and potential for high mortality and major health impact. These agents/diseases include Nipah virus, hantavirus, tickborne hemorrhagic fever viruses, tickborne encephalitis viruses, yellow fever, and tuberculosis.

Cellular immunity, cell-mediated immunity   a type of immune response in which subpopulations of T cells (helper T cells and killer T cells) cooperate to destroy cells in the body that bear foreign antigens, such as bacteria.

Cephalosporin   a class of antibiotic.

Chemokine   any of a group of chemotactic cytokines that are produced by various cells (as at sites of inflammation), that are thought to provide directional cues for the movement of white blood cells (as T cells, monocytes, and neutrophils), and that include some playing a role in HIV infection because the cell surface receptors to which they bind are also used by specific strains of HIV for entry into cells.

Chronic disease   diseases that have one or more of the following characteristics: they are permanent, leave residual disability, are caused by nonreversible pathological alteration, require special training of the patient for rehabilitation, or may be expected to require a long period of supervision, observation, or care.

Clonal   of or pertaining to a group of genetically identical organisms derived from a single parent or a DNA population derived from a single DNA molecule by replication in a bacterial or eukaryotic host cell.

Coding sequence   the order of nucleotide bases in a nucleic acid that speci-
fies the production of a particular product, such as a protein. A change
in the coding sequence (e.g., as a result of mutation) can result in a
change in the product.

Communicable disease   an illness due to a specific infectious agent or its
toxic products that arises though transmission of that agent or its
products from an infected person, animal, or inanimate reservoir to a
susceptible host; either directly or indirectly through an intermediate
plant or animal host, vector, or inanimate environment; infectious disease.

Contagious   communicable by contact; bearing contagion.

Cytokine   any of a class of immunoregulatory proteins (as interleukin,
tumor necrosis factor, and interferon) that are secreted by cells, especially of the immune system.

DDT   1,1,1-trichloro-2,2-bis(*p*-chlorophenyl)ethane or chlorophenothane,
a pesticide.

Deletion mutation   a mutation that results from the deletion of one or
more amino acids present in the genetic material of the organism undergoing the mutation.

Disease   as used in this report, refers to a situation in which infection has
elicited signs and symptoms in the infected individual; the infection has
become clinically apparent.

DNA   deoxyribonucleic acid, a carrier of genetic information (i.e., heredi-
tary characteristics) found chiefly in the nucleus of cells.

DNA virus   a virus that contains only DNA as its genetic material.

Droplet nuclei   the very small particles of moisture expelled when a person
coughs, sneezes, or speaks that may transfer infectious organisms to
another person who inhales the droplets.

Ecology   a branch of science concerned with the interrelationship of organisms and their environments.

Ecosystem   the complex of a community and its environment functioning
as an ecological unit in nature.

Emerging infection   either a newly recognized, clinically distinct infectious
disease, or a known infectious disease whose reported incidence is
increasing in a given place or among a specific population.

Encephalitis   inflammation of the brain.

Endemic   the constant presence of a disease or infectious agent within a
given geographic area; it may also refer to the usual prevalence of a
given disease within such area.

Endogenous   developing or originating from within the individual.

Endophilic   ecologically associated with humans and their domestic environment (mosquitoes that are *endophilic* vectors of malaria).

Entomology   a branch of zoology that deals with insects.

Enzootic refers to a disease (can be either low or high morbidity) that is endemic in an animal community.

Epidemic the occurrence in a community or region of cases of an illness (or outbreak) with a frequency clearly in excess of normal expectancy.

Epidemiology branch of science that deals with the incidence, distribution, and control of disease in a population; the sum of the factors controlling the presence or abundance of a disease or pathogen.

Epizootic a disease of generally high morbidity that rapidly spreads through an animal population.

Etiological agent the organism that causes a disease.

Etiology the cause or origin of a disease.

Fluoroquinolone a class of antibiotic.

Foodborne illness a sickness caused by food contaminated with microorganisms, chemicals, or other substances hazardous to human health.

Genetic adaptability the ability of a microorganism to adapt to its environment, often allowing it to avoid detection or an immune response generated against it.

Genome the complete genetic composition of an organism (e.g., human, bacterium, protozoan, helminth, or fungus), contained in a chromosome or set of chromosomes or in a DNA or RNA molecule (e.g., virus).

Genomics a branch of biotechnology concerned with applying the techniques of genetics and molecular biology to the genetic mapping and DNA sequencing of sets of genes or the complete genomes of selected organisms using high-speed methods, organizing the results in databases, and with applications of the data (as in medicine or biology).

Glycoprotein a conjugated protein in which the nonprotein group is a carbohydrate.

Gram-negative refers to the inability of a microorganism to accept a certain stain. This inability is related to the cell wall composition of the microorganism and has been useful in classifying bacteria.

Gram-positive refers to the ability of a microorganism to retain a certain stain. This ability is related to the cell wall composition of the microorganism and has been useful in classifying bacteria.

Haplotype a group of alleles of different genes (as of the major histocompatibility complex) on a single chromosome that are closely enough linked to be inherited usually as a unit.

Hemagglutinin a molecule, such as an antibody or lectin, that agglutinates red blood cells.

Hemoglobin iron-containing respiratory pigment of vertebrate red blood cells that functions primarily in the transport of oxygen from the lungs to the tissues of the body.

Hemoglobinopathy   a blood disorder (such as sickle cell anemia) caused by a genetically determined change in the molecular structure of hemoglobin.

Hemorrhagic fever   a group of diverse, severe epidemic viral infections of worldwide distribution but occurring especially in tropical countries, that are usually transmitted to humans by arthropod bites or contact with virus-infected rodents or monkeys and that share common clinocopathological features (e.g., fever, hemorrhaging, shock, thrombocytopenia, neurological disturbances). Examples are Argentine, Bolivian, and Venezuelan hemorrhagic fevers; chikungunya; Rift Valley fever; and Ebola and Marburg virus diseases.

Heterozygous   having the two genes at corresponding loci on homologous chromosomes different for one or more loci.

HIV disease   the broad spectrum of opportunistic infections and diseases that occur in an individual infected with the human immunodeficiency virus.

Homozygous   having the two genes at corresponding loci on homologous chromosomes identical for one or more loci.

Host   a person or other living creature, including birds and arthropods, that affords subsistence or lodgment to an infectious agent under natural (as opposed to experimental) conditions.

Humoral immunity   antibody-mediated immunity; one of the mechanisms, using antibodies found in the blood and other body fluids, that the body uses to fight off infections.

Hyperendemic   the condition in which a disease is present in a community at all times and with a high incidence.

Iatrogenic   any consequence of treatment by a physician.

Immunity   that resistance usually associated with the presence of antibodies or cells having a specific action on the microorganism concerned with a particular infectious disease or on its toxin.

Immunization   a process that increases an organism's reaction to antigen and therefore improves its ability to resist or overcome infection.

Immunocompromised   a condition (caused, for example, by the administration of immunosuppressive drugs or irradiation, malnutrition, aging, or a condition such as cancer or HIV disease) in which an individual's immune system is unable to respond adequately to a foreign substance.

Immunosuppression   the retardation or cessation of an immune response as a result of, for example, anticancer drugs.

Incidence rate   the number of new cases of a specified disease during a defined period of time divided by the number of persons in a stated population in which the cases occurred.

Infection   the entry and development (of many parasites) or a multiplication of an infectious agent in the body of persons or animals.

Infectious   capable of causing infection; communicable by invasion of the body of a susceptible organism.

Infectious agent   an organism (virus, rickettsia, bacteria, fungus, protozoan, or helminth) that is capable of producing infection or infectious disease.

Microbe   any microorganism or biologic agent that can replicate in humans (including bacteria, viruses, protozoa, fungi, and prions); in other usage, any multicellular organism.

Microbial traffic   the transfer of existing microbes to new host populations.

Microbiome   the ensemble of microbes that may share the body space of a multicellular host, in health or disease; may be intra- or extracellular.

Monoclonal antibody   immunoglobulins derived from a single clone of plasma cells. Monoclonal antibodies constitute a pure population because they are produced by a single clone in vitro and are chemically and structurally identical.

Mutation   a transmissible change in the genetic material of an organism, usually in a single gene.

Neuraminidase   sialidase; an enzyme that catalyzes the hydrolysis of glucosidic linkages between a sialic acid residue and a hexose or hexosamine residue in glycoproteins, glycolipids, and proteoglycans. Neuraminidase is a major antigen of myxoviruses.

Nosocomial infection   an infection occurring in a patient in a hospital or other health care facility in whom it was not present or incubating at the time of admission; or the residual infection acquired during a previous admission.

Opportunistic infection   an infection caused by an organism that ordinarily does not cause disease but under circumstances such as impaired immunity becomes pathogenic.

Pandemic   an epidemic that occurs worldwide.

Parasite   organism living in, with, or on another organism.

Pathogen   a microorganism that causes disease.

Pathogenic   capable of causing disease.

PCR   see polymerase chain reaction.

Pharmacokinetics   the study of bodily absorption, distribution, metabolism, and excretion of drugs; the characteristic interactions of a drug and the body in terms of its absorption, distribution, metabolism, and excretion.

Plasmid   an extrachromosomal, self-replicating structure found in cells that carries genes for a variety of functions not essential for cell growth. Plasmids are any extranuclear genetic particle.

Point mutation   a mutation resulting from a change in a single base pair in the DNA molecule, resulting from the substitution of one nucleotide for another.

Polymerase chain reaction   a laboratory method of amplifying low levels of specific microbial DNA or RNA sequences.

Prevalence rate   the total number of persons sick or portraying a certain condition in a stated population at a particular time or during a stated period of time, regardless of when that illness or condition began, divided by the population at risk of having the disease or condition at the point in time midway through the period in which they occurred.

Probiotic   general term for a substance that promotes growth of microorganisms; an organism that changes health of carrier.

Public health   the art and science of dealing with the protection and improvement of community health by organized community effort and including preventive medicine and sanitary and social health.

Receptor   a cell or group of cells that receive(s) stimuli; a chemical group or molecule (such as a protein) on the cell surface or in the cell interior that has an affinity for a specific chemical group, molecule, or virus.

Recombination   the formation of new combinations of genes as a result of crossing over (exchange of genes) between structurally similar chromosomes, resulting in progeny with different gene combinations than in the parents.

Reservoir   any person, animal, arthropod, plant, soil, or substance (or combination of these) in which an infectious agent normally lives and multiplies, on which it depends primarily for survival, and where it reproduces itself in such a manner that it can be transmitted to a susceptible host.

Resistance   the sum total of body mechanisms that interpose barriers to the invasion or multiplication of infectious agents, or to damage by their toxic products.

Retrovirus   any of large family of RNA viruses that includes lentiviruses and oncoviruses, so called because they carry reverse transcriptase.

Reverse transcriptase   RNA-directed DNA polymerase; an enzyme, such as is found in the human immunodeficiency virus, that catalyzes the reaction that uses RNA as a template for double-stranded DNA synthesis.

RNA   ribonucleic acid.

RNA virus   a virus that contains RNA as its genetic material.

Rodent-borne   disease spread by rodents.

Selective pressure   pressure exerted on an organism by its environment that causes a change in the organism's ability to cope with that environment.

Septicemia, septicemic   systemic disease associated with the presence and persistence of microorganisms in the blood.

Seroconversion   the change of a serological test result from negative to positive as a result of antibodies induced by the introduction of microorganisms into the host.

Serological   the use of immune serum in any number of tests (agglutination, precipitation, enzyme-linked immunosorbent assay, etc.) used to measure the response (antibody titer) to infectious disease; the use of serological reactions to detect antigen.

Seronegative   negative result in a serological test; that is, the inability to detect the antibodies or antigens being tested for.

Seropositive   positive results in a serological test.

Serotype   the characterization of a microorganism based on the kinds and combinations of constituent antigens present in that organism; a taxonomic subdivision of bacteria based on the above.

Slow virus   any virus (or virus-like agent) causing a disease characterized by a very long preclinical course and a very gradual progression of symptoms; many examples are prions.

Strain   a subgrouping of organisms within a species, characterized by some particular quality.

Surveillance   the continuing scrutiny of all aspects of occurrence and spread of a disease that are pertinent to effective control.

Syndrome   a set of symptoms that may occur concurrently.

T cell   any of several lymphocytes (such as a helper T cell) that differentiate in the thymus, process highly specific cell-surface antigen receptors, and include some that control the initiation or suppression of cell-mediated and humoral immunity and others that lyse antigen-bearing cells.

Tetramer   molecule (such as an enzyme or polymer) that consists of four structural subunits.

Toll   the Toll signaling pathway, which is required for the establishment of the dorsal ventral axis in *Drosophila* embryos, plays an important role in the response of larval and adult *Drosophila* to microbial infections.

Toll-like receptor   a system of innate immunity originally discovered in *Drosophila*.

Transovarially   relating to or being transmission of a pathogen from an organism (such as a tick) to its offspring by infection of eggs in its ovary.

Vaccine   a preparation of purified polypeptide, protein or polysaccharide, or DNA or of killed microorganisms, living attenuated organisms, or living virulent or crude or purified organisms that is administered to produce or artificially increase immunity to a particular disease.

Vector   a carrier, especially an arthropod, that transfers an infective agent from one host (which can include itself) to another.

Vector-borne   (i) Mechanical: includes simple mechanical carriage by a crawling or flying insect through soiling of its feet or proboscis, or by passage of organisms through its gastrointestinal tract. This does not require multiplication or development of the organism. (ii) Biological: propagation (multiplication), cyclic development, or a combination of these (cyclopropagative) is required before the arthropod can transmit the infective form of the agent to humans. An incubation period (extrinsic) is required following infection before the arthropod becomes infective. The infectious agent may be passed vertically to succeeding generations (transovarian transmission); transstadial transmission indicates its passage from one stage of life cycle to another, as nymph to adult. Transmission may be by injection of salivary gland fluid during biting, or by regurgitation or deposition on the skin of feces or other material capable of penetrating through the bite wound or through an area of trauma from scratching or rubbing. This transmission is by an infected nonvertebrate host and not simple mechanical carriage by a vector or vehicle. However, an arthropod in either role is termed a vector.

Virulence   the degree of pathogenicity of an organism as evidenced by the severity of resulting disease and the organism's ability to invade the host tissues.

Virus   causative agent of an infectious disease.

Xenogeneic infection   derived from, originating in, or being a member of another species.

Xenotransplantation   transplantation of an organ, tissue, or cells between two different species (such as a human and a domestic swine).

Zoonosis   an infection or infectious disease transmissible under natural conditions from vertebrate animals to humans. May be enzootic or epizootic.

References

Aarestrup FM, Seyfarth AM, Emborg HD, Pedersen K, Hendriksen RS, Bager F. 2001. Effect of abolishment of the use of antimicrobial agents for growth promotion on occurrence of antimicrobial resistance in fecal enterococci from food animals in Denmark. *Antimicrob Agents Chemother* 45(7):2054–9.

Abdel-Wahab MF. 1982. *Schistosomiasis in Egypt*. Boca Raton, FL: CRC Press, Inc.

Acosta CJ, Galindo CM, Kimario J, Senkoro K, Urassa H, Casals C, Corachan M, Eseko N, Tanner M, Mshinda H, Lwilla F, Vila J, Alonso PL. 2001. Cholera outbreak in southern Tanzania: risk factors and patterns of transmission. *Emerg Infect Dis* 7(3 Suppl):583–7.

Adelman ZN, Blair CD, Carlson JO, Beaty BJ, Olson KE. 2001. Sindbis virus-induced silencing of dengue viruses in mosquitoes. *Insect Mol Biol* 10(3):265–73.

Adeyi O, Hecht R, Njobvu E, Soucat A. 2001. AIDS, Poverty Reduction and Debt Relief: Toolkit for Mainstreaming HIV/AIDS Programmes into Development Instruments. UNAIDS/01.01E. Geneva: UNAIDS.

Afonso CL, Tulman ER, Lu Z, Balinsky CA, Moser BA, Becnel JJ, Rock DL, Kutish GF. 2001. Genome sequence of a baculovirus pathogenic for *Culex nigripalpus*. *J Virol* 75(22):11157–65.

Ahmad K. 2000. More deaths from Rift Valley fever in Saudi Arabia and Yemen. *Lancet* 356(9239):1422.

Alibek K. 1999. The Soviet Union's anti-agricultural biological weapons. *Ann N Y Acad Sci* 894:18–9.

Alibek K., Handelman S. 2000. Biohazard. New York: Delta Books.

Alliance for the Prudent Use of Antibiotics (APUA). 2001. Antibiotic resistance: synthesis of recommendations by expert policy groups. WHO/CDS/CSR/DRS/2001.10. Geneva: WHO.

APUA. 2002. The Need to Improve Antimicrobial Use in Agriculture: Ecological and Human Health Consequences. Executive Summary. [Online]. Available: http://www.healthsci.tufts.edu/apua/Ecology/faairExec Sum_6–02.html#ExSum [accessed June 13, 2002].

241

Almroth G, Ekermo B, Mansson AS, Svensson G, Widell A. 2002. Detection and prevention of hepatitis C in dialysis patients and renal transplant recipients. A long–term follow up (1989–January 1997). *J Intern Med* 251(2):119–28.

Alphey L, Beard CB, Billingsley P, Coetzee M, Crisanti A, Curtis C, Eggleston P, Godfray C, Hemingway J, Jacobs–Lorena M, James AA, Kafatos FC, Mukwaya LG, Paton M, Powell JR, Schneider W, Scott TW, Sina B, Sinden R, Sinkins S, Spielman A, Toure Y, Collins FH. 2002. Malaria control with genetically manipulated insect vectors. *Science* 298(5591):119–21.

Alterholt TB, LeChevalier MW, Norton WD, Rosen JS. 1998. Effect of rainfall on giardia and crypto. *J Am Water Works Assoc* 90:66–80.

American Social Health Association. 1998. Sexually Transmitted Disease in America: How Many Cases and at What Cost? Menlo Park, CA: Kaiser Family Foundation.

American Social Health Association. 2001. HPV Background Information. [Online]. Available: http://www.ashastd.org/hpvccrc/background.html [accessed March 5, 2003].

Animal and Plant Health Inspection Service (APHIS). 1992. The Foreign Animal Disease Diagnostic Laboratory at Plum Island Animal Disease Center. [Online]. Available: http://www.aphis.usda.gov/oa/pubs/ fsfadlab.html [accessed January 29, 2003].

APHIS. 1999a. Poultry and Eggs. Washington, DC: U.S. Department of Agriculture.

APHIS. 1999b. Factsheet: Invasive Species. Washington, DC: U.S. Department of Agriculture.

APHIS. 2002. Chronic Wasting Disease. [Online]. Available: http://www.aphis.usda.gov/lpa/issues/cwd/cwd.html [accessed February 22, 2003].

Aoki T. 1988. Drug-resistant plasmids from fish pathogens. *Microbiol Sci* 5(7):219–23.

Aral S. 1999. Elimination and reintroduction of a sexually transmitted disease: lessons to be learned? *Am J Public Health* 89(7):995–7.

Armstrong GL, Conn LA, Pinner RW. 1999. Trends in infectious disease mortality in the United States during the 20th century. *JAMA* 281(1):61–6.

Arnon SS, Schechter R, Inglesby TV, Henderson DA, Bartlett JG, Ascher MS, Eitzen E, Fine AD, Hauer J, Layton M, Lillibridge S, Osterholm MT, O'Toole T, Parker G, et al. 2001. Botulinum toxin as a biological weapon: medical and public health management. *JAMA* 285(8):1059–70.

Asthana S, Oostvogels R. 1996. Community participation in HIV prevention: problems and prospects for community-based strategies among female sex workers in Madras. *Soc Sci Med* 43(2):133–48.

Attaran A, Roberts DR, Curtis CF, Kilama WL. 2000. Balancing risks on the backs of the poor. *Nat Med* 6(7):729–31.

Baier EG. 1997. The Impact of HIV/AIDS on Rural Households/Communities and the Need for Multisectoral Prevention and Mitigation Strategies to Combat the Epidemic in Rural Areas. Rome: Food and Agriculture Organization of the United Nations.

Ball TM, Holberg CJ, Aldous MB, Martinez FD, Wright AL. 2002. Influence of attendance at day care on the common cold from birth through 13 years of age. *Arch Pediatr Adolesc Med* 156(2):121–6.

Barbour AG, Fish D. 1993. The biological and social phenomenon of Lyme disease. *Science* 260(5114):1610–6.

Barclay AJ, Foster A, Sommer A. 1987. Vitamin A supplements and mortality related to measles: a randomised clinical trial. *Br Med J (Clin Res Ed)* 294(6567):294–6.

Barragan A, Kremsner PG, Wahlgren M, Carlson J. 2000. Blood group A antigen is a coreceptor in *Plasmodium falciparum* rosetting. *Infect Immun* 68(5):2971–5.

Bartlett JG, Breiman RF, Mandell LA, File TM Jr. 1998. Community-acquired pneumonia in adults: guidelines for management. The Infectious Diseases Society of America. *Clin Infect Dis* 26(4):811–38.

Bartlett JG, Dowell SF, Mandell LA, File Jr TM, Musher DM, Fine MJ. 2000. Practice guidelines for the management of community-acquired pneumonia in adults. Infectious Diseases Society of America. *Clin Infect Dis* 31(2):347–82.

Beard CB, Cordon–Rosales C, Durvasula RV. 2002. Bacterial symbionts of the triatominae and their potential use in control of Chagas disease transmission. *Annu Rev Entomol* 47:123–41.

Beaty BJ. 2000. Genetic manipulation of vectors: a potential novel approach for control of vector-borne diseases. *Proc Natl Acad Sci U S A* 97(19):10295–7.

Belgrader P, Benett W, Hadley D, Long G, Mariella R Jr, Milanovich F, Nasarabadi S, Nelson W, Richards J, Stratton P. 1998. Rapid pathogen detection using a microchip PCR array instrument. *Clin Chem* 44(10):2191–4.

Belgrader P, Hansford D, Kovacs GT, Venkateswaran K, Mariella R Jr, Milanovich F, Nasarabadi S, Okuzumi M, Pourahmadi F, Northrup MA. 1999a. A minisonicator to rapidly disrupt bacterial spores for DNA analysis. *Anal Chem* 71(19):4232–6.

Belgrader P, Benett W, Hadley D, Richards J, Stratton P, Mariella R Jr, Milanovich F. 1999b. PCR detection of bacteria in seven minutes. *Science* 284(5413):449–50.

Bellini WJ, Rota PA. 1998. Genetic diversity of wild-type measles viruses: implications for global measles elimination programs. *Emerg Infect Dis* 4(1):29–35.

Bender JB, Hedberg CW, Besser JM, Boxrud DJ, MacDonald KL, Osterholm MT. 1997. Surveillance by molecular subtype for *Escherichia coli* O157:H7 infections in Minnesota by molecular subtyping. *N Engl J Med* 337(6):388–94.

Beninati C, Oggioni MR, Boccanera M, Spinosa MR, Maggi T, Conti S, Magliani W, De Bernardis F, Teti G, Cassone A, Pozzi G, Polonelli L. 2000. Therapy of mucosal candidiasis by expression of an anti-idiotype in human commensal bacteria. *Nat Biotechnol* 18(10):1060–4.

Bergeron MG, Ouellette M. 1998. Preventing antibiotic resistance using rapid DNA-based diagnostic tests. *Infect Control Hosp Epidemiol* 19(8):560–4.

Berkman LF, Kawachi I, eds. 2000. *Social Epidemiology*. New York: Oxford University Press.

Bernstein E, Kaye D, Abrutyn E, Gross P, Dorfman M, Murasko DM. 1999. Immune response to influenza vaccination in a large healthy elderly population. *Vaccine* 17(1):82–94.

Bez C, Lodi G, Scully C, Porter SR. 2000. Genoprevalence of TT virus among clinical and auxiliary UK dental healthcare workers: a pilot study. *Br Dent J* 189(10):554–5.

Bhargava A, Jamison DT, Lau LJ, Murray CJ. 2001. Modeling the effects of health on economic growth. *J Health Econ* 20(3):423–40.

Black WC 4th, Baer CF, Antolin MF, DuTeau NM. 2001. Population genomics: genome-wide sampling of insect populations. *Annu Rev Entomol* 46:441–69.

Bloland PB. Drug Resistance in Malaria. 2001. Geneva: World Health Organization.

Bloom BR. 2002. Tuberculosis—the global view. *N Engl J Med* 346(19):1434–5.

Bloom DE, Sachs J. 1998. Geography, Demography, and Economic Growth in Africa. *Brookings Papers on Economic Activity* 2:207–295.

Blusch JH, Patience C, Martin U. 2002. Pig endogenous retroviruses and xenotransplantation. *Xenotransplantation* 9(4):242–51.

Boeing. 2002. Jetliner Safety: How Safe Is Flying. [Online]. Available: http://www.boeing.com/commercial/safety/pf/pf_howsafe.html.

Boete C, Koella JC. 2003. Evolutionary ideas about genetically manipulated mosquitoes and malaria control. *Trends Parasitol* 19(1):32–8.

Boone JD, Otteson EW, McGwire KC, Villard P, Rowe JE, St Jeor SC. 1998. Ecology and demographics of hantavirus infections in rodent populations in the Walker River Basin of Nevada and California. *Am J Trop Med Hyg* 59(3):445–51.

Braude R, Kon SK, Porter J. 1953. Antibiotics in nutrition. *Nutr Abstr Rev* 23:473–95.

Braunwald E, Fauci A, Kasper DL, Hauser SL, Longo DL, Jameson JL, eds. 2001. *Harrison's Principles of Internal Medicine*. 15th ed. New York: McGraw–Hill Companies.

Brinton LA. 1992. The epidemiology of cervical cancer—overview. In: Munoz N, Bosch FX, Shah KV, Meheus A, eds. *The Epidemiology of Cervical Cancer and Human Papillomavirus*. Lyon, France: International Agency for Research in Cancer. Pp. 3–23.

Brinton LA, Reeves WC, Brenes MM, Herrero R, Gaitan E, Tenorio F, de Britton RC, Garcia M, Rawls WE. 1989a. The male factor in the etiology of cervical cancer among sexually monogamous women. *Int J Cancer* 44(2):199–203.

Brinton LA, Reeves WC, Brenes MM, Herrero R, de Britton RC, Gaitan E, Tenorio F, Garcia M, Rawls WE. 1989b. Parity as a risk factor for cervical cancer. *Am J Epidemiol* 130(3):486–96.

Bryan FL. 1982. Diseases transmitted by foods (A classification and summary). 2nd edition. U.S. Department of Heath and Human Services, Centers for Disease Control. Atlanta: HHS Pub No. (CDC) 84–8237.

Burton EC, Nemetz PN. 2000. Medical error and outcomes measures: where have all the autopsies gone? *MedGenMed* E8.

Buzby JC, Roberts T. 1997. Economic costs and trade impacts of microbial foodborne illness. *World Health Stat Q* 50(1–2):57–66.

Cairns L, Blythe D, Kao A, Pappagianis D, Kaufman L, Kobayashi J, Hajjeh R. 2000. Outbreak of coccidioidomycosis in Washington state residents returning from Mexico. *Clin Infect Dis* 30(1):61–4.

Calhoun ES, McGovern RM, Janney CA, Cerhan JR, Iturria SJ, Smith DI, Gostout BS, Persing DH. 2002. Host genetic polymorphism analysis in cervical cancer. *Clin Chem* 48(8): 1218–24.

Calisher CH, Root JJ, Mills JN, Beaty BJ. 2002. Assessment of ecologic and biologic factors leading to hantavirus pulmonary syndrome, Colorado, U.S.A. *Croat Med J* 43(3):330–7.

Campbell LA, Kuo CC, Grayston JT. 1998. *Chlamydia pneumoniae* and cardiovascular disease. *Emerg Infect Dis* 4(4):571–9.

Campsmith ML, Nakashima AK, Jones JL. 2000. Association between crack cocaine use and high-risk sexual behaviors after HIV diagnosis. *J Acquir Immune Defic Syndr* 25(2):192–8.

Candinas D, Adams DH. 2000. Xenotransplantation: postponed by a millennium? *QJM* 93(2):63–6.

Carpenter C, Fayer R, Trout J, Beach MJ. 1999. Chlorine disinfection of recreational water for *Cryptosporidium parvum*. *Emerg Infect Dis* 5(4):579–84.

Carter R. 2001. Transmission blocking malaria vaccines. *Vaccine* 19(17–19):2309–14.

Cassell GH. 1998. Infectious causes of chronic inflammatory diseases and cancer. *Emerg Infect Dis* 4(3):475–87.

Cassell GH, Waites KB, Crouse DT. 1994. Mycoplasmal infections. In: Remington JS, KLein JO, eds. *Infectious Diseases of the Fetus and Newborn Infant*. 4th ed. Philadelphia: WB Saunders Co. Pp. 619-656.

Castro-Leal F, Dayton J, Demery L, Mehra K. 2000. Public spending on health care in Africa: do the poor benefit? *Bull World Health Org* 78(1):66–74.

CDC. 1983. Epidemiologic notes and reports interstate importation of measles following transmission in an airport—California, Washington, 1982. *MMWR* 32(16):215–216.

CDC. 1984. Cryptosporidiosis among children attending day care centers—Georgia, Pennsylvania, Michigan, California, New Mexico. *MMWR* 33(42):599–601.

CDC. 1994a. Coccidioidomycosis following the Northridge Earthquake—California, 1994. *MMWR* 43(10):194–5.

CDC. 1994b. Outbreak of pneumonia associated with a cruise ship, 1994. *MMWR* 43(28): 521.

CDC. 1994c. Update: outbreak of Legionnaires' disease associated with a cruise ship, 1994. *MMWR* 43(31):574–5.

CDC. 1994d. Update: human plague—India, 1994. *MMWR* 43(41):761–2.

CDC. 1995a. Outbreak of Ebola viral hemorrhagic fever—Zaire, 1995. *MMWR* 44(19):381–2.

CDC. 1995b. Update: outbreak of Ebola viral hemorrhagic fever—Zaire, 1995. *MMWR* 44(25):468–9, 475.

CDC. 1997a. Reduced susceptibility of *Staphylococcus aureus* to vancomycin—Japan, 1996. *MMWR* 46(27):624–6.

CDC. 1997b. Update: *Staphylococcus aureus* with reduced susceptibility to vancomycin—United States, 1997. *MMWR* 46(35):813–5.

CDC. 1997c. Update: influenza activity—United States, 1997–1998 season. *MMWR* 46(46): 1094–8.

CDC. 1998a. Outbreak of *Vibrio parahaemolyticus* infections associated with eating raw oysters—Pacific Northwest, 1997. *MMWR* 47(22):457–62.

CDC. 1998b. Report to the State of Iowa Department of Public Health on the Investigation of the Chemical and Microbial Constituents of Ground and Surface Water Proximal to Large-Scale Swine Operations. Atlanta, GA: Centers for Disease Control and Prevention.

CDC. 1998c. Preventing emerging infectious diseases: a strategy for the 21st century. Overview of the updated CDC plan. *MMWR* 47(No. RR-15):1–14.

CDC. 1998d. Rubella among crew members of commercial cruise ships—Florida, 1997. *MMWR* 46(52–53):1247–50.

CDC. 1999a. Resurgent bacterial sexually transmitted disease among men who have sex with men—King County, Washington, 1997–1999. *MMWR* 48(35):773–7.

CDC. 1999b. Increases in unsafe sex and rectal gonorrhea among men who have sex with men—San Francisco, California, 1994–1997. *MMWR* 48(3):45–8.

CDC. 1999c. Outbreaks of *Shigella sonnei* infection associated with eating fresh parsley—United States and Canada, July–August 1998. *MMWR* 48(14):285–9.

CDC. 2000a. HIV/AIDS Surveillance Report. Atlanta, GA: Centers for Disease Control and Prevention. 12(2):1–44.

CDC. 2000b. Biological and chemical terrorism: strategic plan for preparedness and response. Recommendations of the CDC Strategic Planning Workgroup. *MMWR Recomm Rep* 49(RR-4):1–14.

CDC. 2000c. Outbreak of Rift Valley fever—Yemen, August–October 2000. *MMWR* 49(47): 1065–6.

CDC. 2000d. Serogroup W135 meningococcal disease among travelers returning from Saudi Arabia—United States, 2000. *MMWR* 49(16):345–6.

CDC. 2000e. Monitoring hospital-acquired infections to promote patient safety—United States, 1990–1999. *MMWR* 49(8):149–53.

CDC. 2000f. Integration Project: National Electronic Disease Surveillance System. [Online]. Available: http://www.cdc.gov/od/hissb/act_int.htm [accessed January 31, 2003].

CDC. 2001a. HIV/AIDS Surveillance Report. Atlanta, GA: Centers for Disease Control and Prevention. *MMWR* 13(2):1–44.

CDC. 2001b. Methicillin-resistant *Staphylococcus aureus* skin or soft tissue infections in a state prison—Mississippi, 2000. *MMWR* 50(42):919–22.

CDC. 2001c. Cancer Prevention and Control: Breast and Cervical Cancer Facts. The National Breast and Cervical Cancer Early Detection Program. [Online]. Available: http://www.cdc.gov/cancer/nbccedp/anniversary/ facts.htm [accessed February 21, 2003].

CDC. 2001d. Outbreak of acute respiratory febrile illness among college students—Acapulco, Mexico, March 2001. *MMWR* 50(14):261–2.

CDC. 2001e. Mycotic Disease Listing. National Center for Infectious Diseases–Division of Bacterial and Mycotic Diseases. [Online]. Available: http://www.cdc.gov/ncidod/dbmd/ [accessed February 21, 2003].

CDC. 2001f. Sexually Transmitted Diseases Surveillance, 2000. Atlanta: U.S. Department of Health and Human Services, Centers for Disease Control and Prevention.

CDC. 2001g. Risk for meningococcal disease associated with the Hajj 2001. *MMWR* 50(6): 97–8.

CDC. 2001h. Update: assessment of risk for meningococcal disease associated with the Hajj 2001. *MMWR* 50(12):221–2.

CDC. 2001i. Influenza B virus outbreak on a cruise ship—Northern Europe, 2000. *MMWR* 50(8):137–40.

CDC. 2001j. Importation of Nonhuman Primates: Foreign Quarantine regulations Relating to NHP (42CFR71.53). [Online]. Available: http://www.cdc.gov/ncidod/dq/nonhuman. htm [accessed February 18, 2003].

CDC. 2001k. Measles History. National Immunization Program. [Online]. Available: http:// www.cdc.gov/nip/diseases/measles/history.htm [accessed February 18, 2003].

CDC. 2001l. Unexplained deaths following knee surgery—Minnesota, November 2001. *MMWR* 50(46):1035–6.

CDC. 2001m. Dengue Fever: CDC Dengue Fever Home Page. [Online]. Available: http:// www.cdc.gov/ncidod/dvbid/dengue/ [accessed February 18, 2003].

CDC. 2001n. The Autopsy, Medicine, and Mortality Statistics. National Center for Health Statistics. *Vital Health Stat* 3(32).

CDC. 2001o. Public Health Action Plan to Combat Antimicrobial Resistance. National Center for Infectious Diseases, Centers for Disease Control and Prevention. Atlanta, GA [Online]. Available: http://www.cdc.gov/drugresistance/actionplan/html/index.htm [accessed January 30, 2003].

CDC. 2002a. Epidemiology and Prevention of Vaccine—Preventable Diseases. Washington, DC: Public Health Foundation.

CDC. 2002b. Smallpox Overview. [Online]. Available: http://www.bt.cdc.gov/agent/small-pox/overview/overview.pdf [accessed February 21, 2003].

CDC. 2002c. Local transmission of *Plasmodium vivax* Malaria—Virginia, 2002. *MMWR* 51:931–923.

CDC. 2002d. *Staphylococcus aureus* resistant to vancomycin—United States, 2002. *MMWR* 51(26):565–7.

CDC. 2002e. Increases in *fluoroquinolone-resistant Neisseria gonorrhoeae*—Hawaii and California, 2001. *MMWR* 51(46):1041–1044.

CDC. 2002f. Drug-Associated HIV Transmission Continues in the United States. National Center for HIV, STD and TB Prevention–Division of HIV/AIDS Prevention. [Online]. Available: http://www.cdc.gov/hiv/ pubs/facts/idu.htm [accessed February 14, 2003].

CDC. 2002g. Trends in sexual risk behaviors among high school students—United States, 1991–2001. *MMWR* 51(38):856–9.

CDC. 2002h. Sexually Transmitted Disease Surveillance, 2001. Atlanta: U.S. Department of Health and Human Services.

CDC. 2002i. Investigations of West Nile virus infections in recipients of blood transfusions. *MMWR* 51(43):973–4.

CDC. 2002j. Update: allograft-associated bacterial infections—United States, 2002. *MMWR* 51(10):207–10.

CDC. 2002l. Malaria surveillance—United States, 2000. *MMWR* 51(SS05):9–21.

CDC. 2002m. Outbreaks of gastroenteritis associated with noroviruses on cruise ships—United States, 2002. *MMWR* 51(49):1112–5.

CDC. 2002n. The National Molecular Subtyping Network for Foodborne Disease Surveillance. [Online]. Available: http://www.cdc.gov/pulsenet/ index.htm [accessed February 18, 2003].

CDC. 2002o. Press Release: CDC Releases New Hand-Hygiene Guidelines. [Online]. Available: www.cdc.gov/od/oc/media/pressrel/r021025.htm [accessed February 18, 2003].

CDC. 2002p. Measles—United States, 2000. *MMWR* 51(6):120–3.

CDC. 2002q. Press Release: Measles no longer endemic in the United States. [Online]. Available: http://www.cdc.gov/od/oc/media/pressrel/r020429.htm [accessed February 21, 2003].

CDC. 2002r. Protecting the Nation's health in an Era of Globalization. CDC's Global Infectious Disease Strategy. Atlanta, GA: Center for Disease Control and Prevention.

CDC. 2002s. Programs in Brief Epidemic Information Exchange (Epi–X). [Online]. Available: http://www.cdc.gov/programs/research5.htm [accessed January 30, 2003].

CDC. 2002t. National Electronic Disease Surveillance System. [Online]. Available: http://www.cdc.gov/nedss/ [accessed January 31, 2003].

CDC. 2002u. National Center for Infectious Diseases: Surveillance Resources, Emerging Infections Program. [Online]. Available: http://www.cdc.gov /ncidod/osr/EIP.htm [accessed January 30, 2003].

CDC. 2002v. Special Pathogens Branch, Division of Viral and Rickettsial Diseases, unpublished data.

CDC. 2002w. New Variant CJD: Fact Sheet. [Online]. Available: http://www.cdc.gov/od/oc/media/pressrel/fs020418.htm [accessed February 27, 2003].

CDC. 2002x. All About Hantavirus. National Center for Infectious Diseases–Special Pathogens Branch. [Online]. Available: http://www.cdc.gov/ncidod/diseases/hanta/hps/noframes/hpsslideset/index.htm [accessed March 4, 2003].

CDC. 2003a. Biological Diseases/Agents. [Online]. Available: http://www.bt. cdc.gov/ agent/agentlist.asp#categoryadiseases [accessed February 21, 2003].

CDC. 2003b. Nationally Notifiable Infectious Diseases. [Online]. Available: http://www.cdc. gov/epo/dphsi/PHS/infdis.htm [accessed January 30, 2003].

CDC. 2003c. West Nile Virus Update: Current Case Count. [Online]. Available: http://www.cdc.gov/od/oc/media/wncount.htm [accessed February 27, 2003].

Center for Infectious Disease Research and Policy (CIDRAP). 2002. Providing a Framework for Public Health Bioterrorism Preparedness: Public Health Workforce, Collaboration, and Infrastructure Issues. Washington, DC. [Online]. Available: http://www1.umn.edu/cidrap/center/mission /papers/btworkforce.html [accessed January 30, 2003].

Center for Science in the Public Interest (CSPI). 1998. Protecting the Crown Jewels: A Strategic Plan to Preserve the Effectiveness of Antibiotics. [Online]: Available: http://www.cspinet.org/reports/abiotic.htm [accessed January 30, 2003].

Chamberland ME, Epstein J, Dodd RY, Persing D, Will RG, DeMaria A Jr, Emmanuel JC, Pierce B, Khabbaz R. 1998. Blood safety. *Emerg Infect Dis* 4(3):410–1.

Chamberland ME, Alter HJ, Busch MP, Nemo G, Ricketts M. 2001. Emerging infectious disease issues in blood safety. *Emerg Infect Dis* 7(3 Suppl):552–3.

Chambers HF. 2001. The changing epidemiology of *Staphylococcus aureus*? *Emerg Infect Dis* 7(2):178–82.

Chandra RK. 1997. Nutrition and the immune system: an introduction. *Am J Clin Nutr* 66(2):460S–463S.

Chandrasekaran S, Lalithakumari D. 1998. Plasmid-mediated rifampicin resistance in *Pseudomonas fluorescens*. *J Med Microbiol* 47(3):197–200.

Chapman LE, Bloom ET. 2001. Clinical xenotransplantation. *JAMA* 285(18):2304–6.

Chee–Sanford JC, Aminov RI, Krapac IJ, Garrigues–Jeanjean N, Mackie RI. 2001. Occurrence and diversity of tetracycline resistance genes in lagoons and groundwater underlying two swine production facilities. *Appl Environ Microbiol* 67(4):1494–502.

Chen DK, McGeer A, de Azavedo JC, Low DE. 1999. Decreased susceptibility of *Streptococcus pneumoniae* to fluoroquinolones in Canada. Canadian Bacterial Surveillance Network. *N Engl J Med* 341(4):233–9.

Chen Z, Ge Y, Landman N, Kang JX. 2002a. Decreased expression of the mannose 6-phosphate/insulin-like growth factor-II receptor promotes growth of human breast cancer cells. *BMC Cancer* 2(1):18.

Chen SY, Gibson S, Katz MH, Klausner JD, Dilley JW, Schwarcz SK, Kellogg TA, McFarland W. 2002b. Continuing increases in sexual risk behavior and sexually transmitted diseases among men who have sex with men: San Francisco, Calif, 1999–2001, USA. *Am J Pub Health* 92(9):1387–8.

Childs JE, Ksiazek TG, Spiropoulou CF, Krebs JW, Morzunov S, Maupin GO, Gage KL, Rollin PE, Sarisky J, Enscore RE, et al. 1994. Serologic and genetic identification of *Peromyscus maniculatus* as the primary rodent reservoir for a new hantavirus in the southwestern United States. *J Infect Dis* 169(6):1271–80.

Chin J, ed. 2000. *Control of Communicable Diseases Manual.* 17th ed. Washington, DC: American Public Health Association.

Chua KB, Bellini WJ, Rota PA, Harcourt BH, Tamin A, Lam SK, Ksiazek TG, Rollin PE, Zaki SR, Shieh W, Goldsmith CS, Gubler DJ, Roehrig JT, Eaton B, Gould AR, et al. 2000. Nipah virus: a recently emergent deadly paramyxovirus. *Science* 288(5470):1432–5.

Chukwuani CM. 1999. Socio-economic implication of multi-drug resistant malaria in the community; how prepared is Nigeria for this emerging problem? *West Afr J Med* 18(4): 303–6.

Cohen ML. 2000. Changing patterns of infectious disease. *Nature* 406(6797):762–7.

Coker R. 2001. Control of tuberculosis in Russia. *Lancet* 358(9280):434–5.

Cole LA. 1997. *The Eleventh Plague: The Politics of Biological and Chemical Warfare.* New York: WH Freeman and Company.

Connolly M, Programme on Communicable Diseases in Complex Emergencies. 2002. Communicable diseases. *Action Against Infection: A Newsletter for the World Health Organization and Its Partners* 3(2):1–4.

Conway DJ, Roper C. 2000. Micro-evolution and emergence of pathogens. *Int J Parasitol* 30(12–13):1423–30.

Cooper RS, Osotimehin B, Kaufman JS, Forrester T. 1998. Disease burden in sub-Saharan Africa: what should we conclude in the absence of data? *Lancet* 351(9097):208–10.

Coughlan E, Mindel A, Estcourt CS. 2001. Male clients of female commercial sex workers: HIV, STDs and risk behaviour. *Int J STD AIDS* 12(10):665–9.

Cox NJ, Subbarao K. 2000. Global epidemiology of influenza: past and present. *Annu Rev Med* 51:407–21.

Cunningham-Rundles S and Nesin M. 2000. Bacterial infections in the immunocompromised host. In: Nataro J, Blaser M, Cunningham-Rundles S, eds. *Persistent Bacterial Infections.* Washington, DC: ASM Press. Pp. 145–163.

Daar AS. 1999. Animal-to-human organ transplants—a solution or a new problem? *Bull World Health Organ* 77(1):54–61.

Danesh J, Newton R, Beral V. 1997. Epidemiology. A human germ project? *Nature* 389(6646):21, 23–4.

Davis CJ. 1999. Nuclear blindness: An overview of the biological weapons programs of the former Soviet Union and Iraq. *Emerg Infect Dis* 5(4):509–12.

Davis R, Kimball AM. 2001. The economics of emerging infections in the Asia Pacific region: what do we know and what do we need to know? In: Price-Smith AT, ed. *Plagues and Politics: Infectious Disease and International Policy.* New York: Palgrave Macmillan.

Day JF, Duxbury CV, Glasscock S, Pganessi JE. 2001. Removal trapping for the control of coastal biting midge populations. *Technical Bulletin Florida Control Association* 3:15–16.

De Grandis SA, Stevenson RM. 1985. Antimicrobial susceptibility patterns and R plasmid–mediated resistance of the fish pathogen *Yersinia ruckeri. Antimicrob Agents Chemother* 27(6):938–42.

de The G. 1995. Viruses and human cancers: challenges for preventive strategies. *Environ Health Perspect* 103 Suppl 8:269–73.

De Tott F. 1973. *Memoirs of Baron De Tott.* New York: Arno Press.

Dennis DT, Inglesby TV, Henderson DA, Bartlett JG, Ascher MS, Eitzen E, Fine AD, Friedlander AM, Hauer J, Layton M, Lillibridge SR, McDade JE, Osterholm MT, et al. 2001. Tularemia as a biological weapon: medical and public health management. *JAMA* 285(21):2763–73.

Denver Summit of the Eight. 1997. Communique. Denver, June 22, 1997. [Online] Available: http://usinfo.state.gov/topical/econ/group8/summit97/document.htm [accessed January 30, 2003].

Department of Defense–Global Emerging Infections System (DoD–GEISWeb). 2002. ESSENCE: Web Instructions. Electronic Surveillance System for the Early Notification of Community–Based Epidemics. [Online]. Available: http://www.geis.ha.osd.mil/GEIS/SurveillanceActivities/ESSENCE/ESSENCEinstructions.asp [accessed January 30, 2003].

DHHS (U.S. Department of Health and Human Services). 2000a. HHS Fact Sheet. HHS Guidelines for Xenotransplantation Safety. [Online]. Available: http://www.hhs.gov/news/press/2000pres/20000526.html [accessed March 4, 2003].

DHHS. 2000b. Healthy People 2010: 2nd ed. With Understanding and Improving Health and Objectives for Improving Health. 2 vols. Washington, DC: U.S. Government Printing Office.

DHHS, CDC, NIH. 1999. Biosafety in Microbiological and Biomedical Laboratories. 4th ed. HHS Publication No. (CDC) 93–8395. Washington, DC: U.S. Government Printing Office.

Diaz-Bonilla E, Babinard J, Pinstrup–Anderson P. 2001. Globalization and Health: A Survey of Opportunities and Risks for the Poor in Developing Counties. CMH Working Paper Series No. WG4: 11. Cambridge, MA: Commission on Globalization and Health.

DiMasi JA, Hansen RW, Grabowski HG, Lasagna L. 1991. Cost of innovation in the pharmaceutical industry. *J Health Econ* 10(2):107–42.

Dixon DM, McNeil MM, Cohen ML, Gellin BG, La Montagne JR. 1996. Fungal infections: a growing threat. *Public Health Rep* 111(3):226–35.

Dixon S, McDonald S, Roberts J. 2002. The impact of HIV and AIDS on Africa's economic development. *BMJ* 324(7331):232–4.

Doebbeling BN, Stanley GL, Sheetz CT, Pfaller MA, Houston AK, Annis L, Li N, Wenzel RP. 1992. Comparative efficacy of alternative hand–washing agents in reducing nosocomial infections in intensive care units. *N Engl J Med* 327(2):88–93.

Dumler JS, Valsamakis A. 1999. Molecular diagnostics for existing and emerging infections. Complementary tools for a new era of clinical microbiology. *Am J Clin Pathol* 112(Suppl 1):S33–9.

Dye C, Scheele S, Dolin P, Pathania V, Raviglione MC. 1999. Consensus statement. Global burden of tuberculosis: estimated incidence, prevalence, and mortality by country. WHO Global Surveillance and Monitoring Project. *JAMA* 282(7):677–86.

Dyke MP, Grauaug A, Kohan R, Ott K, Andrews R. 1993. *Ureaplasma urealyticum* in a neonatal intensive care population. *J Paediatr Child Health* 29(4):295–7.

Eandi M, Zara GP. 1998. Economic impact of resistance in the community. *Int J Clin Pract Suppl* 95:27–38.

Economic Research Service. 2001. U.S. Department of Agriculture. Research Emphasis–food safety: features. [Online]. Available: http://www.ers.usda.gov/emphases/safefood/features. htm [accessed February 3, 2003].

Edlin BR, Irwin KL, Faruque S, McCoy CB, Word C, Serrano Y, Inciardi JA, Bowser BP, Schilling RF, Holmberg SD. 1994. Intersecting epidemics—crack cocaine use and HIV infection among inner–city young adults. Multicenter Crack Cocaine and HIV Infection Study Team. *N Engl J Med* 331(21):1422–7.

Edmond MB, Wallace SE, McClish DK, Pfaller MA, Jones RN, Wenzel RP. 1999. Nosocomial bloodstream infections in United States hospitals: a three–year analysis. *Clin Infect Dis* 29(2):239–44.

Effler P, Ching–Lee M, Bogard A, Ieong MC, Nekomoto T, Jernigan D. 1999. Statewide system of electronic notifiable disease reporting from clinical laboratories: comparing automated reporting with conventional methods. *JAMA* 282(19):1845–50.

Ekeus R. 1999. Biological inspections in Iraq. In: Drell SD, Sofaer AD, Wilson GD, eds. *The New Terror: Facing the Threat of Biological and Chemical Weapons.* Stanford, CA: Hoover Institution Press. Pp. 237–254.

El Alamy MA, Cline BL. 1977. Prevalence and intensity of *Schistosoma haematobium* and *S. mansoni* infection in Qalyub, Egypt. *Am J Trop Med Hyg* 26(3):470–2.

Elder RO, Keen JE, Siragusa GR, Barkocy–Gallagher GA, Koohmaraie M, Laegreid WW. 2000. Correlation of enterohemorrhagic *Escherichia coli* O157 prevalence in feces, hides, and carcasses of beef cattle during processing. *Proc Natl Acad Sci U S A* 97(7):2999–3003.

Elliott LH, Ksiazek TG, Rollin PE, Spiropoulou CF, Morzunov S, Monroe M, Goldsmith CS, Humphrey CD, Zaki SR, Krebs JW, et al. 1994. Isolation of the causative agent of hantavirus pulmonary syndrome. *Am J Trop Med Hyg* 51(1):102–8.

Emborg H, Ersboll AK, Heuer OE, Wegener HC. 2001. The effect of discontinuing the use of antimicrobial growth promoters on the productivity in the Danish broiler production. *Prev Vet Med* 50(1–2):53–70.

Epstein SE, Zhou YF, Zhu J. 1999. Infection and atherosclerosis: emerging mechanistic paradigms. *Circulation* 100(4):e20–8.

Esiobu N, Armenta L, Ike J. 2002. Antibiotic resistance in soil and water environments. *Int J Environ Health Res* 12(2):133–44.

FAO (Food and Agriculture Organization of the United Nations). 2001. FAO Global Information and Early Warning System (GIEWS). Food supply situation and crop prospects in sub-Saharan Africa. Africa Report. No.1. Rome: FAO/GIEWS.

Farmer P. 1996. Social inequalities and emerging infectious diseases. *Emerg Infect Dis* 2(4): 259–69.

Fauci AS. 2001. Infectious diseases: considerations for the 21st century. *Clin Infect Dis* 32(5):675–85.

Fayer R. 2000. Presidential address. Global change and emerging infectious diseases. *J Parasitol* 86(6):1174–81.

Fayer R, Ungar BL. 1986. *Cryptosporidium* spp. and cryptosporidiosis. *Microbiol Rev* 50(4): 458–83.

FDA (Food and Drug Administration). 2000. FDA Task Force on Antimicrobial Resistance: Key Recommendations and Report. Washington, DC. [Online]. Available: http://www. fda.gov/oc/antimicrobial/taskforce 2000.html [accessed January 30, 2003].

FDA. 2001. Antibiotic resistance from down on the chicken farm. FDA Consumer Magazine. [Online]. Available: http://www.fda.gov/fdac/ features/2001/101_chic.html [accessed March 4, 2003].

Federation of American Scientists (FAS). 2002. Crimean–Congo Hemorrhagic Fever and America's War on Terrorism. [Online]. Available: http://www.fas.org/ahead/disease/cchf/ outbreak/2001afg.htm [accessed February 10, 2003].

Feldman M, Cryer B, McArthur KE, Huet BA, Lee E. 1996. Effects of aging and gastritis on gastric acid and pepsin secretion in humans: a prospective study. *Gastroenterology* 110(4):1043–52.

Fey PD, Safranek TJ, Rupp ME, Dunne EF, Ribot E, Iwen PC, Bradford PA, Angulo FJ, Hinrichs SH. 2000. Ceftriaxone-resistant salmonella infection acquired by a child from cattle. *N Engl J Med* 342(17):1242–9.

Field AK, Laughlin CA. 1999. In: Granoff A, Webster R, eds. *Encyclopedia of Virology*, vol. 1. 2nd ed. San Diego, CA: Academic Press. Pp. 54–68.

Fine A, Layton M. 2001. Lessons from the West Nile viral encephalitis outbreak in New York City, 1999: implications for bioterrorism preparedness. *Clin Infect Dis* 32(2):277–82.

Fisher-Hoch SP, Tomori O, Nasidi A, Perez–Oronoz GI, Fakile Y, Hutwagner L, McCormick JB. 1995. Review of cases of nosocomial Lassa fever in Nigeria: the high price of poor medical practice. *BMJ* 311(7009):857–9.

Fleming DT, Wasserheit JN. 1999. From epidemiological synergy to public health policy and practice: the contribution of other sexually transmitted diseases to sexual transmission of HIV infection. *Sex Transm Infect* 75(1):3–17.

Flint J, Harding RM, Boyce AJ, Clegg JB. 1993. The population genetics of the haemo-globinopathies. *Baillieres Clin Haematol* 6(1):215–62.

Focks DA, Daniels E, Haile DG, Keesling JE. 1995. A simulation model of the epidemiology of urban dengue fever: literature analysis, model development, preliminary validation, and samples of simulation results. *Am J Trop Med Hyg* 53(5):489–506.

Fonseca DM, Campbell S, Crans WJ, Mogi M, Miyagi I, Toma T, Bullians M, Andreadis TG, Berry RL, Pagac B, Sardelis MR, Wilkerson RC. 2001. *Aedes* (Finlaya) *japonicus* (Diptera: Culicidae), a newly recognized mosquito in the United States: analyses of genetic variation in the United States and putative source populations. *J Med Entomol* 38(2): 135–46.

Foy BD, Killeen GF, Magalhaes T, Beier JC. In press. Immunological targeting of critical insect antigens. *Amer Entomol*.

Francis E. 1921. Tularaemia: Francis 1921. I. The occurrence of tularemia in nature as a disease of Man. *Public Helth Rep* 36:1731–8.

Franco EL, Duarte–Franco E, Ferenczy A. 2001. Cervical cancer: epidemiology, prevention and the role of human papillomavirus infection. *CMAJ* 164(7):1017–25.

Frank B. 2000. An overview of heroin trends in New York City: past, present and future. *Mt Sinai J Med* 67(5–6):340–6.

French GL, Ling J, Chow KL, Mark KK. 1987. Occurrence of multiple antibiotic resistance and R–plasmids in gram–negative bacteria isolated from faecally contaminated freshwater streams in Hong Kong. *Epidemiol Infect* 98(3):285–99.

Fuller R. 1989. Probiotics in man and animals. *J Appl Bacteriol* 66(5):365–78.

Galambos L, Sewell JE. 1995. *Networks of Innovation: Vaccine Development at Merck, Sharp & Dohme, and Mulford, 1895–1995*. New York: Cambridge University Press.

Galimand M, Guiyoule A, Gerbaud G, Rasoamanana B, Chanteau S, Carniel E, Courvalin P. 1997. Multidrug resistance in *Yersinia pestis* mediated by a transferable plasmid. *N Engl J Med* 337(10):677–80.

Gant V, Parton S. 2000. Community-acquired pneumonia. *Curr Opin Pulm Med* 6(3):226–33.

GAO (U.S. General Accounting Office). 1995. Animal agriculture: information on waste management and water quality issues. GAO/RCED–95–200BR. Washington, DC: GAO.

GAO. 1999. Food Safety: The Agricultural Use of Antibiotics and Its Implications for Human Health. GAO/RCED–99–74. Washington, DC: GAO.

GAO. 2002. Childhood Vaccines: Challenges in Preventing Future Shortages. Statement of Janet Heinrich, Director, Health Care–Public Health Issues. Testimony before the Subcommittee on Public Health, Committee on Health, Education, Labor, and Pensions, US Senate. GAO–02–1105T. Washington, DC: GAO

Gao X, Nelson GW, Karacki P, Martin MP, Phair J, Kaslow R, Goedert JJ, Buchbinder S, Hoots K, Vlahov D, O'Brien SJ, Carrington M. 2001. Effect of a single amino acid change in MHC class I molecules on the rate of progression to AIDS. *N Engl J Med* 344(22):1668–75.

Garcia–Sastre A. 2002. Mechanisms of inhibition of the host interferon alpha/beta–mediated antiviral responses by viruses. *Microbes Infect* 4(6):647–55.

Garrett ES, dos Santos CL, Jahncke ML. 1997. Public, animal, and environmental health implications of aquaculture. *Emerg Infect Dis* 3(4):453–7.

Garrett L. 1989. Emerging viruses, growing concerns. *Newsday* 30:1.

Garrett L. 1995. *The Coming Plague*. New York: Penguin Books.

Garrett L. 1998. Social, behavioral, and demographic factors in emerging infections. *J Urban Health* 75(3):492–500.

Gewolb J, ed. 2001. Random samples: the perils of pilgrimage. *Science* 294(5550):2285.

Gilmore Commission. 2000. Second Annual Report of the Advisory Panel to Assess Domestic Response Capabilities for Terrorism Involving Weapons of Mass Destruction. Toward a National Strategy for Combating Terrorism. Arlington, VA: RAND.

Gionchetti P, Rizzello F, Venturi A, Brigidi P, Matteuzzi D, Bazzocchi G, Poggioli G, Miglioli M, Campieri M. 2000. Oral bacteriotherapy as maintenance treatment in patients with chronic pouchitis: a double–blind, placebo-controlled trial. *Gastroenterology* 119(2):305–9.

Glass GE, Watson AJ, LeDuc JW, Childs JE. 1994. Domestic cases of hemorrhagic fever with renal syndrome in the United States. *Nephron* 68(1):48–51.

Glass GE, Cheek JE, Patz JA, Shields TM, Doyle TJ, Thoroughman DA, Hunt DK, Enscore RE, Gage KL, Irland C, Peters CJ, Bryan R. 2000. Using remotely sensed data to identify areas at risk for hantavirus pulmonary syndrome. *Emerg Infect Dis* 6(3):238–47.

Goh KJ, Tan CT, Chew NK, Tan PS, Kamarulzaman A, Sarji SA, Wong KT, Abdullah BJ, Chua KB, Lam SK. 2000. Clinical features of Nipah virus encephalitis among pig farmers in Malaysia. *N Engl J Med* 342(17):1229–35.

GOMA Epidemiology Group. 1995. Public health impact of Rwandan refugee crisis: what happened in Goma, Zaire, in July, 1994? Goma Epidemiology Group. *Lancet* 345(8946):339–44.

Gonzales R, Malone DC, Maselli JH, Sande MA. 2001. Excessive antibiotic use for acute respiratory infections in the United States. *Clin Infect Dis* 33(6):757–62.

Gorbach SL. 2001. Antimicrobial use in animal feed-time to stop. *N Engl J Med* 345(16):1202–3.

Gorrochotequi-Escalante N, Gomez-Machorro C, Lozano-Fuentes S, Fernandez-Salas I, De Lourdes, Munoz M, Farfan-Ale J, Beaty BJ, Black WC. 2002. The breeding structure of *Aedes aegypti* populations in Mexico varies by region. *Am J Trop Med Hyg* 66(2):213-22.

Gostin LO. 2001a. Public health law reform. *Am J Pub Health* 91(9):1365–8.

Gostin LO. 2001b. *Public Health Law: Power, Duty, Restraint*. Berkeley and New York: University of California Press and Milbank Memorial Fund.

Gostin LO. 2002. *Public Health Law and Ethics: A Reader*. Berkeley and New York: University of California Press and Milbank Memorial Fund.

Gostin LO, Burris S, Lazzarini Z. 1999. The law and the public's health: a study of infectious disease law in the United States. *Columbia Law Rev* 99(1):59–128.

Gostin LO, Sapsin JW, Teret SP, Burris S, Mair JS, Hodge JG Jr, Vernick JS. 2002. The Model State Emergency Health Powers Act: planning for and response to bioterrorism and naturally occurring infectious diseases. *JAMA* 288(5):622–8.

Grattan LM, Oldach D, Perl TM, Lowitt MH, Matuszak DL, Dickson C, Parrott C, Shoemaker RC, Kauffman CL, Wasserman MP, Hebel JR, Charache P, Morris JG Jr. 1998. Learning and memory difficulties after environmental exposure to waterways containing toxin–producing *Pfiesteria* or *Pfiesteria*–like dinoflagellates. *Lancet* 352(9127):532–9.

Gratz NG. 1999. Emerging and resurging vector-borne diseases. *Annu Rev Entomol* 44:51–75.

Gray MW, Burger G, Lang BF. 1999. Mitochondrial evolution. *Science* 283(5407):1476–81.

Greenberg BL, Semba RD, Vink PE, Farley JJ, Sivapalasingam M, Steketee RW, Thea DM, Schoenbaum EE. 1997. Vitamin A deficiency and maternal–infant transmissions of HIV in two metropolitan areas in the United States. *AIDS* 11(3):325–32.

Greenko JA, Mostashari F, Fine A, Layton M. 2002 (March 24–27). Clinical validation study of the EMS 911 syndromic surveillance system for bioterrorism or pandemic influenza in New York City. International Conference on Emerging Infectious Diseases. Atlanta. CDC.

Griffin DW, Kellogg CA, Shinn EA. 2001. Dust in the wind: Long range transport of dust in the atmosphere and its implications for global public and ecosystem health. *Global Change and Human Health* 2(1):20–33.

Groisman EA, Ochman H. 1996. Pathogenicity islands: bacterial evolution in quantum leaps. *Cell* 87(5):791–4.

Groom AV, Wolsey DH, Naimi TS, Smith K, Johnson S, Boxrud D, Moore KA, Cheek JE. 2001. Community-acquired methicillin-resistant *Staphylococcus aureus* in a rural American Indian community. *JAMA* 286(10):1201–5.

Gruebler A, Nakicenovic N. 1991. The Evolution of Transport Systems: Past and Future. Research Report RR–91–008. Laxenburg, Vienna: International Institute for Applied Systems Analysis.

Gryseels B, Stelma FF, Talla I, van Dam GJ, Polman K, Sow S, Diaw M, Sturrock RF, Doehring–Schwerdtfeger E, Kardorff R, et al. 1994. Epidemiology, immunology and chemotherapy of *Schistosoma mansoni* infections in a recently exposed community in Senegal. *Trop Geogr Med* 46(4 Spec No):209–19.

Gubareva LV, Robinson MJ, Bethell RC, Webster RG. 1997. Catalytic and framework mutations in the neuraminidase active site of influenza viruses that are resistant to 4-guanidino–Neu5Ac2en. *J Virol* 71(5):3385–90.

Gubareva LV, Matrosovich MN, Brenner MK, Bethell RC, Webster RG. 1998. Evidence for zanamivir resistance in an immunocompromised child infected with influenza B virus. *J Infect Dis* 178(5):1257–62.

Gubareva LV, Kaiser L, Hayden FG. 2000. Influenza virus neuraminidase inhibitors. *Lancet* 355(9206):827–35.

Gubler DJ. 1998. Resurgent vector-borne diseases as a global health problem. *Emerg Infect Dis* 4(3):442–50.

Gubler DJ. 2001. Human arbovirus infections worldwide. *Ann N Y Acad Sci* 951:13–24.

Gubler DJ. 2002. Epidemic dengue/dengue hemorrhagic fever as a public health, social and economic problem in the 21st century. *Trends Microbiol* 10(2):100–3.

Guermonprez P, Valladeau J, Zitvogel L, Thery C, Amigorena S. 2002. Antigen presentation and T cell stimulation by dendritic cells. *Annu Rev Immunol* 20:621–67.

Guerrant RL, Schorling JB, McAuliffe JF, de Souza MA. 1992. Diarrhea as a cause and an effect of malnutrition: diarrhea prevents catch-up growth and malnutrition increases diarrhea frequency and duration. *Am J Trop Med Hyg* 47(1 Pt 2):28–35.

Gunn RA, Montes JM, Toomey KE, Rolfs RT, Greenspan JR, Spitters CE, Waterman SH. 1995. Syphilis in San Diego County 1983–1992: crack cocaine, prostitution, and the limitations of partner notification. *Sex Transm Dis* 22(1):60–6.

Gustafson P, Gomes VF, Vieira CS, Jensen H, Seng R, Norberg R, Samb B, Naucler A, Aaby P. 2001. Tuberculosis mortality during a civil war in Guinea–Bissau. *JAMA* 286(5):599–603.

Gwatkin DR. 2000. Health inequalities and the health of the poor: what do we know? What can we do? *Bull World Health Organ* 78(1):3–18.

Gwatkin DR, Guillot M, Heuveline P. 1999. The burden of disease among the global poor. *Lancet* 354(9178):586–9.

Hacker J, Kaper JB. 2000. Pathogenicity islands and the evolution of microbes. *Annu Rev Microbiol* 54:641–79.

Hacker J, Blum–Oehler G, Muhldorfer I, Tschape H. 1997. Pathogenicity islands of virulent bacteria: structure, function and impact on microbial evolution. *Mol Microbiol* 23(6):1089–97.

Haldane JBS. 1949. Disease and Evolution. *La Ricerca Scientifica* Suppl A(19):68–76.

Hamblin MT, Thompson EE, Di Rienzo A. 2002. Complex signatures of natural selection at the Duffy blood group locus. *Am J Hum Genet* 70(2):369–83.

Hamscher G, Sczesny S, Hoper H, Nau H. 2002. Determination of persistent tetracycline residues in soil fertilized with liquid manure by high-performance liquid chromatography with electrospray ionization tandem mass spectrometry. *Anal Chem* 74(7):1509–18.

Handszuh, HF, Chief, Quality of Tourism Development. 2001 (February 22–23). Symposium on Tourism Services. Geneva. World Tourism Organization (WTO-OMT).

Hansen RW. 1979. The pharmaceutical development process: estimates of current development costs and times and the effects of regulatory changes. In: Chien RI, ed. *Issues in Pharmaceutical Economics.* Lexington, MA: Lexington Books. Pp.151–187.

Hanzlick R, Baker P. 1998. Case of the month: institutional autopsy rates. Autopsy Committee of the College of American Pathologists. *Arch Intern Med* 158(11):1171–2.

Harries AD, Maher D. 1996. *TB/HIV A Clinical Manual.* Geneva: WHO.

Haruma K, Kamada T, Kawaguchi H, Okamoto S, Yoshihara M, Sumii K, Inoue M, Kishimoto S, Kajiyama G, Miyoshi A. 2000. Effect of age and *Helicobacter pylori* infection on gastric acid secretion. *J Gastroenterol Hepatol* 15(3):277–83.

Hasson J, Schneiderman H. 1995. Autopsy training programs. To right a wrong. *Arch Pathol Lab Med* 119(3):289–91.

Hay AJ, Wolstenholme AJ, Skehel JJ, Smith MH. 1985. The molecular basis of the specific anti-influenza action of amantadine. *EMBO J* 4(11):3021–4.

Hayden FG. 2001. Perspectives on antiviral use during pandemic influenza. *Philos Trans R Soc Lond B Biol Sci* 356(1416):1877–84.

Hayden FG, Hay AJ. 1992. Emergence and transmission of influenza A viruses resistant to amantadine and rimantadine. *Curr Top Microbiol Immunol* 176:119–30.

Hayden FG, Treanor JJ, Fritz RS, Lobo M, Betts RF, Miller M, Kinnersley N, Mills RG, Ward P, Straus SE. 1999. Use of the oral neuraminidase inhibitor oseltamivir in experimental human influenza: randomized controlled trials for prevention and treatment. *JAMA* 282(13):1240–6.

Hearst N, Mandel JS, Coates TJ. 1995. Collaborative AIDS prevention research in the developing world: the CAPS experience. *AIDS* 9 Suppl 1:S1–5.

Hedberg CW, MacDonald KL, Osterholm MT. 1994. Changing epidemiology of food-borne disease: a Minnesota perspective. *Clin Infect Dis* 18(5):671–80; quiz 681–2.

Helminen ME, Kilpinen S, Virta M, Hurme M. 2001. Susceptibility to primary Epstein–Barr virus infection is associated with interleukin-10 gene promoter polymorphism. *J Infect Dis* 184(6):777–80.

Henderson DA. 1999. The looming threat of bioterrorism. *Science* 283(5406):1279–82.

Henderson DA, Moss B. 1999. Smallpox and vaccinia. In: Plotkin SA, Orenstein O, eds. *Vaccines*. 3rd ed. Philadelphia: WB Saunders Company.

Henderson DA, Inglesby TV, Bartlett JG, Ascher MS, Eitzen E, Jahrling PB, Hauer J, Layton M, McDade J, Osterholm MT, O'Toole T, Parker G, Perl T, Russell PK, Tonat K. 1999. Smallpox as a biological weapon: medical and public health management. Working Group on Civilian Biodefense. *JAMA* 281(22):2127–37.

Henderson FW, Clyde WA Jr, Collier AM, Denny FW, Senior RJ, Sheaffer CI, Conley WG 3rd, Christian RM. 1979. The etiologic and epidemiologic spectrum of bronchiolitis in pediatric practice. *J Pediatr* 95(2):183–90.

Herlocher ML, Carr J, Ives J, Elias S, Truscon R, Roberts N, Monto AS. 2002. Influenza virus carrying an R292K mutation in the neuraminidase gene is not transmitted in ferrets. *Antiviral Res* 54(2):99–111.

Herrero IA, Issa NC, Patel R. 2002. Nosocomial spread of linezolid-resistant, vancomycin-resistant *Enterococcus faecium*. *N Engl J Med* 346(11):867–9.

Herrero R. 1996. Epidemiology of cervical cancer. *J Natl Cancer Inst Monogr* (21):1–6.

Hersh SM. 1968. *Chemical and Biological Warfare: America's Hidden Arsenal*. New York: Bobbs–Merrill Company, Inc.

Herwaldt BL, Ackers ML. 1997. An outbreak in 1996 of cyclosporiasis associated with imported raspberries. The Cyclospora Working Group. *N Engl J Med* 336(22):1548–56.

Herwaldt BL, Beach MJ. 1999. The return of cyclospora in 1997: another outbreak of cyclosporiasis in North America associated with imported raspberries. Cyclospora Working Group. *Ann Intern Med* 130(3):210–20.

Heymann DL. 2001 (September 5). Strengthening Global Preparedness for Defense Against Infectious Disease Threats. Statement by Executive Director for Communicable Diseases WHO.

Hill AV. 1998. The immunogenetics of human infectious diseases. *Annu Rev Immunol* 16: 593–617.

Hill AV. 2001. The genomics and genetics of human infectious disease susceptibility. *Annu Rev Genomics Hum Genet* 2:373–400.

Hill AV, Allsopp CE, Kwiatkowski D, Anstey NM, Twumasi P, Rowe PA, Bennett S, Brewster D, McMichael AJ, Greenwood BM. 1991. Common west African HLA antigens are associated with protection from severe malaria. *Nature* 352(6336):595–600.

Hill CA, Fox AN, Pitts RJ, Kent LB, Tan PL, Chrystal MA, Cravchik A, Collins FH, Robertson HM, Zwiebel LJ. 2002. G protein-coupled receptors in *Anopheles gambiae*. *Science* 298(5591):176–8.

Hjelle B, Glass GE. 2000. Outbreak of hantavirus infection in the Four Corners region of the United States in the wake of the 1997–1998 El Nino–southern oscillation. *J Infect Dis* 181(5):1569–73.

Ho GY, Kadish AS, Burk RD, Basu J, Palan PR, Mikhail M, Romney SL. 1998. HPV 16 and cigarette smoking as risk factors for high-grade cervical intra-epithelial neoplasia. *Int J Cancer* 78(3):281–5.

Hodge JG Jr. 2002. West Nile Virus in the United States: A State of the Art Assessment of Law and Policy. Baltimore and Washington, DC: Center for Law and the Public's Health.

Holly EA. 1996. Cervical intraepithelial neoplasia, cervical cancer, and HPV. *Annu Rev Public Health* 17:69–84.

Holt RA, Subramanian GM, Halpern A, Sutton GG, Charlab R, Nusskern DR, Wincker P, Clark AG, Ribeiro JM, Wides R, Salzberg SL, Loftus B, Yandell M, et al. 2002. The genome sequence of the malaria mosquito *Anopheles gambiae*. *Science* 298(5591):129–49.

Holtgrave DR, Pinkerton SD. 2000. Consequences of HIV prevention interventions and programs: spectrum, selection, and quality of outcome measures. *AIDS* 14 Suppl 2:S27–33.

Holtz TH, Kachur SP, MacArthur JR, Roberts JM, Barber AM, Steketee RW, Parise ME. 2001. Malaria surveillance–United States, 1998. *MMWR CDC Surveill Summ* 50(5):1–20.

Hooper LV, Gordon JI. 2001. Commensal host–bacterial relationships in the gut. *Science* 292(5519):1115–8.

Houweling TA, Kunst AE, Mackenbach JP. 2001. World Health Report 2000: inequality index and socioeconomic inequalities in mortality. *Lancet* 357(9269):1671–2.

Hoxie NJ, Davis JP, Vergeront JM, Nashold RD, Blair KA. 1997. Cryptosporidiosis-associated mortality following a massive waterborne outbreak in Milwaukee, Wisconsin. *Am J Public Health* 87(12):2032–5.

Huebner DM, Gerend MA. 2001. The relation between beliefs about drug treatments for HIV and sexual risk behavior in gay and bisexual men. *Ann Behav Med* 23(4):304–12.

Humane Society of the United States. 2001. The trade in live reptiles: imports to the United States. Washington, DC: Humane Society.

Humane Society of the United States. 2002. Fast–Food Restaurants Curbing Antibiotics in Poultry. [Online]. Available: http://www.hsus.org/ace/13383 [accessed March 5, 2003].

Humphrey RW, Davis DA, Newcomb FM, Yarchoan R. 1998. Human herpesvirus 8 (HHV–8) in the pathogenesis of Kaposi's sarcoma and other diseases. *Leuk Lymphoma* 28(3–4):255–64.

Hunter CA, Reiner SL. 2000. Cytokines and T cells in host defense. *Curr Opin Immunol* 12(4):413–8.

Hyder AA, Morrow RH. 2000. Applying burden of disease methods in developing countries: a case study from Pakistan. *Am J Pub Health* 90(8):1235–40.

Inglesby TV, Dennis DT, Henderson DA, Bartlett JG, Ascher MS, Eitzen E, Fine AD, Friedlander AM, Hauer J, Koerner JF, Layton M, McDade J, Osterholm MT, et al. 2000. Plague as a biological weapon: medical and public health management. Working Group on Civilian Biodefense. *JAMA* 283(17):2281–90.

Inglesby TV, O'Toole T, Henderson DA, Bartlett JG, Ascher MS, Eitzen E, Friedlander AM, Gerberding J, Hauer J, Hughes J, McDade J, Osterholm MT, Parker G, et al. 2002. Anthrax as a biological weapon, 2002: updated recommendations for management. *JAMA* 287(17):2236–52.

Intergovernmental Panel on Climate Change (IPCC). 2001a. Climate Change 2001: The Scientific Basis. Contribution of Working Group I to the Third Assessment Report of the Intergovernmental Panel on Climate Change. Cambridge, UK: Cambridge University Press.

IPCC. 2001b. Climate Change 2001: Impacts, Adaptation and Vulnerability. Contribution of Working Group II to the Third Assessment Report of the Intergovernmental Panel on Climate Change. Cambridge, UK: Cambridge University Press.

International Agency for Research on Cancer Working Group. 1995. Human Papillomaviruses. IARC Monographs on the Evaluation of Carcinogenic Risks to Humans. Vol. 64. Lyon: International Agency for Research on Cancer.

International Society for Infectious Diseases (ISID). 2001. ProMED–mail. [Online]. Available: http://www.promedmail.org/pls/askus/f?p=2400:1000 [accessed January 30, 2003].

IOM. 1988. *The Future of Public Health*. Washington, DC: National Academy Press.

IOM. 1991. *Malaria: Obstacles and Opportunities.* Washington, DC: National Academy Press.

IOM. 1992. *Emerging Infections: Microbial Threats to Health in the United States.* Washington, DC: National Academy Press.

IOM. 1996. *Xenotransplantation: Science, Ethics, and Public Policy.* Washington, DC: National Academy Press.

IOM. 1997. *The Hidden Epidemic: Confronting Sexually Transmitted Diseases.* Washington, DC: National Academy Press.

IOM. 1999a. *Assessment of Future Needs for Live Variola Virus.* Washington, DC: National Academy Press.

IOM. 1999b. *The Use of Drugs in Food Animals: Benefits and Risks.* Washington, DC: National Academy Press.

IOM. 2000. *Managed Care Systems and Emerging Infections: Challenges and Opportunities for Strengthening Surveillance, Research, and Prevention, Workshop Summary.* Washington, DC: National Academy Press.

IOM. 2001b. *Emerging Infectious Diseases from the Global to the Local Perspective.* Washington, DC: National Academy Press.

IOM. 2001c. *Firepower in the Lab: Automation in the Fight Against Infectious Disease and Bioterrorism.* Washington, DC: National Academy Press.

IOM. 2001d. *Vaccines for the 21st Century: A Tool for Decisionmaking.* Washington, DC: National Academy Press.

IOM. 2001e. *Perspectives on the Department of Defense Global Emerging Infections Surveillance and Response System: A Program Review.* Washington, DC: National Academy Press.

IOM. 2002a. *Biological Threats and Terrorism: Assessing the Science and Response Capabilities, Workshop Summary.* Washington, DC: National Academy Press.

IOM. 2002b. *Considerations for Viral Disease Eradication.* Washington, DC: National Academy Press.

IOM. 2002c. *Dietary Reference Intake for Vitamin A, Vitamin K, Arsenic, Boron, Chromium, Copper, Iodine, Iron, Manganese, Molybdenum, Nickel, Silicon, Vanadium, and Zinc.* Washington, DC: National Academy Press.

IOM. 2002d. *The Emergence of Zoonotic Diseases: Understanding the Impact on Animal and Human Health.* Washington, DC: National Academy Press.

IOM. 2002e. *Who Will Keep the Public Healthy? Educating Public Health Professionals for the 21st Century.* Washington, DC: National Academy Press.

IOM. 2003. *Review of the Centers for Disease Control and Prevention's Smallpox Vaccination Program Implementation, Letter Report #1.* Washington, DC: National Academy Press.

Ito J, Ghosh A, Moreira LA, Wimmer EA, Jacobs-Lorena M. 2002. Transgenic anopheline mosquitoes impaired in transmission of a malaria parasite. *Nature* 417(6887):452–455.

Jaax N, Jahrling P, Geisbert T, Geisbert J, Steele K, McKee K, Nagley D, Johnson E, Jaax G, Peters C. 1995. Transmission of Ebola virus (Zaire strain) to uninfected control monkeys in a biocontainment laboratory. *Lancet* 346(8991–8992):1669–71.

Jaramillo E. 2002. DOTS–Plus & the Green Light Committee. Presentation at "Meet the Expert" Session of the 33rd IUATLD World Conference on Lung Health, Montreal. Palais de Congres. WHO/CDS/STB/TBS.

Jarvis WR. 1994. Handwashing—the Semmelweis lesson forgotten? *Lancet* 344(8933):1311–2.

Jernigan DB, Raghunathan PL, Bell BP, Brechner R, Bresnitz EA, Butler JC, Cetron M, Cohen M, Doyle T, Fischer M, Greene C, Griffith KS, Guarner J, Hadler JL et al. 2002. Investigation of bioterrorism-related anthrax, United States, 2001: epidemiologic findings. *Emerg Infect Dis* 8(10):1019–28.

Jeronimo SM, Oliveira RM, Mackay S, Costa RM, Sweet J, Nascimento ET, Luz KG, Fernandes MZ, Jernigan J, Pearson RD. 1994. An urban outbreak of visceral leishmaniasis in Natal, Brazil. *Trans R Soc Trop Med Hyg* 88(4):386–8.

Jones OA, Voulvoulis N, Lester JN. 2001. Human pharmaceuticals in the aquatic environment a review. *Environ Technol* 22(12):1383–94.

Jones TF, Kellum ME, Porter SS, Bell M, Schaffner W. 2002. An outbreak of community-acquired foodborne illness caused by methicillin-resistant *Staphylococcus aureus*. *Emerg Infect Dis* 8(1):82–4.

Junger S. 1998. *The Perfect Storm*. New York: HarperPaperbacks, A Division of Harper CollinsPublishers.

Kadlec RP, Zelicoff AP, Vrtis AM. 1999. Biological weapons control: prospects and implications for the future. In: Lederberg J, ed. *Biological Weapons: Limiting the Threat*. Cambridge, MA: MIT Press. Pp. 95–111.

Kalipeni E, Oppong J. 1998. The refugee crisis in Africa and implications for health and disease: a political ecology approach. *Soc Sci Med* 46(12):1637–53.

Kamhawi S, Belkaid Y, Modi G, Rowton E, Sacks D. 2000. Protection against cutaneous leishmaniasis resulting from bites of uninfected sand flies. *Science* 290(5495):1351–4.

Kapadia F, Vlahov D, Des Jarlais DC, Strathdee SA, Ouellet L, Kerndt P, Morse EV, Williams I, Garfein RS. 2002. Does bleach disinfection of syringes protect against hepatitis C infection among young adult injection drug users? *Epidemiology* 13(6):738–41.

Karon JM, Fleming PL, Steketee RW, De Cock KM. 2001. HIV in the United States at the turn of the century: an epidemic in transition. *Am J Public Health* 91(7):1060–8.

Kaslow RA, Carrington M, Apple R, Park L, Munoz A, Saah AJ, Goedert JJ, Winkler C, O'Brien SJ, Rinaldo C, Detels R, Blattner W, Phair J, Erlich H, Mann DL. 1996. Influence of combinations of human major histocompatibility complex genes on the course of HIV–1 infection. *Nat Med* 2(4):405–11.

Katz MH, Schwarcz SK, Kellogg TA, Klausner JD, Dilley JW, Gibson S, McFarland W. 2002. Impact of highly active antiretroviral treatment on HIV seroincidence among men who have sex with men: San Francisco. *Am J Pub Health* 92(3):388–94.

Kelch WJ, Lee JS. 1978. Antibiotic resistance patterns of gram–negative bacteria isolated from environmental sources. *Appl Environ Microbiol* 36(3):450–6.

Kemp E. 1996. Xenotransplantation. *J Intern Med* 239(4):287–97.

Kenny GE, Kuo C. 2000. Infection and chronic disease. *Washington Public Health*:1–4.

Kenyon TA, Valway SE, Ihle WW, Onorato IM, Castro KG. 1996. Transmission of multidrug-resistant *Mycobacterium tuberculosis* during a long airplane flight. *N Engl J Med* 334(15):933–8.

Khan IM, Laaser U. 2002. Burden of tuberculosis in Afghanistan: update on a war-stricken country. *Croat Med J* 43(2):245–7.

Kilbourne ED, Cerini CP, Khan MW, Mitchell JW Jr, Ogra PL. 1987. Immunologic response to the influenza virus neuraminidase is influenced by prior experience with the associated viral hemagglutinin. I. Studies in human vaccinees. *J Immunol* 138(9):3010–3.

Kilmarx PH, Knapp JS, Xia M, St Louis ME, Neal SW, Sayers D, Doyle LJ, Roberts MC, Whittington WL. 1998. Intercity spread of gonococci with decreased susceptibility to fluoroquinolones: a unique focus in the United States. *J Infect Dis* 177(3):677–82.

Kim J, Nietfeldt J, Ju J, Wise J, Fegan N, Desmarchelier P, Benson AK. 2001. Ancestral divergence, genome diversification, and phylogeographic variation in subpopulations of sorbitol-negative, beta-glucuronidase-negative enterohemorrhagic *Escherichia coli* O157. *J Bacteriol* 183(23):6885–97.

Kim JY, Shakow ADA, Bayona J. 1999. The privatization of health care in Peru. *Development* 42(4):121–125.

Kinsella K, Velkoff VA. 2001. An Aging World: 2001. U.S. Census Bureau, Series P95/01–1. Washington, DC: U.S. Government Printing Office.

Klein G, Powers A, Croce C. 2002. Association of SV40 with human tumors. *Oncogene* 21(8):1141–9.

Klein JO. 1986. Infectious diseases and day care. *Rev Infect Dis* 8(4):521–6.

Klenerman P, Cerundolo V, Dunbar PR. 2002. Tracking T cells with tetramers: new tales from new tools. *Nat Rev Immunol* 2(4):263–72.

Klug SJ, Wilmotte R, Santos C, Almonte M, Herrero R, Guerrero I, Caceres E, Peixoto–Guimaraes D, Lenoir G, Hainaut P, Walboomers JM, Munoz N. 2001. TP53 polymorphism, HPV infection, and risk of cervical cancer. *Cancer Epidemiol Biomarkers Prev* 10(9):1009–12.

Koumans EH, Katz DJ, Malecki JM, Kumar S, Wahlquist SP, Arrowood MJ, Hightower AW, Herwaldt BL. 1998. An outbreak of cyclosporiasis in Florida in 1995: a harbinger of multistate outbreaks in 1996 and 1997. *Am J Trop Med Hyg* 59(2):235–42.

Koutsky LA, Holmes KK, Critchlow CW, Stevens CE, Paavonen J, Beckmann AM, DeRouen TA, Galloway DA, Vernon D, Kiviat NB. 1992. A cohort study of the risk of cervical intraepithelial neoplasia grade 2 or 3 in relation to papillomavirus infection. *N Engl J Med* 327(18):1272–8.

Koutsky LA, Ault KA, Wheeler CM, Brown DR, Barr E, Alvarez FB, Chiacchierini LM, Jansen KU. 2002. A controlled trial of a human papillomavirus type 16 vaccine. *N Engl J Med* 347(21):1645–51.

Kummerer K. 2000. Drugs, diagnostic agents and disinfectants in wastewater and water—a review. *Schriftenr Ver Wasser Boden Lufthyg* 105:59–71.

Kurstak E, ed. 1993. *Control of Virus Diseases.* New York: Marcel Dekker, Inc.

Lamb RA, Krug RM. 2001. Orthomyxoviridae: the viruses and their replication. In: Knipe DM, Howley PM, eds. *Fields Virology.* 4th ed. Philadelphia: Lippincott Williams & Wilkins.

Lander ES, Linton LM, Birren B, Nusbaum C, Zody MC, Baldwin J, Devon K, Dewar K, Doyle M, FitzHugh W, Funke R, Gage D, Harris K, Heaford A, Howland J, et al. 2001. Initial sequencing and analysis of the human genome. *Nature* 409(6822):860–921.

Lange WR, Ball JC, Pfeiffer MB, Snyder FR, Cone EJ. 1989. The Lexington addicts, 1971–1972: demographic characteristics, drug use patterns, and selected infectious disease experience. *Int J Addict* 24(7):609–26.

Lederberg J. 1999. J.B.S. Haldane (1949) on infectious disease and evolution. *Genetics* 153(1):1–3.

Lederberg J. 2000. Infectious history. *Science* 288(5464):287–93.

Levander OA. 1997. Nutrition and newly emerging viral diseases: an overview. *J Nutr* 127(5 Suppl):948S–950S.

Leverstein–van Hall MA, Box AT, Blok HE, Paauw A, Fluit AC, Verhoef J. 2002. Evidence of extensive interspecies transfer of integron-mediated antimicrobial resistance genes among multidrug-resistant enterobacteriaceae in a clinical setting. *J Infect Dis* 186(1):49–56.

Liang AP, Koopmans M, Doyle MP, Bernard DT, Brewer CE. 2001. Teaming up to prevent foodborne disease. *Emerg Infect Dis* 7(3 Suppl):533–4.

Liaw KL, Glass AG, Manos MM, Greer CE, Scott DR, Sherman M, Burk RD, Kurman RJ, Wacholder S, Rush BB, Cadell DM, Lawler P, Tabor D, Schiffman M. 1999. Detection of human papillomavirus DNA in cytologically normal women and subsequent cervical squamous intraepithelial lesions. *J Natl Cancer Inst* 91(11):954–60.

Lima AA, Fang G, Schorling JB, de Albuquerque L, McAuliffe JF, Mota S, Leite R, Guerrant RL. 1992. Persistent diarrhea in northeast Brazil: etiologies and interactions with malnutrition. *Acta Paediatr Suppl* 381:39–44.

Linthicum KJ, Anyamba A, Tucker CJ, Kelley PW, Myers MF, Peters CJ. 1999. Climate and satellite indicators to forecast Rift Valley fever epidemics in Kenya. *Science* 285(5426): 397–400.

LoGiudice K, Ostfeld RS, Schmidt KA, Keesing F. 2003. The ecology of infectious disease: effects of host diversity and community composition on Lyme disease risk. *Proc Natl Acad Sci U S A* 100(2):567–71.

Lounibos LP. 2002. Invasions by insect vectors of human disease. *Annu Rev Entomol* 47:233–66.

MacKenzie WR, Hoxie NJ, Proctor ME, Gradus MS, Blair KA, Peterson DE, Kazmierczak JJ, Addiss DG, Fox KR, Rose JB. 1994. A massive outbreak in Milwaukee of cryptosporidium infection transmitted through the public water supply. *N Engl J Med* 331(3): 161–7.

Maciag PC, Schlecht NF, Souza PS, Franco EL, Villa LL, Petzl–Erler ML. 2000. Major histocompatibility complex class II polymorphisms and risk of cervical cancer and human papillomavirus infection in Brazilian women. *Cancer Epidemiol Biomarkers Prev* 9(11): 1183–91.

Mahon BE, Mintz ED, Greene KD, Wells JG, Tauxe RV. 1996. Reported cholera in the United States, 1992–1994: a reflection of global changes in cholera epidemiology. *JAMA* 276(4):307–12.

Mansergh G, Colfax GN, Marks G, Rader M, Guzman R, Buchbinder S. 2001. The Circuit Party Men's Health Survey: findings and implications for gay and bisexual men. *Am J Public Health* 91(6):953–8.

Mansky LM, Temin HM. 1995. Lower in vivo mutation rate of human immunodeficiency virus type 1 than that predicted from the fidelity of purified reverse transcriptase. *J Virol* 69(8):5087–94.

Marinella MA, Pierson C, Chenoweth C. 1997. The stethoscope. A potential source of nosocomial infection? *Arch Intern Med* 157(7):786–90.

Marshall BJ. 1989. History of the discovery of C. pylori. In: Blaser MJ, ed. *Camplobacter Pylori in Gastritis and Peptic Ulcer Disease.* New York: Igaku-Shoin. Pp. 7–23.

Martens P, Hall L. 2000. Malaria on the move: human population movement and malaria transmission. *Emerg Infect Dis* 6(2):103–9.

Mata L. 1992. Diarrheal disease as a cause of malnutrition. *Am J Trop Med Hyg* 47(1 Pt 2):16–27.

Mata LJ, Kromal RA, Urrutia JJ, Garcia B. 1977. Effect of infection on food intake and the nutritional state: perspectives as viewed from the village. *Am J Clin Nutr* 30(8):1215–27.

Mattison AM, Ross MW, Wolfson T, Franklin D. 2001. Circuit party attendance, club drug use, and unsafe sex in gay men. *J Subst Abuse* 13(1–2):119–26.

Mavroidi A, Tzouvelekis LS, Tassios PT, Flemetakis A, Daniilidou M, Tzelepi E. 2000. Characterization of *Neisseria gonorrhoeae* strains with decreased susceptibility to fluoroquinolones isolated in Greece from 1996 to 1999. *J Clin Microbiol* 38(9):3489–91.

Mayer JD. 2000. Geography, ecology and emerging infectious diseases. *Soc Sci Med* 50(7–8):937–52.

McCarthy M. 2002. US FDA orders transplant tissue recall. *Lancet* 360(9333):623.

McDaniel TK, Kaper JB. 1997. A cloned pathogenicity island from enteropathogenic *Escherichia coli* confers the attaching and effacing phenotype on *E. coli* K–12. *Mol Microbiol* 23(2):399–407.

McDermott J. 1987. *The Killing Winds: The Menace of Biological Warfare.* New York: Arbor House.

McDonald LC, Rossiter S, Mackinson C, Wang YY, Johnson S, Sullivan M, Sokolow R, DeBess E, Gilbert L, Benson JA, Hill B, Angulo FJ. 2001. Quinupristin–dalfopristin-resistant *Enterococcus faecium* on chicken and in human stool specimens. *N Engl J Med* 345(16):1155–60.

McEwen SA, Fedorka-Cray PJ. 2002. Antimicrobial use and resistance in animals. *Clin Infect Dis* 34 (Suppl 3):S93–S106.

McIlhaney JS Jr. 2000. Sexually transmitted infection and teenage sexuality. *Am J Obstet Gynecol* 183(2):334–9.

McKimm-Breschkin JL, McDonald M, Blick TJ, Colman PM. 1996. Mutation in the influenza virus neuraminidase gene resulting in decreased sensitivity to the neuraminidase inhibitor 4–guanidino–Neu5Ac2en leads to instability of the enzyme. *Virology* 225(1): 240–2.

Mead PS, Slutsker L, Dietz V, McCaig LF, Bresee JS, Shapiro C, Griffin PM, Tauxe RV. 1999. Food-related illness and death in the United States. *Emerg Infect Dis* 5(5):607–25.

Mercado R. 1975. Rodent control programmes in areas affected by Bolivian haemorrhagic fever. *Bull World Health Org* 52(4–6):691–6.

Meselson M, Guillemin J, Hugh–Jones M, Langmuir A, Popova I, Shelokov A, Yampolskaya O. 1994. The Sverdlovsk anthrax outbreak of 1979. *Science* 266(5188):1202–8.

Miller JM, Tam TW, Maloney S, Fukuda K, Cox N, Hockin J, Kertesz D, Klimov A, Cetron M. 2000. Cruise ships: high–risk passengers and the global spread of new influenza viruses. *Clin Infect Dis* 31(2):433–8.

Miller LH. 1994. Impact of malaria on genetic polymorphism and genetic diseases in Africans and African Americans. *Proc Natl Acad Sci U S A* 91(7):2415–9.

Mills JN, Childs JE. 1998. Ecologic studies of rodent reservoirs: their relevance for human health. *Emerg Infect Dis* 4(4):529–37.

Mills JN, Ellis BA, McKee KT Jr, Calderon GE, Maiztegui JI, Nelson GO, Ksiazek TG, Peters CJ, Childs JE. 1992. A longitudinal study of Junin virus activity in the rodent reservoir of Argentine hemorrhagic fever. *Am J Trop Med Hyg* 47(6):749–63.

Mills JN, Yates T.L., Ksiazek TG, Peters CJ, Childs JE. 1999. Long–term studies of hantavirus reservoir populations in the southwestern United States: a synthesis. *Emerg Infect Dis* 5(1):135–42.

Moller H, Heseltine E, Vainio H. 1995. Working group report on schistosomes, liver flukes and *Helicobacter pylori*. *Int J Cancer* 60(5):587–9.

Monath TP. 1993. Arthropod–borne viruses. In: Morse SS, ed. *Emerging Viruses.* New York: Oxford University Press.

Monath TP. 2001. Yellow fever: an update. *Lancet Infect Dis* 1(1):11–20.

Monath TP, Cetron MS. 2002. Prevention of yellow fever in persons traveling to the tropics. *Clin Infect Dis* 34(10):1369–78.

Monitoring the AIDS Pandemic Network. 2000 (July 9-14). The Status and Trends of the HIV/AIDS in the World Symposium of the XIIIth International AIDS Conference. Washington, DC: MAP.

Monroe MC, Morzunov SP, Johnson AM, Bowen MD, Artsob H, Yates T, Peters CJ, Rollin PE, Ksiazek TG, Nichol ST. 1999. Genetic diversity and distribution of *Peromyscus*-borne hantaviruses in North America. *Emerg Infect Dis* 5(1):75–86.

Moore CG. 1999. *Aedes albopictus* in the United States: current status and prospects for further spread. *J Am Mosq Control Assoc* 15(2):221–7.

Morris CN, Burdge DR, Cheevers EJ. 2000. Economic impact of HIV infection in a cohort of male sugar mill workers in South Africa from the perspective of industry. Unpublished.

Morris JG, Potter M. 1997. Emergence of new pathogens as a function of changes in host susceptibility. *Emerg Infect Dis* 3(4):435–41.

Morse D, Brothwell DR, Ucko PJ. 1964. Tuberculosis in ancient Egypt. *Ann Rev Respir Dis* 90:524–541.

Morse SS. 1995. Factors in the emergence of infectious diseases. *Emerg Infect Dis* 1(1):7–15.

Moscicki AB, Hills N, Shiboski S, Powell K, Jay N, Hanson E, Miller S, Clayton L, Farhat S, Broering J, Darragh T, Palefsky J. 2001. Risks for incident human papillomavirus infection and low–grade squamous intraepithelial lesion development in young females. *JAMA* 285(23):2995–3002.

Moser MR, Bender TR, Margolis HS, Noble GR, Kendal AP, Ritter DG. 1979. An outbreak of influenza aboard a commercial airliner. *Am J Epidemiol* 110(1):1–6.

Moss B. 1996. Genetically engineered poxviruses for recombinant gene expression, vaccination, and safety. *Proc Natl Acad Sci U S A* 93(21):11341–8.

Moss B, Shisler JL. 2001. Immunology 101 at poxvirus U: immune evasion genes. *Semin Immunol* 13(1):59–66.

Mostashari F, Bunning ML, Kitsutani PT, Singer DA, Nash D, Cooper MJ, Katz N, Liljebjelke KA, Biggerstaff BJ, Fine AD, Layton MC, Mullin SM, Johnson AJ, Martin DA, Hayes EB, Campbell GL. 2001. Epidemic West Nile encephalitis, New York, 1999: results of a household-based seroepidemiological survey. *Lancet* 358(9278):261–4.

Mukadi YD, Maher D, Harries A. 2001. Tuberculosis case fatality rates in high HIV prevalence populations in sub-Saharan Africa. *AIDS* 15(2):143–52.

Mukamolova GV, Kaprelyants AS, Young DI, Young M, Kell DB. 1998. A bacterial cytokine. *Proc Natl Acad Sci U S A* 95(15):8916–21.

Munoz N, Bosch FX, de Sanjose S, Tafur L, Izarzugaza I, Gili M, Viladiu P, Navarro C, Martos C, Ascunce N, et al. 1992. The causal link between human papillomavirus and invasive cervical cancer: a population-based case-control study in Colombia and Spain. *Int J Cancer* 52(5):743–9.

Murray CJ, Lopez AD. 1997. Mortality by cause for eight regions of the world: Global Burden of Disease Study. *Lancet* 349(9061):1269–76.

Murray CJ, King G, Lopez AD, Tomijima N, Krug EG. 2002. Armed conflict as a public health problem. *BMJ* 324(7333):346–9.

Myung PS, Boerthe NJ, Koretzky GA. 2000. Adapter proteins in lymphocyte antigen-receptor signaling. *Curr Opin Immunol* 12(3):256–66.

Nadel S, Newport MJ, Booy R, Levin M. 1996. Variation in the tumor necrosis factor–alpha gene promoter region may be associated with death from meningococcal disease. *J Infect Dis* 174(4):878–80.

Nash D, Mostashari F, Fine A, Miller J, O'Leary D, Murray K, Huang A, Rosenberg A, Greenberg A, Sherman M, Wong S, Layton M. 2001. The outbreak of West Nile virus infection in the New York City area in 1999. *N Engl J Med* 344(24):1807–14.

Nasta P, Donisi A, Cattane A, Chiodera A, Casari S. 1997. Acute Histoplasmosis in spelunkers returning from Mato Grosso, Peru. *J Travel Med* 4(4):176–8.

National Commission on Terrorism. 2000. Countering the Changing Threat of International Terrorism, Report of the Natinal Commission on Terrorism, Pursuant to Public Law 277, 105th Congress, Ambassador L. Paul Bremer III, Chairman.

National Intelligence Council. 2000. National Intelligence Estimate: The Global Infectious Disease Threat and Its Implications for the United States. NIE 99–17D. Washington, DC: NIC.

National Intelligence Council. 2002. The Next Wave of HIV/AIDS: Nigeria, Ethiopia, Russia, India, and China. McLean, VA : Central Intelligence Agency.

National Nosocomial Infections Surveillance System. 2001. National Nosocomial Infections Surveillance (NNIS) System Report, Data Summary from January 1992–June 2001, issued August 2001. *Am J Infect Control* 29(6):404–21.

National Science and Technology Council (NSTC). 1995. National Science and Technology Council Accomplishments (November 1993–September 1995). [Online] Available: http://www.ostp.gov/NSTC/html/accomp–novsept.html [accessed January 30, 2003].

Navin TR, Juranek DD. 1984. Cryptosporidiosis: clinical, epidemiologic, and parasitologic review. *Rev Infect Dis* 6(3):313–27.

Nchinda TC. 1998. Malaria: a reemerging disease in Africa. *Emerg Infect Dis* 4(3):398–403.

NCHS (National Center for Health Statistics). 2001. Health, United States, 2001 with Urban and Rural Health Chartbook. Hyattsville, MD: National Center for Health Statistics.

Nerlich AG, Haas CJ, Zink A, Szeimies U, Hagedorn HG. 1997. Molecular evidence for tuberculosis in an ancient Egyptian mummy. *Lancet* 350(9088):1404.

Netesov SV, Conrad JL. 2001. Emerging infectious diseases in Russia, 1990–1999. *Emerg Infect Dis* 7(1):1–5.

Neu HC. 1992. The crisis in antibiotic resistance. *Science* 257(5073):1064–73.

Neumann G, Kawaoka Y. 2001. Reverse genetics of influenza virus. *Virology* 287(2):243–50.

Nichol ST, Spiropoulou CF, Morzunov S, Rollin PE, Ksiazek TG, Feldmann H, Sanchez A, Childs J, Zaki S, Peters CJ. 1993. Genetic identification of a hantavirus associated with an outbreak of acute respiratory illness. *Science* 262(5135):914–7.

Niel C, de Oliveira JM, Ross RS, Gomes SA, Roggendorf M, Viazov S. 1999. High prevalence of TT virus infection in Brazilian blood donors. *J Med Virol* 57(3):259–63.

NIH (National Institutes of Health). 1999. Annual Report of International Activities. [Online]. Available: http://www.nih.gov/fic/textonly/news/annrpt99.html [accessed January 30, 2003].

NIH. 2001. Human Papillomavirus and Genital Warts Fact Sheet. [Online]. Available: http://www.niaid.nih.gov/factsheets/stdhpv.htm [accessed March 4, 2003].

Nishizawa T, Okamoto H, Konishi K, Yoshizawa H, Miyakawa Y, Mayumi M. 1997. A novel DNA virus (TTV) associated with elevated transaminase levels in posttransfusion hepatitis of unknown etiology. *Biochem Biophys Res Commun* 241(1):92–7.

Nobbenhuis MA, Walboomers JM, Helmerhorst TJ, Rozendaal L, Remmink AJ, Risse EK, van der Linden HC, Voorhorst FJ, Kenemans P, Meijer CJ. 1999. Relation of human papillomavirus status to cervical lesions and consequences for cervical-cancer screening: a prospective study. *Lancet* 354(9172):20–5.

Nohynek H, Eskola J, Laine E, Halonen P, Ruutu P, Saikku P, Kleemola M, Leinonen M. 1991. The causes of hospital-treated acute lower respiratory tract infection in children. *Am J Dis Child* 145(6):618–22.

NRC (National Research Council). 1983. *Manpower Needs and Career Opportunities in the Field Aspects of Vector Biology: Report of a Workshop.* Washington, DC: National Academy Press.

NRC. 1999. *The Use of Drugs in Food Animals Benefits and Risks.* Washington, DC: National Academy Press.

NRC. 2001. *Under the Weather: Climate, Ecosystems, and Infectious Disease.* Washington, DC: National Academy Press.

O'Brien FG, Pearman JW, Gracey M, Riley TV, Grubb WB. 1999. Community strain of methicillin–resistant *Staphylococcus aureus* involved in a hospital outbreak. *J Clin Microbiol* 37(9):2858–62.

O'Brien TF. 2002. Emergence, spread, and environmental effect of antimicrobial resistance: how use of an antimicrobial anywhere can increase resistance to any antimicrobial anywhere else. *Clin Infect Dis* 34 Suppl 3:S78–84.

Ochman H, Moran NA. 2001. Genes lost and genes found: evolution of bacterial pathogenesis and symbiosis. *Science* 292(5519):1096–9.

Okeke IN, Lamikanra A, Edelman R. 1999. Socioeconomic and behavioral factors leading to acquired bacterial resistance to antibiotics in developing countries. *Emerg Infect Dis* 5(1):18–27.

Olliaro P, Cattani J, Wirth D. 1996. Malaria, the submerged disease. *JAMA* 275(3):230–3.

Olson KB. 1999. Aum Shinrikyo: once and future threat? *Emerg Infect Dis* 5(4):513–6.

Olson KE, Higgs S, Gaines PJ, Powers AM, Davis BS, Kamrud KI, Carlson JO, Blair CD, Beaty BJ. 1996. Genetically engineered resistance to dengue-2 virus transmission in mosquitoes. *Science* 272(5263):884–6.

Osterholm MT. 1997. Cyclosporiasis and raspberries—lessons for the future. *N Engl J Med* 336(22):1597–9.

Osterholm MT, Reves RR, Murph JR, Pickering LK. 1992. Infectious diseases and child day care. *Pediatr Infect Dis J* 11(8 Suppl):S31–41.

Ostrow DE, Fox KJ, Chmiel JS, Silvestre A, Visscher BR, Vanable PA, Jacobson LP, Strathdee SA. 2002. Attitudes towards highly active antiretroviral therapy are associated with sexual risk taking among HIV-infected and uninfected homosexual men. *AIDS* 16(5): 775–80.

Overby KJ, Kegeles SM. 1994. The impact of AIDS on an urban population of high-risk female minority adolescents: implications for intervention. *J Adolesc Health* 15(3):216–27.

Overhage JM, Tierney WM, Zhou XH, McDonald CJ. 1997. A randomized trial of "corollary orders" to prevent errors of omission. *J Am Med Inform Assoc* 4(5):364–75.

Padula PJ, Edelstein A, Miguel SD, Lopez NM, Rossi CM, Rabinovich RD. 1998. Hantavirus pulmonary syndrome outbreak in Argentina: molecular evidence for person-to-person transmission of Andes virus. *Virology* 241(2):323–30.

Pain A, Urban BC, Kai O, Casals–Pascual C, Shafi J, Marsh K, Roberts DJ. 2001. A non–sense mutation in Cd36 gene is associated with protection from severe malaria. *Lancet* 357(9267):1502–3.

Panackal AA, Hajjeh RA, Cetron MS, Warnock DW. 2002. Fungal infections among returning travelers. *Clin Infect Dis* 35(9):1088–95.

Paquet C, van Soest M. 1994. Mortality and malnutrition among Rwandan refugees in Zaire. *Lancet* 344(8925):823–4.

Parsonnet J. 1998. *Helicobacter pylori. Infect Dis Clin North Am* 12(1):185–97.

Pater MM, Mittal R, Pater A. 1994. Role of steroid hormones in potentiating transformation of cervical cells by human papillomaviruses. *Trends Microbiol* 2(7):229–34.

Patz JA, Graczyk TK, Geller N, Vittor AY. 2000. Effects of environmental change on emerging parasitic diseases. *Int J Parasitol* 30(12–13):1395–405.

Patz JA, McGeehin MA, Bernard SM, Ebi KL, Epstein PR, Grambsch A, Gubler DJ, Reiter P, Romieu I, Rose JB, Samet JM, Trtanj J. 2001. Potential consequences of climate variability and change for human health in the United States. In: *Climate Change Impacts on the United States: The Potential Consequences of Climate Variability and Change.* Washington, DC: U.S. Global Change Research Program. Cambridge, MA: Cambridge University Press. Pp. 620.

Paul VK, Singh M, Gupta U, Buckshee K, Bhargava VL, Takkar D, Nag VL, Bhan MK, Deorari AK. 1999. *Chlamydia trachomatis* infection among pregnant women: prevalence and prenatal importance. *Natl Med J India* 12(1):11–4.

Peeling RW, Brunham RC. 1996. Chlamydiae as pathogens: new species and new issues. *Emerg Infect Dis* 2(4):307–19.

Peng MM, Xiao L, Freeman AR, Arrowood MJ, Escalante AA, Weltman AC, Ong CS, Mac Kenzie WR, Lal AA, Beard CB. 1997. Genetic polymorphism among *Cryptosporidium parvum* isolates: evidence of two distinct human transmission cycles. *Emerg Infect Dis* 3(4):567–73.

Penman AD, Kohn MA, Fowler M. 1997. A shipboard outbreak of tuberculosis in Mississippi and Louisiana, 1993 to 1994. *Am J Public Health* 87(7):1234.

Perelson AS, Neumann AU, Markowitz M, Leonard JM, Ho DD. 1996. HIV-1 dynamics in vivo: virion clearance rate, infected cell life–span, and viral generation time. *Science* 271(5255):1582–6.

Persing DH, Prendergast FG. 1999. Infection, immunity, and cancer. *Arch Pathol Lab Med* 123(11):1015–22.

Peters CJ, Johnson ED, Jahrling PB, Ksiazek TG, Rollin PE, White J, Hall W, Trotter R, Jaax. 1991. Filoviruses. In: Morse S, ed. *Emerging Viruses*. New York: Oxford University Press. Pp. 159–75.

Petersen LR, Roehrig JT. 2001. West Nile virus: a reemerging global pathogen. *Emerg Infect Dis* 7(4):611–4.

PhRMA. 2002. New Medicines in Development for Infectious Diseases. 2002 Survey. Washington, DC: Pharmaceutical Research and Manufacturers of America.

Pickering LK, Evans DG, DuPont HL, Vollet JJ 3rd, Evans DJ Jr. 1981. Diarrhea caused by *Shigella*, rotavirus, and *Giardia* in day-care centers: prospective study. *J Pediatr* 99(1): 51–6.

Piot P, Coll Seck AM. 2001. International response to the HIV/AIDS epidemic: planning for success. *Bull World Health Org* 79(12):1106–12.

Pisani P, Parkin DM, Munoz N, Ferlay J. 1997. Cancer and infection: estimates of the attributable fraction in 1990. *Cancer Epidemiol Biomarkers Prev* 6(6):387–400.

Pisani P, Parkin DM, Bray F, Ferlay J. 1999. Estimates of the worldwide mortality from 25 cancers in 1990. *Int J Cancer* 83(1):18–29.

Pittendrigh BR, Gaffney PJ. 2001. Pesticide resistance: can we make it a renewable resource? *J Theor Biol* 211(4):365–75.

Pittet D, Dharan S, Touveneau S, Sauvan V, Perneger TV. 1999. Bacterial contamination of the hands of hospital staff during routine patient care. *Arch Intern Med* 159(8):821–6.

Platonov AE. 2001. West Nile encephalitis in Russia 1999–2001: were we ready? Are we ready? *Ann N Y Acad Sci* 951:102–16.

Platonov AE, Shipulin GA, Shipulina OY, Tyutyunnik EN, Frolochkina TI, Lanciotti RS, Yazyshina S, Platonova OV, Obukhov IL, Zhukov AN, Vengerov YY, Pokrovskii VI. 2001. Outbreak of West Nile virus infection, Volgograd Region, Russia, 1999. *Emerg Infect Dis* 7(1):128–32.

Plotkin SA, Mortimer EA, eds. 1994. *Vaccines*. 2nd ed. Philadelphia: WB Saunders Co.

Polyak CS, Macy JT, Irizarry-De La Cruz M, Lai JE, McAuliffe JF, Popovic T, Pillai SP, Mintz ED. 2002. Bioterrorism-related anthrax: international response by the Centers for Disease Control and Prevention. *Emerg Infect Dis* 8(10):1056–9.

Poovorawan Y, Theamboonlers A, Jantaradsamee P, Kaew-in N, Hirsch P, Tangkitvanich P. 1998. Hepatitis TT virus infection in high-risk groups. *Infection* 26(6):355–8.

Popovic T, Sacchi CT, Reeves MW, Whitney AM, Mayer LW, Noble CA, Ajello GW, Mostashari F, Bendana N, Lingappa J, Hajjeh R, Rosenstein NE. 2000. *Neisseria meningitidis* serogroup W135 isolates associated with the ET-37 complex. *Emerg Infect Dis* 6(4):428–9.

Potischman N, Brinton LA. 1996. Nutrition and cervical neoplasia. *Cancer Causes Control* 7(1):113–26.

Prusiner SB. 1995. The prion diseases. *Sci Am* 272(1):48–51, 54–7.

Qiu H, Jun HW, McCall JW. 1998. Pharmacokinetics, formulation, and safety of insect repellent N,N-diethyl-3-methylbenzamide (deet): a review. *J Am Mosq Control Assoc* 14(1):12–27.

Ramalingaswami V. 1996. The plague outbreaks of India, 1994—a prologue. *Current Science* 71:781–806.

Ramers C, Billman G, Hartin M, Ho S, Sawyer MH. 2000. Impact of a diagnostic cerebrospinal fluid enterovirus polymerase chain reaction test on patient management. *JAMA* 283(20):2680–5.

Rappuoli R, Miller HI, Falkow S. 2002. Medicine. The intangible value of vaccination. *Science* 297(5583):937–9.

Rastogi S, Kapur S, Salhan S, Mittal A. 1999. *Chlamydia trachomatis* infection in pregnancy: risk factor for an adverse outcome. *Br J Biomed Sci* 56(2):94–8.

Ray AJ, Hoyen CK, Taub TF, Eckstein EC, Donskey CJ. 2002. Nosocomial transmission of vancomycin-resistant enterococci from surfaces. *JAMA* 287(11):1400–1.

Raymond M, Chevillon C, Guillemaud T, Lenormand T, Pasteur N. 1998. An overview of the evolution of overproduced esterases in the mosquito *Culex pipiens*. *Philos Trans R Soc Lond B Biol Sci* 353(1376):1707–11.

Read RC, Camp NJ, di Giovine FS, Borrow R, Kaczmarski EB, Chaudhary AG, Fox AJ, Duff GW. 2000. An interleukin-1 genotype is associated with fatal outcome of meningococcal disease. *J Infect Dis* 182(5):1557–60.

Redfield RR, Wright DC, James WD, Jones TS, Brown C, Burke DS. 1987. Disseminated vaccinia in a military recruit with human immunodeficiency virus (HIV) disease. *N Engl J Med* 316(11):673–6.

Regis L, Silva-Filha MH, Nielsen-LeRoux C, Charles JF. 2001. Bacteriological larvicides of dipteran disease vectors. *Trends Parasitol* 17(8):377–80.

Rembacken BJ, Snelling AM, Hawkey PM, Chalmers DM, Axon AT. 1999. Non-pathogenic *Escherichia coli* versus mesalazine for the treatment of ulcerative colitis: a randomised trial. *Lancet* 354(9179):635–9.

Ribera E, Miro JM, Cortes E, Cruceta A, Merce J, Marco F, Planes A, Pare JC, Moreno A, Ocana I, Gatell JM, Pahissa A. 1998. Influence of human immunodeficiency virus 1 infection and degree of immunosuppression in the clinical characteristics and outcome of infective endocarditis in intravenous drug users. *Arch Intern Med* 158(18):2043–50.

Rice AL, Sacco L, Hyder A, Black RE. 2000. Malnutrition as an underlying cause of childhood deaths associated with infectious diseases in developing countries. *Bull World Health Organ* 78(10):1207–21.

Richman DD. 2001. HIV chemotherapy. *Nature* 410(6831):995–1001.

Ritzinger FR. 1965. Disease transmission by aircraft. *Aeromed Rev* 4:1–10.

Roberts DR, Laughlin LL, Hsheih P, Legters LJ. 1997. DDT, global strategies, and a malaria control crisis in South America. *Emerg Infect Dis* 3(3):295–302.

Roberts DR, Alecrim WD, Hshieh P, Grieco JP, Bangs M, Andre RG, Chareonviriphap T. 2000. A probability model of vector behavior: effects of DDT repellency, irritancy, and toxicity in malaria control. *J Vector Ecol* 25(1):48–61.

Roberts L. 2001. Mortality in Eastern Republic of Congo: Results from Eleven Mortality Surveys. [Online]. Available: www.intrescom.org/docs/ mortality_2001/ mortII_report. pdf [accessed February 8, 2002].

Roivainen M, Rasilainen S, Ylipaasto P, Nissinen R, Ustinov J, Bouwens L, Eizirik DL, Hovi T, Otonkoski T. 2000. Mechanisms of coxsackievirus-induced damage to human pancreatic beta-cells. *J Clin Endocrinol Metab* 85(1):432–40.

Rosebury T. 1947. Experimental Airborne Infection. Baltimore: Williams and Wilkins.

Rousseau JJ. 1993. *The Social Contract*, 3rd ed. Trans. Henry J. Tozer. London: J.M. Dent.

Rubin RJ, Harrington CA, Poon A, Dietrich K, Greene JA, Moiduddin A. 1999. The economic impact of *Staphylococcus aureus* infection in New York City hospitals. *Emerg Infect Dis* 5(1):9–17.

Ruwende C, Khoo SC, Snow RW, Yates SN, Kwiatkowski D, Gupta S, Warn P, Allsopp CE, Gilbert SC, Peschu N, et al. 1995. Natural selection of hemi- and heterozygotes for G6PD deficiency in Africa by resistance to severe malaria. *Nature* 376(6537):246–9.

Saade C, Bateman M, Bendahmane D. The Story of a Successful Public–Private Partnership in Central America: Handwashing for Diarrheal Disease Prevention. 2001. Arlington, VA: Basic Support for Child Survival Project (BASICS II), Environmental Health Project, United Nations Children's Fund, United States Agency for International Development, World Bank.

Sabato AR, Martin AJ, Marmion BP, Kok TW, Cooper DM. 1984. *Mycoplasma pneumoniae*: acute illness, antibiotics, and subsequent pulmonary function. *Arch Dis Child* 59(11): 1034–7.

Saikku P, Leinonen M, Mattila K, Ekman MR, Nieminen MS, Makela PH, Huttunen JK, Valtonen V. 1988. Serological evidence of an association of a novel *Chlamydia*, TWAR, with chronic coronary heart disease and acute myocardial infarction. *Lancet* 2(8618): 983–6.

Saikku P, Leinonen M, Tenkanen L, Linnanmaki E, Ekman MR, Manninen V, Manttari M, Frick MH, Huttunen JK. 1992. Chronic *Chlamydia pneumoniae* infection as a risk factor for coronary heart disease in the Helsinki Heart Study. *Ann Intern Med* 116(4): 273–8.

Sanchez J, Comerford M, Chitwood DD, Fernandez MI, McCoy CB. 2002. High risk sexual behaviours among heroin sniffers who have no history of injection drug use: implications for HIV risk reduction. *AIDS Care* 14(3):391–8.

Sandia National Laboratories. 2002. Rapid Syndrome Validation Project (RSVP). User's Manual and Description. DRAFT Version 2.3, 7/21/02. Albuquerque, New Mexico. [Online]. Available: http://rsvp.sandia.gov/ [accessed January 30, 2003].

Sbarbaro J. 2000. Trade Liberalization in Health Insurance: Opportunities and Challenges: The Potential Impact of Introducing or Expanding the Availability of Private Health Insurance Within Low and Middle Income Countries. Commission on Macro Economics and Health. Geneva: WHO.

Schiffman MH, Brinton LA. 1995. The epidemiology of cervical carcinogenesis. *Cancer* 76(10 Suppl):1888–901.

Schmaljohn C, Hjelle B. 1997. Hantaviruses: a global disease problem. *Emerg Infect Dis* 3(2):95–104.

Schneider E, Hajjeh RA, Spiegel RA, Jibson RW, Harp EL, Marshall GA, Gunn RA, McNeil MM, Pinner RW, Baron RC, Burger RC, Hutwagner LC, Crump C, Kaufman L, Reef SE, Feldman GM, Pappagianis D, Werner SB. 1997. A coccidioidomycosis outbreak following the Northridge, Calif, earthquake. *JAMA* 277(11):904–8.

Schoepf BG. 2001. International AIDS research in anthropology: taking a critical perspective on the crisis. *Ann Rev Anthropol* 30:335–61.

Schrag SJ, Zywicki S, Farley MM, Reingold AL, Harrison LH, Lefkowitz LB, Hadler JL, Danila R, Cieslak PR, Schuchat A. 2000. Group B streptococcal disease in the era of intrapartum antibiotic prophylaxis. *N Engl J Med* 342(1):15–20.

Schuchat A, Hilger T, Zell E, Farley MM, Reingold A, Harrison L, Lefkowitz L, Danila R, Stefonek K, Barrett N, Morse D, Pinner R. 2001. Active bacterial core surveillance of the emerging infections program network. *Emerg Infect Dis* 7(1):92–9.

Schwarcz SK, Kellogg TA, McFarland W, Louie B, Klausner J, Withum DG, Katz MH. 2002. Characterization of sexually transmitted disease clinic patients with recent human immunodeficiency virus infection. *J Infect Dis* 186(7):1019–22.

Scott TW, Takken W, Knols BG, Boete C. 2002. The ecology of genetically modified mosquitoes. *Science* 298(5591):117–9.

Sealy DP, Schuman SH. 1983. Endemic giardiasis and day care. *Pediatrics* 72(2):154–8.

Seas C, Gotuzzo E. 2000. Gram-negative bacilli. In: Mandell GL, Bennett JE, Dolin R, eds. *Principles and Practice of Infectious Diseases.* 5th ed. Philadelphia: Churchill Livingstone.

Seggev JS, Lis I, Siman-Tov R, Gutman R, Abu–Samara H, Schey G, Naot Y. 1986. *Mycoplasma pneumoniae* is a frequent cause of exacerbation of bronchial asthma in adults. *Ann Allergy* 57(4):263–5.

Semba RD, Miotti PG, Chiphangwi JD, Saah AJ, Canner JK, Dallabetta GA, Hoover DR. 1994. Maternal vitamin A deficiency and mother-to-child transmission of HIV–1. *Lancet* 343(8913):1593–7.

Sen A. 1981. *Poverty and Famines: An Essay on Entitlement and Deprivation.* Oxford and New York: Oxford University Press.

Sen A. 1999. *Development as Freedom.* New York: Anchor.

Seppala H, Klaukka T, Lehtonen R, Nenonen E, Huovinen P. 1997. Erythromycin resistance of group A streptococci from throat samples is related to age. *Pediatr Infect Dis J* 16(7):651–6.

Shah KV. 1997. Human papillomaviruses and anogenital cancers. *N Engl J Med* 337(19):1386–8.

Shaman J, Day JF, Stieglitz M. 2002. Drought-induced amplification of Saint Louis encephalitis virus, Florida. *Emerg Infect Dis* 8(6):575–80.

Shaw DM, Gaerthe B, Leer RJ, Van Der Stap JG, Smittenaar C, Heijne Den Bak–Glashouwer M, Thole JE, Tielen FJ, Pouwels PH, Havenith CE. 2000. Engineering the microflora to vaccinate the mucosa: serum immunoglobulin G responses and activated draining cervical lymph nodes following mucosal application of tetanus toxin fragment C-expressing lactobacilli. *Immunology* 100(4):510–8.

Shieh WJ, Guarner J, Layton M, Fine A, Miller J, Nash D, Campbell GL, Roehrig JT, Gubler DJ, Zaki SR. 2000. The role of pathology in an investigation of an outbreak of West Nile encephalitis in New York, 1999. *Emerg Infect Dis* 6(4):370–2.

Shoemaker NB, Vlamakis H, Hayes K, Salyers AA. 2001. Evidence for extensive resistance gene transfer among *Bacteroides* spp. and among *Bacteroides* and other genera in the human colon. *Appl Environ Microbiol* 67(2):561–8.

Sidell FR, Takafuji ET, Franz DR, eds. 1997. *Medical Aspects of Chemical and Biological Warfare.* Washington, DC: Office of the Surgeon General, United States Army.

Simon PA, Thometz E, Bunch JG, Sorvillo F, Detels R, Kerndt PR. 1999. Prevalence of unprotected sex among men with AIDS in Los Angeles County, California 1995–1997. *AIDS* 13(8):987–90.

Simor AE, Ofner-Agostini M, Bryce E, Green K, McGeer A, Mulvey M, Paton S. 2001. The evolution of methicillin-resistant *Staphylococcus aureus* in Canadian hospitals: 5 years of national surveillance. *CMAJ* 165(1):21–6.

Simpson VR. 1992. Cryptosporidiosis in newborn red deer (*Cervus elaphus*). *Vet Rec* 130(6):116–8.

Sina BJ, Aultman K. 2001. Resisting resistance. *Trends Parasitol* 17(7):305–6.

Sinard JH. 2001. Factors affecting autopsy rates, autopsy request rates, and autopsy findings at a large academic medical center. *Exp Mol Pathol* 70(3):333–43.

Singh N. 2000. Infections in solid organ transplant recipients. *Curr Opin Infect Dis* 13(4):343–347.

Smith DL, Harris AD, Johnson JA, Silbergeld EK, Morris JG Jr. 2002. Animal antibiotic use has an early but important impact on the emergence of antibiotic resistance in human commensal bacteria. *Proc Natl Acad Sci U S A* 99(9):6434–9.

Smithson AE. 2000. Rethinking the Lessons of Tokyo. In: Smithson AE, Levy LA, eds. Ataxia: The Chemical and Biological Terrorism Threat and the US Response. Stimson Center Report No. 35. Washington, DC: The Henry L. Stimson Center.

Spielman A. 1994. A commentary on research needs for monitoring and containing emergent vector-borne infections. Disease in Evolution: Global Changes and Emergence of Infectious Diseases. *Ann NY Acad Sci* 740:457–461.

Spika JS, Facklam RR, Plikaytis BD, Oxtoby MJ. 1991. Antimicrobial resistance of *Streptococcus pneumoniae* in the United States, 1979–1987. The Pneumococcal Surveillance Working Group. *J Infect Dis* 163(6):1273–8.

Srivastava P. 2002. Interaction of heat shock proteins with peptides and antigen presenting cells: chaperoning of the innate and adaptive immune responses. *Annu Rev Immunol* 20:395–425.

Steidler L, Hans W, Schotte L, Neirynck S, Obermeier F, Falk W, Fiers W, Remaut E. 2000. Treatment of murine colitis by *Lactococcus lactis* secreting interleukin–10. *Science* 289(5483):1352–5.

Stephens DS, Levin B, Halloran ME. 1998. Symposium on population biology, evolution, and control of infectious diseases. Introduction. *Am J Med Sci* 315(2):63.

Stocker K, Waitzkin H, Iriart C. 1999. The exportation of managed care to Latin America. *N Engl J Med* 340(14):1131–6.

Strausbaugh LJ. 2001. Emerging health care-associated infections in the geriatric population. *Emerg Infect Dis* 7(2):268–71.

Stuver SO, Boschi–Pinto C, Trichopoulos D. 1997. Infection with hepatitis B and C viruses, social class and cancer. *IARC Sci Publ* (138):319–24.

Su X. 2002. Gonococcal resistance to ciprofloxacin and its clinical significance. 12th IUSTI Asia–Pacific Congress on STI, HIV/AIDS. Beijing, 2002. Abstract no. SY103. Pp. 55–56.

Su X, Lind I. 2001. Molecular basis of high-level ciprofloxacin resistance in *Neisseria gonorrhoeae* strains isolated in Denmark from 1995 to 1998. *Antimicrob Agents Chemother* 45(1):117–23.

Sullivan AD, Wigginton J, Kirschner D. 2001. The coreceptor mutation CCR5Delta32 influences the dynamics of HIV epidemics and is selected for by HIV. *Proc Natl Acad Sci U S A* 98(18):10214–9.

Summerfield D. 1997. The social, cultural and political dimensions of contemporary war. *Med Confl Surviv* 13(1):3–25.

Swaminathan B, Barrett TJ, Hunter SB, Tauxe RV. 2001. PulseNet: the molecular subtyping network for foodborne bacterial disease surveillance, United States. *Emerg Infect Dis* 7(3):382–9.

Swartz MN. 2002. Human diseases caused by foodborne pathogens of animal origin. *Clin Infect Dis* 34 (Suppl 3):S111–22.

Szucs T. 2000. Cost–benefits of vaccination programmes. *Vaccine* 18 (Suppl 1):S49–51.

Tabachnick WJ, Wallis GP, Aitken TH, Miller BR, Amato GD, Lorenz L, Powell JR, Beaty BJ. 1985. Oral infection of *Aedes aegypti* with yellow fever virus: geographic variation and genetic considerations. *Am J Trop Med Hyg* 34(6):1219–24.

Taha MK, Achtman M, Alonso JM, Greenwood B, Ramsay M, Fox A, Gray S, Kaczmarski E. 2000. Serogroup W135 meningococcal disease in Hajj pilgrims. *Lancet* 356(9248):2159.

Taubenberger JK, Reid AH, Janczewski TA, Fanning TG. 2001. Integrating historical, clinical and molecular genetic data in order to explain the origin and virulence of the 1918 Spanish influenza virus. *Philos Trans R Soc Lond B Biol Sci* 356(1416):1829–39.

Taylor LH, Latham SM, Woolhouse ME. 2001a. Risk factors for human disease emergence. *Philos Trans R Soc Lond B Biol Sci* 356(1411):983–9.

Taylor MT, Belgrader P, Furman BJ, Pourahmadi F, Kovacs GT, Northrup MA. 2001b. Lysing bacterial spores by sonication through a flexible interface in a microfluidic system. *Anal Chem* 73(3):492–6.

Thiery I, Baldet T, Barbazan P, Becker N, Junginger B, Mas JP, Moulinier C, Nepstad K, Orduz S, Sinegre G. 1997. International indoor and outdoor evaluation of *Bacillus sphaericus* products: complexity of standardizing outdoor protocols. *J Am Mosq Control Assoc* 13(3):218–26.

Threlfall EJ, Ward LR, Frost JA, Willshaw GA. 2000. The emergence and spread of antibiotic resistance in food-borne bacteria. *Int J Food Microbiol* 62(1–2):1–5.

Titus RG, Ribeiro JM. 1988. Salivary gland lysates from the sand fly *Lutzomyia longipalpis* enhance *Leishmania* infectivity. *Science* 239(4845):1306–8.

Tokars JI, Frank M, Alter MJ, Arduino MJ. 2002. National surveillance of dialysis–associated diseases in the United States, 2000. *Semin Dial* 15(3):162–71.

Toole MJ, Waldman RJ. 1990. Prevention of excess mortality in refugee and displaced populations in developing countries. *JAMA* 263(24):3296–302.

Toole MJ, Galson S, Brady W. 1993. Are war and public health compatible? *Lancet* 341(8854):1193–6.

Topcu Z, Chiba I, Fujieda M, Shibata T, Ariyoshi N, Yamazaki H, Sevgican F, Muthumala M, Kobayashi H, Kamataki T. 2002. CYP2A6 gene deletion reduces oral cancer risk in betel quid chewers in Sri Lanka. *Carcinogenesis* 23(4):595–8.

Topouzis D, du Guerny J. 1999. Sustainable Agriculture/Rural Development and Vulnerability to the AIDS Epidemic. Geneva: UNAIDS/FAO.

Topouzis D, Hemrich G. 2000. Multi-sectoral responses to HIV/AIDS: constraints and opportunities for technical cooperation. *J Intern Dev* 12:85–99.

Torok TJ, Tauxe RV, Wise RP, Livengood JR, Sokolow R, Mauvais S, Birkness KA, Skeels MR, Horan JM, Foster LR. 1997. A large community outbreak of salmonellosis caused by intentional contamination of restaurant salad bars. *JAMA* 278(5):389–95.

Tsiodras S, Gold HS, Sakoulas G, Eliopoulos GM, Wennersten C, Venkataraman L, Moellering RC, Ferraro MJ. 2001. Linezolid resistance in a clinical isolate of *Staphylococcus aureus*. *Lancet* 358(9277):207–8.

Tuazon CU, Sheagren JN. 1974. Increased rate of carriage of *Staphylococcus aureus* among narcotic addicts. *J Infect Dis* 129(6):725–7.

Tzipori S, Angus KW, Campbell I, Sherwood D. 1981. Diarrhea in young red deer associated with infection with *Cryptosporidium*. *J Infect Dis* 144(2):170–5.

Umemura T, Alter HJ, Tanaka E, Yeo AE, Shih JW, Orii K, Matsumoto A, Yoshizawa K, Kiyosawa K. 2001. Association between SEN virus infection and hepatitis C in Japan. *J Infect Dis* 184(10):1246–51.

UNAIDS. 2000. Report on the Global HIV/AIDS Epidemic: June 2000. UNAIDS/00.13E. Geneva: Joint United Nations Programme on HIV/AIDS.

UNAIDS. 2001. Twenty years of HIV/AIDS in graphics. [Online]. Available: http://www.unaids.org/fact_sheets/files/AIDStwenty_en.html#graphics [accessed March 4, 2003].

UNAIDS. 2002. Report on the Global HIV/AIDS Epidemic: July 2002. UNAIDS/02.26E. Geneva: Joint United Nations Programme on HIV/AIDS.

UNAIDS, WHO. 2001. AIDS Epidemic Update: December 2001. UNAIDS/01.74E—WHO/CDS/NCS/2001.2. Geneva: Joint United Nations Programme on HIV/AIDS/World Health Organization.

UNAIDS, WHO. 2002. AIDS epidemic update. UNAIDS/02.46E. Geneva Switzerland: World Health Organization.

Union of Concerned Scientists (UCS). 2002. Food and Environment: Antibiotic Resistance. http://www.ucsusa.org/food_and_environment/antibiotic_resistance/index.cfm?pageID=10.

United Nations Economic Commission for Africa. 2000. African Development Forum 2000, AIDS: the Greatest Leadership Challenge HIV/AIDS and Economic Development in Sub–Saharan Africa. United Nations Economic Commission for Africa. [Online]. Available: http://www.uneca.org/adf2000/theme1.htm#1 [accessed March 5, 2003].

United Nations Popuation Division. 1999. The World at Six Billion. ESA/P/WP.154. New York: Population Division, Department of Economic and Social Affairs.

United Nations Population Division. 2001. World Population Prospects: The 2000 Revision. ESA/P/WP.165. New York: United Nations.

United Nations Population Division. 2002. World Urbanization Prospects: The 2001 Revision. ESA/P/WP.173. New York: Population Division, Department of Economic and Social Affairs.

United Nations Population Fund (UNFPA). 1999. The State of World Population 1999. [Online]. Available: http://www.unfpa.org/swp/1999/ contents.htm [accessed February 14, 2003].

UNFPA. 2001. The State of World Population 2001. [Online]. Available: http://www.unfpa.org/swp/swpmain.htm [accessed February 14, 2003].

United States Commission on National Security/21st Century. 2001. Road Map for National Security: Imperative for Change. The Phase III Report of the U.S. Commission on National Security/21st Century.

University Renal Research and Education Association, United Network for Organ Sharing. 2003. 2002 Annual Report of the U.S. Organ Procurement and Transplantation Network and the Scientific Registry of Transplant Recipients: Transplant Data 1992–2001. Rockville, MD: Department of Health and Human Services, Health Resources and Services Administration, Office of Special Programs, Division of Transplantation.

Uppal PK. 2000. Emergence of Nipah virus in Malaysia. *Ann N Y Acad Sci* 916:354–7.

U.S. Census Bureau. 2001. Population Profile of the United States: 2000 (Internet Release). [Online]. Available: http://www.census.gov/population/ www/pop–profile/profile2000.html [accessed March 5, 2003].

U.S. Census Bureau. 2002a. United States Census 2000. [Online]. Available: http://www.census.gov/main/www/cen2000.html [accessed February 14, 2003].

U.S. Census Bureau. 2002b. Current Population Reports, P60–219, Poverty in the United States: 2001. Washington, DC: U.S. Government Printing Office.

U.S. Congress, Office of Technology Assessment. 1993a. Technologies Underlying Weapons of Mass Destruction, OTA–BP–ISC–115. Washington, DC: U.S. Government Printing Office.

U.S. Congress, Office of Technology Assessment. 1993b. Proliferation of Weapons of Mass Destruction: Assessing the Risks, OTA–ISC–559. Washington, DC: U.S. Government Printing Office.

USDA. 1997. Part III: Changes in the U.S. Pork Industry 1990–1995 Fort Collins, CO: U.S. Department of Agriculture.

USDA. 2000a. Changes in the U.S. Feedlot Industry, 1994–1999. #N327.0800. Fort Collins, CO: USDA:APHIS:VS, CEAH, National Animal Health Monitoring System.

USDA. 2000b. Part III: Health Management and Biosecurity in U.S. Feedlots, 1999. #N336.1200. Fort Collins, CO: USDA:APHIS:VS, CEAH, National Animal Health Monitoring System.

USDA. 2001. Part I: Reference of Swine Health and Management in the United States, 2000, National Health Monitoring System. #N338.0801. Fort Collins, CO: U.S. Department of Agriculture.

USDA, EPA. 1999. Unified National Strategy for Animal Feeding Operations. Washington, DC: U.S. Department of Agriculture, Environmental Protection Agency.

Usera MA, Aladuena A, Gonzalez R, De la Fuente M, Garcia–Pena J, Frias N, Echeita MA. 2002. Antibiotic resistance of *Salmonella* spp. from animal sources in Spain in 1996 and 2000. *J Food Prot* 65(5):768–73.

Valencia GB, Banzon F, Cummings M, McCormack WM, Glass L, Hammerschlag MR. 1993. *Mycoplasma hominis* and *Ureaplasma urealyticum* in neonates with suspected infection. *Pediatr Infect Dis J* 12(7):571–3.

Valenzuela JG, Belkaid Y, Garfield MK, Mendez S, Kamhawi S, Rowton ED, Sacks DL, Ribeiro JM. 2001. Toward a defined anti-*Leishmania* vaccine targeting vector antigens: characterization of a protective salivary protein. *J Exp Med* 194(3):331–42.

van Belkum A, Verbrugh H. 2001. 40 years of methicillin resistant *Staphylococcus aureus*. *BMJ* 323(7314):644–5.

Venczel LV, Desai MM, Vertz PD, England B, Hutin YJ, Shapiro CN, Bell BP. 2001. The role of child care in a community-wide outbreak of hepatitis A. *Pediatrics* 108(5):E78.

Vicca AF. 1999. Nursing staff workload as a determinant of methicillin–resistant *Staphylococcus aureus* spread in an adult intensive therapy unit. *J Hosp Infect* 43(2):109–13.

Vitek CR, Wharton M. 1998. Diphtheria in the former Soviet Union: reemergence of a pandemic disease. *Emerg Infect Dis* 4(4):539–50.

Volmink J, Garner P. 2001. Directly observed therapy for treating tuberculosis. *Cochrane Database Syst Rev* (4):CD003343.

Volmink J, Matchaba P, Garner P. 2000. Directly observed therapy and treatment adherence. *Lancet* 355(9212):1345–50.

Walker JB, Hussey EK, Treanor JJ, Montalvo A Jr, Hayden FG. 1997. Effects of the neuraminidase inhibitor zanamavir on otologic manifestations of experimental human influenza. *J Infect Dis* 176(6):1417–22.

Wallensteen P, Sollenberg M. 1999. Armed conflict, 1989–1998. *J Peace Res* 36(5):593–606.

Wallensteen P, Sollenberg M. 2001. Armed conflict, 1989–2000. *J Peace Res* 38(5):629–644.

Weatherall DJ. 1996a. The genetics of common diseases: the implications of population variability. *Ciba Found Symp* 197:300–8; discussion 308–11.

Weatherall DJ. 1996b. Host genetics and infectious disease. *Parasitology* 112 Suppl:S23–9.

Webster RG, Bean WJ, Gorman OT, Chambers TM, Kawaoka Y. 1992. Evolution and ecology of influenza A viruses. *Microbiol Rev* 56(1):152–79.

Wegener HC, Aarestrup FM, Jensen LB, Hammerum AM, Bager F. 1999. Use of antimicrobial growth promoters in food animals and *Enterococcus faecium* resistance to therapeutic antimicrobial drugs in Europe. *Emerg Infect Dis* 5(3):329–35.

Wellems TE, Plowe CV. 2001. Chloroquine-resistant malaria. *J Infect Dis* 184(6):770–6.

Wenzel RP, Edmond MB. 2001. The impact of hospital-acquired bloodstream infections. *Emerg Infect Dis* 7(2):174–7.

Wenzel RP, Nettleman MD, Jones RN, Pfaller MA. 1991. Methicillin-resistant *Staphylococcus aureus*: implications for the 1990s and effective control measures. *Am J Med* 91(3B): 221S–227S.

West CE. 2000. Vitamin A and measles. *Nutr Rev* 58(2 Pt 2):S46–54.

Westendorp RG, Langermans JA, Huizinga TW, Elouali AH, Verweij CL, Boomsma DI, Vandenbroucke JP, Vandenbroucke JP. 1997. Genetic influence on cytokine production and fatal meningococcal disease. *Lancet* 349(9046):170–3.

White DG, Zhao S, Sudler R, Ayers S, Friedman S, Chen S, McDermott PF, McDermott S, Wagner DD, Meng J. 2001. The isolation of antibiotic-resistant salmonella from retail ground meats. *N Engl J Med* 345(16):1147–54.

Whitehead Institute. 2002. Whitehead—Who We Are. [Online]. Available: www.wi.mit.edu/who/who.html [accessed February 10, 2003].

Whitney CG, Farley MM, Hadler J, Harrison LH, Lexau C, Reingold A, Lefkowitz L, Cieslak PR, Cetron M, Zell ER, Jorgensen JH, Schuchat A. 2000. Increasing prevalence of multidrug-resistant *Streptococcus pneumoniae* in the United States. *N Engl J Med* 343(26):1917–24.

WHO. 1970. Health Aspects of Chemical and Biological Weapons. Geneva: World Health Organization.

WHO. 1996. Fighting Disease, Fostering Development. The World Health Report 1996. Geneva: World Health Organization.

WHO. 1997. Vitamin A Supplements: A Guide to Their Use in the Treatment of Vitamin A Deficiency and Xerophthalmia. Geneva: World Health Organization.

WHO. 1998a. World Health Report 1998: Life in the 21st Century: A Vision for All. Geneva: World Health Organization.

WHO. 1998b. Fact Sheets: Global Infectious Disease Surveillance. Fact Sheet No 200. Geneva: WHO.

WHO. 1999a. Removing Obstacles to Healthy Development. Report on Infectious Disease. Geneva: WHO.

WHO. 1999b. World Health Report 1999: Making a Difference. Geneva: World Health Organization.

WHO. 1999c. Food Safety Issues Associated with Products from Aquaculture. Geneva: World Health Organization.

WHO. 1999d. What Is DOTS? A Guide to Understanding the WHO-Recommended TB Control Strategy Known as DOTS. WHO/CDS/CPC/TB/99.270. Geneva: World Health Organization.

WHO. 1999e. Influenza Pandemic Preparedness Plan. The Role of WHO and Guidelines for National and Regional Planning. Geneva: World Health Organization.

WHO. 2000a. World Health Report 2000: Health Systems: Improving Performance. Geneva: World Health Organization.

WHO. 2000b. Infant and young child nutrition, Report by the Director-General. Fifty-third World Health Assembly. A53/7.

WHO. 2000c. Outbreak news: Rift Valley fever, Saudi Arabia, August–October 2000. *Weekly Epidemiological Record* 75(46):369–376.

WHO. 2000d. Cholera Factsheet. Fact Sheet No 107. Geneva: World Health Organization.

WHO. 2000e. Fifty-Third World Health Assembly. Stop Tuberculosis Initiative, Report by the Director General. A53/5. Geneva: World Health Organization.

WHO. 2000f. WHO Global Principles for the Containment of Antimicrobial Resistance in Animals Intended for Food. Report of a WHO consultation with the participation of the Food and Agriculture Organization of the United Nations and the Office International des Epizooties. Geneva, 5–9 June 2000. WHO/CDS/CSR/APH/2000.4.

WHO. 2000g. A major killer in west and central Africa. *Measles Bulletin*. Issue 5. WHO/V&B/00.38.

WHO. 2001a. World Health Report 2001: Global Tuberculosis Control. Geneva: World Health Organization.

WHO. 2001b. Global Prevalence and Incidence of Selected Curable Sexually Transmitted Infections: Overview and Estimates. Geneva: World Health Organization.

WHO. 2001c. Macroeconomics and Health: Investing in Health for Economic Development. Report of the Commission on Macroeconomics and Health. Geneva: World Health Organization.

WHO. 2001d. Global Prevalence and Incidence of Selected Curable Sexually Transmitted Infections, Overview and Estimates. WHO/HIV_AIDS/2001.02. Geneva: World Health Organization.

WHO. 2001e. Nipah Virus Factsheet. Fact Sheet No 262. [Online]. Available: http://www.who.int/inf–fs/en/fact262.html [accessed February 21, 2003].

WHO. 2001f. Cholera, 2000. *Wkly Epidemiol Rec* 76(31):233–40.

WHO. 2001g. WHO Vaccine-Preventable Diseases: Monitoring System. 2001 Global Summary. Department of Vaccines and Biologicals. WHO/V&B/01.34. Geneva: World Health Organization.

WHO. 2001h. WHO and Lyon—A Partnership for Global Health Security. [Online]. Available: http://www.who.int/emc/lyon/ [accessed January30, 2003].

WHO. 2001i. WHO Global Strategy for Containment of Antimicrobial Resistance. WHO/ CDS/CSR/DRS/2001.2a. Geneva: World Health Organization.

WHO. 2002a. Coordinates 2002—Charting progress against AIDS, TB and malaria. [Online]. Available: http://www.who.int/infectious-disease-news/ [accessed February 13, 2003].

WHO. 2002b. World Health Report 2002: Reducing Risks, Promoting Healthy Life. Geneva: World Health Organization.

WHO. 2002c. Tuberculosis. [Online]. Available: http://www.who.int/ mediacentre/factsheets/ who104/en/index.html [accessed February 21, 2003].

WHO. 2002d. Nutrition. [Online]. Available: http://www.who.int/nut/ [accessed February 20, 2003].

WHO. 2002e. Use of Antimicrobials Outside Human Medicine and Resultant Antimicrobial Resistance in Humans. Fact Sheet 268. Geneva: WHO.

WHO. 2002f. Prevention of Hospital-Acquired Infections, A Practical Guide. Geneva: World Health Organization.

WHO. 2002g. An Expanded DOTS Framework for Effective Tuberculosis Control. WHO/ CDS/TB/2002.297. Geneva: World Health Organization.

WHO. 2002h. Global Tuberculosis Control: Surveillance, Planning, Financing. WHO Report 2002. WHO/CDS/TB/2002.295. Geneva: World Health Organization.

WHO. 2002i. Tuberculosis. Fact Sheet No 104. [Online]. Available: http://www.who.int/ mediacentre/factsheets/who104/en/index.html [accessed February 6, 2003].

WHO. 2002j. Scaling up the Response to Infectious Diseases: A Way Out of Poverty. WHO/ CDS/2002.7. Geneva: World Health Organization.

WHO. 2002k. Global measles mortality reduction and regional elimination, 2000–2001. Part II. *Wkly Epidemiol Rec* 77(8):58–61.

WHO. 2003a. TDR Home Page. [Online]. Available: www.who.int/tdr [accessed February 28, 2003].

WHO. 2003b. Communicable Disease Surveillance & Response (CSR): Global Outbreak Alert & Response Network. [Online]. Available: http://www.who.int/csr/ outbreaknetwork/en/ [accessed January 30, 2003].

WHO, UNICEF. 2001. WHO–UNICEF Joint Statement on Strategies to Reduce Measles Mortality Worldwide. Geneva: WHO.

Wick RL Jr, Irvine LA. 1995. The microbiological composition of airliner cabin air. *Aviat Space Environ Med* 66(3):220–4.

Wierup M. 2001. The Swedish experience of the 1986 year ban of antimicrobial growth promoters, with special reference to animal health, disease prevention, productivity, and usage of antimicrobials. *Microb Drug Resist* 7(2):183–90.

Wierzba TF, El–Yazeed RA, Savarino SJ, Mourad AS, Rao M, Baddour M, El–Deen AN, Naficy AB, Clemens JD. 2001. The interrelationship of malnutrition and diarrhea in a periurban area outside Alexandria, Egypt. *J Pediatr Gastroenterol Nutr* 32(2):189–96.

Will RG, Ironside JW, Zeidler M, Cousens SN, Estibeiro K, Alperovitch A, Poser S, Pocchiari M, Hofman A, Smith PG. 1996. A new variant of Creutzfeldt–Jakob disease in the UK. *Lancet* 347(9006):921–5.

Willadsen P. 2001. The molecular revolution in the development of vaccines against ectoparasites. *Vet Parasitol* 101(3–4):353–68.

Willadsen PL, Billingsley PF. 1996. Immune intervention against blood-feeding insects. In: Lehane ML, Billinsley PF, eds. *Biology of the Insect Midgut*. London: Chapman and Hall. Pp. 323–340.

Wilson ME. 1995. Travel and the emergence of infectious diseases. *Emerg Infect Dis* 1(2):39–46.

Wilson ML. 1994. Rift Valley fever virus ecology and the epidemiology of disease emergence. *Ann N Y Acad Sci* 740:169–80.

Wilson ML. 2001. Ecology and infectious disease. In: Aron JL, Patz J, eds. *Ecosystem Change and Public Health: A Global Perspective*. Baltimore: Johns Hopkins University Press.

Wolitski RJ, Valdiserri RO, Denning PH, Levine WC. 2001. Are we headed for a resurgence of the HIV epidemic among men who have sex with men? *Am J Pub Health* 91(6):883–8.

Wong D, Nye K, Hollis P. 1991. Microbial flora on doctors' white coats. *BMJ* 303(6817): 1602–4.

Wood R, Maartens G, Lombard CJ. 2000. Risk factors for developing tuberculosis in HIV–1-infected adults from communities with a low or very high incidence of tuberculosis. *J Acquir Immune Defic Syndr* 23(1):75–80.

World Bank. 2001. *World Development Report: Attacking Poverty 2000/2001*. New York: Oxford University Press.

World Bank. 2002. World Development Indicators 2001. Washington, DC: World Bank.

World Bank Group. 2002. Poverty Trends and Voices of the Poor: Income Poverty. [Online]. Available: www.worldbank.org/poverty/data/trends/ income.htm [accessed February 27, 2003].

World Resources Institute, United Nations Environment Programme, United Nations Development Programme, World Bank. 1996. *World Resources 1996–97*. New York and Oxford: Oxford University Press.

World Tourism Organization. 2002. *Tourism Highlights 2002*. Madrid, Spain: World Tourism Organization.

Wotherspoon AC, Doglioni C, Diss TC, Pan L, Moschini A, de Boni M, Isaacson PG. 1993. Regression of primary low-grade B-cell gastric lymphoma of mucosa–associated lymphoid tissue type after eradication of *Helicobacter pylori*. *Lancet* 342(8871):575–7.

Wright PF, Webster RG. 2001. Orthomyxoviruses. In: Knipe DM, Howley PM, eds. *Fields Virology*, 4th ed. Philadelphia: Lippincott Williams & Wilkins. Pp. 1533–79.

Yang S. 1998. FoodNet and Enter-net: emerging surveillance programs for foodborne diseases. *Emerg Infect Dis* 4(3):457–8.

Yano T, Ichikawa Y, Komatu S, Arai S, Oizumi K. 1994. Association of *Mycoplasma pneumoniae* antigen with initial onset of bronchial asthma. *Am J Respir Crit Care Med* 149(5):1348–53.

Yates T, Mills J, Parmenter C, Ksiazek T, Parmenter R, Calisher C, Nichol S, Abbott K, Young J, Morrison M, Beaty B, Dunnum J, Baker RJ, Peters CJ. 2002a. The ecology and evolutionary history of an emergent disease: hantavirus pulmonry syndrome. *Bioscience* 52(11):989–98.

Yates T, Mills J, Parmenter C, Ksiazek T, Parmenter R, Calisher C, Nichol S, Abbott K, Young J, Morrison M, Beaty B, Dunnum J, Baker RJ, Peters CJ. 2002b. Biocomplexity and hantavirus pulmonary syndrome: the ecology of an outbreak. *Bioscience*. Submitted.

Ylitalo N, Josefsson A, Melbye M, Sorensen P, Frisch M, Andersen PK, Sparen P, Gustafsson M, Magnusson P, Ponten J, Gyllensten U, Adami HO. 2000. A prospective study showing long-term infection with human papillomavirus 16 before the development of cervical carcinoma in situ. *Cancer Res* 60(21):6027–32.

Zielinski GD, Snijders PJ, Rozendaal L, Voorhorst FJ, van der Linden HC, Runsink AP, de Schipper FA, Meijer CJ. 2001. HPV presence precedes abnormal cytology in women developing cervical cancer and signals false negative smears. *Br J Cancer* 85(3):398–404.

Appendix A

Microbial Threats to Health Public Committee Meeting Agendas

Committee Meeting #1
Tuesday, September 4, 2001
Washington, D.C.
AGENDA
OPEN SESSION

1:00   **Welcome and Introductions**
         Dr. Margaret Hamburg, Co-chair
         Dr. Joshua Lederberg, Co-chair

1:15   **Presentations by Sponsoring Agencies**
         CDC/NCID
         NIH/NIAID
         NIH/Fogarty
         USAID
         U.S. Department of Defense
         Ellison Medical Foundation
         FDA
         USDA/FSIS
         USDA/REE

3:00   **Break**

3:15   Open Discussion by Committee

3:45   **Presentations by Co-chairs**
            Dr. Margaret Hamburg, Co-chair
            Dr. Joshua Lederberg, Co-chair

4:15   **Public Meeting Adjourns**

Committee Meeting #2
Tuesday, November 6, 2001
Washington, DC
AGENDA
Surveillance, Laboratory Capacity, and Training
OPEN SESSION

10:00 am   **The Role of the World Health Organization**
            Dr. Ray Arthur
            Communicable Disease Surveillance and Response Department
            Global Alert and Response Team

10:45   **The Role of the U.S. Agency for International Development**
            Dr. Murray Trostle
            Infectious Disease Surveillance Working Group

11:30   **Dr. Mary J.R. Gilchrist**
            Director, University Hygienic Laboratory, University of Iowa

12:15 pm   **Working Lunch**
            The Role of the Department of Defense
            COL Patrick W. Kelley
            DOD Global Emerging Infections Surveillance and Response
            Systems
            Walter Reed Army Institute of Research

1:15   **The Role of the Centers for Disease Control and Prevention**
            Dr. James Hughes (via telephone)
            Director, National Center for Infectious Diseases

            Dr. Julie Gerberding (via telephone)
            Acting Deputy Director, National Center for Infectious Diseases

Alexandra Levitt
Policy Specialist, Office of the Director, NCID

Dr. Douglas Hamilton
Chief, Epidemiology Intelligence Service

2:54   **Research Capacity Building Programs of the Fogarty International Center/NIH**
Dr. Joel Breman
Senior Policy Advisor

3:30   Break

3:45   **Public Health Workforce**
Dr. Claude Earl Fox
Director, Johns Hopkins Urban Health Institute
Former Administrator, Health Resources and Services Administration

4:30   **Dr. Richard Wansley**
Executive Director, Illinois Health Education Consortium, AHEC

5:15   **The Real World**
Dr. Bob England
Director of Health, City of Milford Health Department, Former Arizona State Epidemiologist

6:00   **Open Discussion**

6:30   Open Session Adjourned

Appendix B

Syndromic Surveillance

Kelly J. Henning, M.D.
Department of Medicine,
University of Pennsylvania School of Medicine

BACKGROUND

Infectious disease threats, both naturally occurring and intentional, continue to challenge the medical and public health communities. Even before the tragic events of September 11, 2001, public health officials had begun a search for new and innovative methods to enhance the detection of emerging infections and illness due to bioterrorist agents. In response to a series of Institute of Medicine reports citing deficiencies in the ability of U.S. public health systems to deal with emerging infectious diseases (Institute of Medicine, 1987, 1988, 1992) the Centers for Disease Control and Prevention (CDC) prepared a plan entitled *Preventing Emerging Infectious Diseases* (CDC, 1998). Strengthening surveillance is one of the primary objectives of this plan. Similarly, developing programs that allow for the "early detection and investigation of outbreaks"(CDC, 1998) is cited in Goal One of the 1998 CDC guideline *Preventing Emerging Infectious Diseases: A Strategy for the 21st Century*. And CDC's strategic plan for biological and chemical preparedness calls for early detection by integrating bioterrorism into existing systems and developing "new mechanisms for detecting, evaluating, and reporting suspicious events" (CDC, 2000).

At the local level, public health officials evaluated lessons learned during the 1999 introduction of West Nile virus into New York City, and emphasized the importance of preparing surveillance tools that would allow tracking of emerging infections and simultaneously be available for bioterrorism events (Fine and Layton, 1999). Likewise, a major obstacle identified in Operation Topoff, a simulated plague attack on metropolitan

Denver, was the lack of a surveillance system that could be sustained and available to continuously communicate information to the central command system (Hoffman and Norton, 2000).

Several epidemics of the recent past have illustrated the need for enhanced, more timely reporting of infectious diseases. The 1976 Legionnaires' Disease outbreak in Pennsylvania is an example of a point-source outbreak of an unknown agent with rapid transmission and high mortality associated with the dispersal of exposed persons (Fraser et al., 1977)—an outbreak that today would certainly require evaluation as a potential bioterrorist attack. Yet surveillance and outbreak data related to this investigation were so unwieldy that they had to be evaluated using mainframe computers (Martin and Bean, 1995). The 1993 hantavirus outbreak in the southwestern United States (CDC, 1993) and the West Nile virus encephalitis outbreak in New York City (CDC, 1999) illustrate the importance of prompt reporting by clinicians in triggered public health investigations. The availability of timely, flexible surveillance systems could have aided in characterizing and determining the scope of the outbreaks after their initial reporting.

CDC notes several recent successes in strengthening surveillance efforts and in implementing new surveillance strategies, and has initiated the Epidemiology and Laboratory Capacity program to provide health departments with laboratory and technical capacity in dealing with emerging infections (CDC, 1998). Seven states have initiated emerging infections programs (EIPs) to conduct population-based surveillance and special research on emerging and re-emerging diseases. Creation of the Foodborne Diseases Active Surveillance Network (FoodNet) within EIPs has provided a model program for outbreak detection within EIPs. Provider-based networks have been established to collect information from nontraditional public health venues (CDC, 1998; Binder et al., 1999). Examples include infectious diseases surveillance in 11 academic emergency rooms (EMERGEncy ID NET) (Talan et al., 1998) a network of enhanced communication among 500 infectious disease practitioners via the Internet (the Infectious Diseases Society of America Emergency Infections Network [IDSA EIN]), and a group of 22 linked travel medicine clinics in the United States and abroad to monitor disease among returning travelers (GeoSentinel) (CDC, 1998). With the exception of the unexplained death and severe illness project within selected EIP sites (discussed below), all of these enhanced or innovative systems rely on the reporting of specific clinically and/or laboratory-confirmed diagnosed cases. None of these systems are based on the reporting of clinical syndromes or groups of clinical signs and symptoms.

Although the need for innovative surveillance techniques had been identified prior to September 11, the U.S. outbreak of anthrax following the intentional delivery of *B. anthracis* spores through the mail in fall 2001,

(CDC, 2001) greatly accelerated the development and initiation of enhanced surveillance systems around the country.

DEFINITIONS AND RATIONALE

The covert aerosol release of a bioterrorist agent, such as anthrax, plague, or botulinum toxin, would require increased surveillance for illness by the public health and medical communities and rapid institution of illness prevention measures (Rotz et al., 2000). With these agents, as well as with numerous naturally occurring emerging infections, people would likely present initially with nonspecific mild illness. Exposed individuals might stay home from work or school, go to the pharmacy to buy over-the-counter remedies, and, as illness progressed, might call their physician's offices to report symptoms.

As their illness worsened, patients might seek appointments with primary care offices or go to emergency rooms for treatment. Even after presenting to a health care provider, many patients might be sent home with prescriptions for various antibiotics, while others would be ill enough to require hospital admission, some to intensive-care units. The rate with which new cases would occur might depend on infectious dose, location at time of agent release or exposure, environmental factors, and host factors. The geographic pattern of cases could be large-scale, widely dispersed, or focal. Surveillance for the above events, before definitive diagnosis, would require innovative, flexible, disease syndrome-based surveillance systems that do not currently exist in the United States.

No published definition of *syndromic surveillance* has been identified by this author. For the purpose of this discussion, syndromic surveillance is defined as the surveillance of disease syndromes (groups of signs and symptoms), rather than specific, clinical, or laboratory-defined diseases.

Syndromic surveillance is a relatively new concept in public health surveillance. Several different terms have been used to denote syndromic systems. Box B-1 lists selected examples. There is considerable overlap in structure and function among these systems, although the source of data collected by each may differ. The lack of an accepted definition for syndromic surveillance and the inconsistent nomenclature in the published literature add to confusion regarding the structure, usefulness, and applicability of this approach.

ATTRIBUTES

Public health surveillance can be described as the ongoing, systematic collection, analysis, interpretation, and dissemination of data regarding a health-related event for use in public health action to reduce morbidity and

---

BOX B-1
Syndromic Surveillance Systems: Nomenclature

The various terms used to denote syndromic systems include the following:

- Syndromic surveillance
- Early warning systems
- Prodromic surveillance
- Outbreak detection systems
- Information system-based sentinel surveillance

SOURCES: Adapted from the following: Brinsfield et al., 2001; Duchin et al., 2001; Harcourt et al., 2001; Lazarus et al., 2001; Lober et al., 2002; Mostashari and Karpati, 2002; Stern and Lightfoot, 1999; Wagner et al., 2001b; Treadwell, CDC, Personal Communication, 2002.

---

mortality and to improve health (CDC, 2001). CDC has identified a list of surveillance system attributes that are useful for evaluation, including usefulness, simplicity, flexibility, data quality, acceptability, sensitivity, predictive value positive, representativeness, timeliness, and stability.

Routinely evaluated surveillance system attributes are relevant to syndromic surveillance systems; however, timeliness and sensitivity may take on added importance (Bravata, 2001). CDC has identified early detection as an essential component for ensuring a prompt response to an intentional biological or chemical attack or the emergence of an unusual or unknown disease (CDC, 2000). Some authors have suggested that, given the level of importance associated with early detection of bioterrorist agents in initiating response, "extreme timeliness of detection" may become a new requirement of at least some public health surveillance systems (Wagner et al., 2001a). For syndromic surveillance, simplicity and acceptability of the system will likely require electronic data transfer that is transparent to providers. Syndromic systems will necessarily be flexible so they can capture a broad range of signs and symptoms that may emerge. Evaluation of the sensitivity of syndromic systems to detect new or emerging health diseases is an evolving science. Most investigators have used naturally occurring, cyclical influenza outbreaks to evaluate existing systems (Tsui et al., 2001; Espino and Wagner, 2001; Canas et al., 2000; CDC, 2002). Because bioterrorism-related events and emerging or reemerging diseases may be spread over very large geographic areas, the representativeness of any one syndromic surveillance system will likely depend on its ability to interact/communicate with other systems in a given locale and with systems in neighboring states or regions.

TYPES OF SYNDROMIC SURVEILLANCE SYSTEMS

Syndromic surveillance systems can be categorized in several ways. Syndromic systems can operate for short-term surveillance projects or they can be designed for ongoing, sustained activities. Some syndromic systems have been designed to "drop in" to a locality, usually to bolster local public health surveillance efforts in response to a defined event. Such drop-in systems have been used to enhance surveillance efforts surrounding large-scale events that are national in scope. Drop-in syndromic surveillance, supported by local health departments and CDC, was implemented in Seattle for the 1999 World Trade Organization Meetings (Duchin, Public Health—Seattle and King County, Personal Communication, 2002), in the Washington metropolitan area for the 2001 presidential inauguration (Blythe, Maryland Department of Health and Mental Hygiene, Personal Communication, 2002; Sockwell, Virginia Department of Health (Northern Region), Personal Communication, 2002), in Philadelphia for the July 31–August 4, 2000, Republican National Convention (Chernak, Philadelphia Department of Health, Personal Communication, 2001), and in Los Angeles County for the August 14–17, 2000, Democratic National Convention (Bancroft, County of Los Angeles, Department of Health Services, Personal Communication, 2002; Peterson, County of Los Angeles, Department of Health Services, Personal Communication, 2002). Drop-in syndromic systems used to date have literally "dropped in" to a local health department, operated during the event and for a few days after (an incubation period), and then "dropped out" of the locality. Drop-in syndromic surveillance systems can be used to lay groundwork for sustained syndromic surveillance by building relationships with hospitals, infection control practitioners, information specialists, and others in the health care environment.

Since early recognition of new or emerging diseases or a bioterrorist release is expected to be an ongoing goal of innovative surveillance systems, sustained syndromic surveillance systems, ideally operating seven days a week throughout the year, are being actively investigated. Most of these systems are in the pilot or development phase. Syndromic systems differ primarily in the way that they capture data. Table B-1 lists several of the broad categories of syndromic systems that are being explored.

Manual systems rely heavily on hospital personnel. A simple, manual system is currently operating in Santa Clara County, California, where a "tally sheet" is used by the emergency department triage nurses in 12 acute care hospitals (Bravata, 2001; Cody, Santa Clara County Department of Health, Personal Communication, 2002). The nurse ticks a mark on the sheet for every patient who has a chief complaint compatible with one of six syndromes: flu-like symptoms, fever with mental status changes, fever with skin rash, diarrhea with dehydration, visual or swallowing difficulties/

TABLE B-1 Syndromic Surveillance: Characteristics, Advantages, and
Disadvantages

	Selected Characteristics	Advantage	Disadvantage
Event-based surveillance			
Drop-In	Defined time period Active Emergency departments (ED) Large clinics	Develop relationships with ED staff, ICPs; transportable to various sites	Labor intensive; not sustainable; not scalable
Sustained surveillance			
Manual	Active/passive FAX-based reporting Usually ED triage logs/tally sheets	Develop relationships with hospital staff; easy to initiate; detailed information obtainable	Labor intensive; difficult to maintain 24/7; not sustainable
Electronic	Passive Auromated transfer of hospital (usually ED triage or diagnosis) or outpatient data; use of data collected for other purposes; data mining for large collections from multiple sources	Can be scalable; minimum or no provider input programming required; data available continuously; data standardized	Need expertise and health dept. informatics expertise; confidentiality
Novel modes of collection	Active Hand-held or touch screen devices	Easy to use; rapid provider feedback; can post alerts/info	Requires providers input; not sustainable
Novel sources of data	Active/passive Medical examiner data; unexplained death or severe illness data	Clearly defined "syndrome"; may be supplemented with laboratory data	Not an early warning; scalable

SOURCES: This table was adapted from the following: Wagner et al., 2001a; Duchin et al., 2001; Pavlin, 2001; Lazarus et al., 2001; Moser et al., 1999; Zelicoff et al., 2001; Stanford report, 2001; Kluger et al., 2001; Rainbow et al., 2000.

slurred speech or dry mouth, and acute respiratory distress syndrome. If the patient's condition does not fit any syndrome, the nurse puts a hash mark in the column "none of the above." The tally marks for each syndrome are totaled at the end of each nursing shift, and the sheet is faxed to the Santa Clara Health Department. No personal identifiers are transmitted. The information is entered into a computer program at the health department, and the totals are reviewed every 24 hours. As noted in Table B-1 and confirmed by the group in Santa Clara, this method is labor-intensive. Participation by hospitals has declined dramatically since the cessation of additional anthrax cases after December 2001, and Santa Clara County is now actively pursuing alternative systems for implementation. Despite the lack of baseline data for comparison and uncertainties regarding when and how to investigate "clusters" of particular syndromes, many local health departments across the country initiated similar efforts immediately following the terrorist attacks of September 11, 2001 (Blythe, Maryland Department of Health and Mental Hygiene, Personal Communication, 2002; Sockwell, Virginia Department of Health (Northern Region), Personal Communication, 2002; Chernak, Philadelphia Department of Health, Personal Communication, 2001; Paladini, Bergen County Department of Health Services, Personal Communication, 2002).

In contrast, several investigators and collaborating health departments have been exploring electronic transfer of data from health facilities to public health departments (Wagner et al., 2001b; Duchin et al., 2001; Pavlin, ESSENCE, Personal Communication, 2001; Mostashari, New York City Department of Health, Personal Communication, 2001; Lazarus et al., 2001; Moser et al., 1999). The key feature of electronic syndromic surveillance is the ability to collect data in an ongoing way without the direct input of health care personnel, so that their operation is transparent to providers. Systems that do not place additional burdens on health care providers are essential for large-scale, sustained syndromic surveillance. Electronic systems have been implemented by the U.S. military (Pavlin, ESSENCE, Personal Communication 2001), regionally within states (Lazarus et al., 2001; RODS; Piposzar, Alleghany County Health Department, Personal Communication, 2002), and at the local level (Mostashari, New York City Department of Health, Personal Communication, 2001). All of these systems are in the pilot or early development stages.

The network developed within the Department of Defense—Global Emerging Infections System (DoD-GEIS)—has initiated surveillance for early detection of infectious disease outbreaks by monitoring seven syndromes (respiratory, fever/malaise/sepsis, gastrointestinal, neurological, dermatological-infectious, dermatological-hemorrhagic, and coma/sudden death) in 313 military treatment facilities worldwide (Pavlin, ESSENCE, Personal Communication, 2001). This system, the Electronic Surveillance

System for the Early Notification of Community-Based Epidemics (ES-SENCE), captures data daily from the standardized ambulatory data record and categorizes syndromes based on *International Classification of Diseases, 9th Revision, Clinical Modification* (ICD-9-CM) diagnoses assigned by providers. The data are routed to a central server in Denver and forwarded to a secure server at Walter Reed Army Institute of Research for analysis and generation of reports. The time delay from visit to data capture and analysis is 2–4 days. Obtaining the syndromic information places no additional requirements on providers or clinic administrators. Regional and local syndromic surveillance systems, such the Real-Time Outbreak and Disease Surveillance (RODS) system in western Pennsylvania (RODS; Wagner et al., 2001b) and the emergency department chief complaint-based system in New York City (Mostashari, New York City Department of Health, Personal Communication, 2001), collect data principally from emergency department visits.

Novel modes of collecting electronic data include several devices that have been developed for direct data entry via touch screens, keypads, or web-based programs (Zelicoff et al., 2001; Stanford Report, 2001; Weiss, Stanford University, Personal Communication, 2001; Coiera, 2001; Zelicoff, Sandia National Laboratories, Personal Communication 2001). These systems simplify the collection of data, but generally require input from health care providers. Although the data transfer can be streamlined by downloading to health authorities via phone lines (Weiss, Stanford University, Personal Communication, 2001) or web-based interfaces (Zelicoff et al., 2001; Coiera, 2001), the systems are not transparent. The Rapid Syndrome Validation Program (RSVP), developed by Sandia National Laboratories, uses a touch-screen-based system to enable health care providers in the emergency department to enter clinical and demographic data on patients with a variety of infectious disease syndromes. The system has network-based reporting that is fast and relatively easy to use. The pilot phase has collected information on six syndromes (flu-like illness, fever with skin findings, fever with altered mental status, acute bloody diarrhea, hepatitis, and adult respiratory distress syndrome) as defined by "physician judgment." The system gives the physician immediate feedback after a syndrome has been entered. These reports include a geographic plot of the syndrome that has been entered, a temporal graph of similar reports over the past several weeks, and alert screens with outbreak information, if indicated. The New Mexico Department of Health can be notified (via beeper, cell phone, or e-mail) of each syndrome report. This system is in the pilot phase, and reports have not yet been received or utilized by the New Mexico Department of Health (Baumbach, New Mexico Department of Health, Personal Communication, 2002).

In 1994, CDC provided funds through state EIPs to Connecticut, California, Minnesota, and Oregon for the conduct of population-based surveillance on unexplained life-threatening illnesses and deaths due to possibly infectious causes among previously healthy persons aged 1 to 49 years (Kluger et al., 2001; Rainbow et al., 2000; Hajjeh et al., 2002). This network was designed to detect emerging infections, and has an extensive laboratory component that includes advanced serological and polymerase chain reaction (PCR) testing to identify novel disease associations or new agents. Reported cases of severe illness or death are assigned clinical syndromes based on the predominant system involved (neurological, cardiac, respiratory, hepatic, or other) (Hajjeh et al., 2002). From 1995 to 1998, 137 cases were identified at the four sites (population 7.7 million), for an overall incidence rate of 0.5 per 100,000 per year. The projects are beginning to report new presentations of known infectious agents. The northern California project has identified a new virus–disease syndrome association, adenovirus Type 3 as an agent of adult toxic shock syndrome (Price et al., 2001), and a novel presentation of Sin Nombre virus (Passaro et al., 2001). The network is not designed for the timely reporting of death or severe illness. Clusters or outbreaks of unexplained death or severe illness have not yet been reported by the network (Hajjeh et al., 2002).

COST-EFFECTIVENESS DATA

There is no published literature on the cost-effectiveness of syndromic surveillance. However, models for estimating the economic impact of a bioterrorist attack due to anthrax, brucellosis, or tularemia have clearly demonstrated that rapid implementation of a post-attack prophylaxis program is the most important means of reducing cost (Kaufmann, 1997). Similarly, modeling of potential responses to the use of smallpox as a biological weapon has emphasized that delay in intervention would be very costly (Meltzer et al., 2001). For a smallpox scenario with 100 initially infected persons, holding the number infected per infectious person, the percent of the population removed by quarantine, and the percent vaccinated constant, a delay in initiation of control measures of 15 days would result in 15,705 excess cases at 1 year (Meltzer et al., 2001). Because outbreak detection must necessarily precede post-attack prophylaxis or other control measures, rapid outbreak detection (by whatever means available) is key. Some authors have used modeled data (Kaufmann et al., 1997) on anthrax to estimate the financial benefit of even 1 hour of earlier detection for an aerosol release of *B. anthracis* affecting 100,000 persons (Dato et al., 2001). Most of the achievable benefit occurs by day 4, and the monetary savings from even 1 hour of earlier detection during days 2 and 3 (the steepest part of the cumulative cost curve) could be as high as $200 million. These estimates assume that postexposure treatment is 90 percent effective, and that treatment is available and administered instantaneously.

KEY STEPS IN DEVELOPMENT OF SYNDROMIC SURVEILLANCE SYSTEMS— QUESTIONS AND UNKNOWNS

Several elements of evaluating a public health surveillance system apply to syndromic surveillance (Centers for Disease Control and Prevention, 2001). A number of features of syndromic surveillance, such as defining specific disease syndromes and ensuring timeliness of reporting, are unique. Most of these components have not been systematically evaluated to date. Box B-2 lists selected practical issues faced by investigators and public health officials as syndromic systems are being developed or contemplated.

Public Health Authority

Most local and state health departments interviewed for this report cited local public health laws that allow the collection of syndromic data (Blythe, Maryland Department of Health and Mental Hygiene, Personal Communication, 2002; Sockwell, Virginia Department of Health (Northern Region), Personal Communication, 2002; Chernak, Philadelphia Department of Health, Personal Communication, 2001; Cody, Santa Clara County Department of Health Services, Personal Communication, 2002;

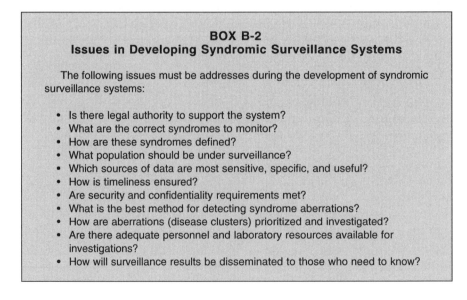

**BOX B-2
Issues in Developing Syndromic Surveillance Systems**

The following issues must be addresses during the development of syndromic surveillance systems:

- Is there legal authority to support the system?
- What are the correct syndromes to monitor?
- How are these syndromes defined?
- What population should be under surveillance?
- Which sources of data are most sensitive, specific, and useful?
- How is timeliness ensured?
- Are security and confidentiality requirements met?
- What is the best method for detecting syndrome aberrations?
- How are aberrations (disease clusters) prioritized and investigated?
- Are there adequate personnel and laboratory resources available for investigations?
- How will surveillance results be disseminated to those who need to know?

Paladini, Bergen County Department of Health Services, Personal Communication, 2002; Mostashari, New York City Department of Health, Personal Communication, 2001; Baumbach, New Mexico Department of Health, Personal Communication, 2002; Barry, Boston Department of Health, Personal Communication, 2002; Klundt, Massachusetts Department of Health, Personal Communication, 2001). The specific areas of public health law viewed by epidemiologists as allowing such jurisdiction varied. Some states cited mandatory reporting of anthrax as sufficient to allow the collection of syndromic data; other localities referred to public health laws designed to allow data collection for clusters of unusual illness. Recent articles have highlighted the special challenges to public health law that would result from a widespread bioterrorist attack (Barbera et al., 2001; Fidler, 2001). However, the degree to which current public health law addresses any of the unique aspects of syndromic surveillance, such as the acquisition of large data sets to search systematically for particular disease syndromes, requires further evaluation and discussion.

Definition of Syndromes

Categorization of clinical symptoms into disease syndromes is the cornerstone of syndromic surveillance. Almost all syndrome categories currently in use are based on expected prodromal symptoms associated with the most likely biological weapon agents. Nevertheless, it is not clear which syndromes are most sensitive for identifying emerging infections or agents of bioterrorism.

Many systems operating since September 11, 2001, have adopted the seven ICD-9-CM code-based syndromes used in the ESSENCE system (Pavlin, ESSENCE, Personal Communication, 2001). As noted earlier, ESSENCE includes seven syndromes: respiratory (common cold, sinus infection), fever/malaise/sepsis, gastrointestinal (vomiting, diarrhea, abdominal pain), neurological (headache, meningitis), dermatological-infectious (vesicular rash), dermatological-hemorrhagic (bruising, petechiae), and coma/sudden death. The drop-in surveillance systems implemented for the 2000 Republican and Democratic National Conventions used somewhat different categories: respiratory infection with fever, diarrhea/gastroenteritis, rash with fever, sepsis or nontraumatic shock, meningitis/encephalitis, botulism-like syndrome, and unexplained death with history of fever (Chernak, Philadelphia Department of Health, Personal Communication, 2001; Bancroft, County of Los Angeles, Department of Health Services, Personal Communication, 2002). Systems that rely on novel collection devices, such as touchscreen or hand-held devices, often query the provider in an algorithm style (e.g., fever present; if yes, rash present; if yes, hemorrhagic, etc.) (Weiss, Stanford University, Personal Communication, 2001). The RSVP touchscreen system relies on the treating physician to decide whether the patient is sick enough to merit data entry into the system (Zeilcoff, Sandia National Laboratories, Personal Communication, 2001).

CDC experience with drop-in surveillance has included limited medical record review to evaluate the accuracy of syndrome categories (Treadwell, CDC, Personal Communication, 2002). Developing definitions for relevant syndromes is a goal for the CDC syndromic surveillance working group. Investigators with the ESSENCE program are currently conducting blinded record review of more than 3,000 charts at three emergency departments to evaluate accuracy of syndrome ICD-9-CM codes (Pavlin, Department of Defense Global Emerging Infections System, Personal Communication, 2002). The results of this evaluation are expected in early 2002. Investigators collecting emergency department-based chief complaint data at Boston Children's and Beth Israel Hospitals have reviewed about 500 medical records and determined that their "respiratory" syndrome category was about 60 percent sensitive in detecting respiratory illness (Mandl, Children's Hospital Boston, Personal Communication, 2002). The Hawaii state health department reviewed retrospective data from a large statewide insurer used to collect ICD-9-CM codes for syndromic surveillance and found only about 20–30 percent accuracy in coding of infectious disease-related syndromes (Chang, Hawaii Department of Health, Personal Communication, 2002). Investigators at the western Pennsylvania syndromic surveillance program evaluated ICD-9-CM-coded emergency department chief complaints by reviewing 800 emergency department records and determined the sensitivity of their acute respiratory illness syndrome codes was only 44 percent (Espino and Wagner, 2001).

Surveillance Population

All syndromic surveillance systems are currently based in states, local health departments, or health systems. There is no national syndromic surveillance system. A large aerosol release of a biological agent would likely affect persons in a region, not within any predetermined jurisdictional boundaries. Similarly, emerging infectious diseases might be expected to occur sporadically across wide geographic areas. The ability of syndromic surveillance systems to communicate within regions and across jurisdictions is therefore desirable. A current example of regional data sharing is the emergency department-based syndromic surveillance system in southern Maryland, Washington, D.C., and northern Virginia. Participants from these three health departments collect emergency department log information electronically or by fax daily. The data are collated for the three sites in Maryland each afternoon, and a daily conference call is held to discuss results of the syndrome totals and any elevations in these totals (Blythe,

Maryland Department of Health and Mental Hygiene, Personal Communication, 2002; Sockwell, Virginia Department of Health (Northern Region), Personal Communication, 2002).

Data Sources

Syndromic surveillance focuses on the early symptom (prodrome) period, prior to development of a clear clinical syndrome or laboratory confirmation of a particular disease. Strictly speaking, syndromic surveillance gathers information about the group of symptoms experienced by cases during the early phase of illness (e.g., cough, fever, shortness of breath). In practice, many so-called syndromic surveillance systems under development are collecting surrogate data for early disease, such as school/work absenteeism or veterinary data.

Box B-3 lists several data sources that are being used or explored for syndromic surveillance, grouped into clinical, laboratory, and surrogate categories. Syndromic data collected from clinical sources, such as emergency department triage logs, generally allow investigators to retrace aberrations or "flags" to specific time periods and potentially to specific patients. The ability to backtrack in response to abnormalities in syndromic data greatly enhances the usefulness of the data. Laboratory sources of syndromic data have not yet been carefully explored. However, many experts express interest in linking clinical syndromic surveillance and laboratory data (Pinner, Centers for Disease Control and Prevention, Personal Communication, 2002; Hirshon, University of Maryland and Baltimore City Department of Health, Personal Communication, 2002). The data sources listed as surrogates include numerous modalities that have not previously been used for public health surveillance. Although several sites are exploring the use of school and work absenteeism (Mostashari, New York City Department of Health, Personal Communication, 2001; Hirshon, University of Maryland and Baltimore City Department of Health, Personal Communication, 2002), as well as patterns of nonprescription medication sales, these data sources have not been validated and should be considered exploratory. Indeed, surrogate data sources have several inherent problems, including a presumed low specificity for the syndromes of interest, high probability of being influenced by factors not related to personal health (e.g., weather, holidays), and difficulty in retracing data aberrations since individual persons are generally not knowable. Despite these shortcomings, however, it may be that a syndromic system encompassing data from clinical, laboratory, and selected surrogate sources is optimal for monitoring emerging infections and bioterrorism events, although the optimal source or combination of sources for this purpose is unknown.

BOX B-3
Potential Data Sources for Syndromic Surveillance Systems

Clinical

Phone calls to emergency department Director/ICP

Emergency department or clinic total patient volume (Barry, Boston Department of Health, Personal Communication, 2002; Brinsfield et al., 2001)

Total hospital or intensive-care unit admissions from emergency department (Chernak, Philadelphia Department of Health, Personal Communication, 2001)

Chief complaints emergency department triage log (Blythe, Maryland Department of Health and Mental Hygiene, Personal Communication, 2002; Sockwell, Virginia Department of Health (Northern Region), Personal Communication, 2002; Cody, Santa Clara County Department of Health Services, Personal Communication, 2002; Paladini, Bergen County Department of Health Services, Personal Communication, 2002; Mostashari, New York City Department of Health, Personal Communication, 2001; Mandl, Children's Hospital Boston, Personal Communication, 2002; Hirshon, University of Maryland and Baltimore City Department of Health, Personal Communication, 2002)

Emergency department visit outcomes (diagnoses) (Duchin, Public Health—Seattle and King County, Personal Communication, 2002; Chang, Hawaii Department of Health, Personal Communication, 2002)

Ambulatory care clinic/HMO outcome (diagnosis) (Duchin, Public Health—Seattle and King County, Personal Communication, 2002; Pavlin, ESSENCE, Personal Communication, 2001; Lazarus et al., 2001; Klundt, Massachusetts Department of Health, Personal Communication, 2001; Kassenborg, Minnesota Department of Health, Personal Communication, 2002; Kleinman, Harvard Pilgrim Health Care and Harvard Vanguard Medical Associates, Personal Communication, 2001; Lazarus, Channing Laboratory, Brigham and Women's Hospital, Harvard medical School, Personal Communication, 2001)

Chief complaints for emergency medical system (911) calls (Mostashari, New York City Department of Health, Personal Communication, 2001; Barry, Boston Department of Health, Personal Communication, 2002; Lober et al., 2002)

Timeliness

Extreme timeliness is a characteristic of surveillance, particularly for bioterrorism, that is currently being explored (Wagner et al., 2001b). Electronic laboratory reporting of notifiable diseases has been shown to decrease the time to reporting by about 4 days as compared with conventional paper reporting, and may be a requirement for early outbreak detection (Kortepeter et al., 2000). Efforts to reduce delays in the transmission of electronic data should improve timeliness. The National Electronic Disease Surveillance System (NEDSS) project at CDC is an attempt to facilitate electronic transfer of data from clinical information systems to public health

Provider call-in line volume, chief complaints (Harcourt et al., 2001)

Poison control center calls (Barry, Boston Department of Health, Personal Communication, 2002)

Unexplained critical illnesses (Hajjeh et al., 2002)

Unexplained deaths (Hajjeh et al., 2002)

Medical examiner case volume, syndromes (Nolte, University of New Mexico, Personal Communication, 2002)

Insurance claims (Chang, Hawaii Department of Health, Personal Communication, 2002)

Laboratory

Radiology reporting

Clinical laboratory ordering volume

Prediagnostic laboratory results (e.g., gram stain, complete blood count)

Surrogate

School absenteeism (Hirshon, University of Maryland and Baltimore City Department of Health, Personal Communication, 2002)

Work absenteeism (Mostashari, New York City Department of Health, Personal Communication, 2001)

Nonprescription medication sales (Mostashari, New York City Department of Health, Personal Communication, 2001; Hirshon, University of Maryland and Baltimore City Department of Health, Personal Communication, 2002)

Usage of health care provider database searches (Jormanainen et al., 2001; Jousimaa et al., 1998)

Volume of web-based health inquiries by the public (Wagner et al., 2001b)

Web-based illness reporting (Woodall, 2001)

Animal illnesses/deaths (animal control programs, American Society for the Prevention of Cruelty to Animals, veterinary medicine) (Hirshon, University of Maryland and Baltimore City Department of Health, Personal Communication, 2002)

surveillance systems (NEDSS, 2001). Under the project, standard vocabularies, standard messages, and definitions to allow for electronic integration are being developed. The eHealth Initiative is a recently formed consortium of 60 health care organizations, including the majority of hardware and software suppliers to hospitals (eHealth Initiative website, 2001). The group, with CDC collaboration, aims to use existing information technology systems to enhance public health data collection—a crucial early step in streamlining data flow.

A few investigators have demonstrated the timeliness of syndromic surveillance methods compared with conventional reporting methods, such as surveillance for national pneumonia and influenza mortality and sentinel physician surveillance for influenza (CDC, 2002; Mostashari, New York City Department of Health, Personal Communication, 2001; Lazarus et al., 2001). The New York City Department of Health, using electronically transmitted data on volume of selected ambulance dispatch call types, has detected each of the last three annual influenza epidemics (1999–2001) 2–3 weeks prior to traditional reporting (CDC, 2002). Figure B-1 shows the respiratory syndrome alarm, at the 99 percent upper confidence level, during 1998–2002.

Security and Confidentiality

Use of password-protected secure servers and removal of identifiers are the security methods most commonly reported by local health departments operating syndromic surveillance systems. Encryption, message authentication, and message nonrepudiation have been incorporated into systems depending on electronic transfer of large clinical data sets, such as the insurance claims data being received by the Hawaii Department of Health (Chang, Hawaii Department of Health, Personal Communication, 2002). A detailed review of the various security measures available and being used at the program level is beyond the scope of this discussion. It is noteworthy,

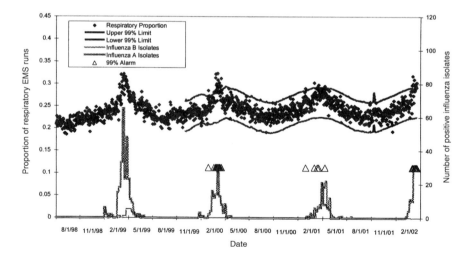

FIGURE B-1 EMS respiratory call syndrome 99 percent threshold precedes influenza sentinel physician surveillance by 2–3 weeks, 1999–2001.
Reproduced with permission. F. Mostashari, New York City Department of Health.

however, that no standard approach to ensuring security is consistently reported.

Confidentiality issues, particularly in light of the 1996 Health Insurance Portability and Accountability Act (HIPAA) (Department of Health and Human Services, 2000) and accompanying regulations, remain a major concern among developers of syndromic surveillance systems. Public health officials in Hawaii, Seattle, and other settings have expressed concerns regarding the inability to access meaningful syndromic data because of HIPAA-related constraints cited by insurers or clinical/laboratory sources (Duchin, Public Health—Seattle and King County, Personal Communication, 2002; Chang, Hawaii Department of Health, Personal Communication, 2002). While health systems may access patient-specific data in response to syndromic aberrations or flags, public health departments may need to rely on clinical investigators on-site to review relevant data and determine the cause of aberrations and the need for additional investigation (Mandl, Children's Hospital Boston, Personal Communication, 2002). Although the new regulations permit the practice of sharing protected health information with public health authorities who are authorized by law to protect the health of the public, further clarification of this rule with health care providers will be needed (NEDSS, 2001). Integration of NEDSS standards into syndromic surveillance projects may facilitate compliance with the rule, as the NEDSS security standards meet the HIPAA requirements.

Aberration Detection Methods

The analytic challenge in outbreak or cluster detection using syndromic data is to isolate a signal of an actual event from the large amount of background "noise" that is present in the data. Syndromic surveillance systems use an array of aberration detection methods to identify increases in the syndrome of interest above some predetermined threshold. Many systems are so new that minimal historical data exist for comparison. Drop-in surveillance systems have generally gathered syndromic data for 3–7 days prior to initiation of the event-related system. Some larger, electronic health system-wide or city-wide emergency medical system (EMS) call systems have several years of historical data for baseline comparison (Institute of Medicine, 1988; RODS).

Time-series analysis has been used to detect outbreaks using surveillance data. CDC has modified a statistical method called cumulative sums (CUSUM) (Hutwagner et al., 1997) that utilizes moving averages for the detection of clusters. This method looks at the day-to-day variability of the data and takes into account patient volume. Modified CUSUM methods have been used by drop-in surveillance systems and some sustained emergency department triage log-based systems (Duchin, Public Health—Seattle and King County, Personal Communication, 2002; Blythe, Maryland Department of Health and Mental Hygiene, Personal Communication, 2002; Sockwell, Virginia Department of Health (Northern Region), Personal Communication, 2002; Chernak, Philadelphia Department of Health, Personal Communication, 2001; Chernak, Philadelphia Department of Health, Personal Communication, 2002). The New York City Department of Health is uses a scan statistic (Kulldorff, 2001), a method that allows for identification of geographic clustering, to evaluate electronically transmitted emergency department triage log data (Mostashari, New York City Department of Health, Personal Communication, 2001). Geographic information system (GIS) data points using mapping functions have been added to several syndromic surveillance systems (Pavlin, ESSENCE, Personal Communication, 2001; Zeilcoff et al., 2001).

Data transfer functions and data analysis have been packaged and integrated with environmental detection systems (PCR-based) by commercial vendors such as Idaho Technology's LEADER (Lightweight Epidemiology and Advanced Detection and Emergency Response System) (Army-technology Website). There is increasing incentive for the development of proprietary packages that incorporate data capture and aberration methodology.

Aberration Response Protocols

The development of protocols for response to aberrations in syndromic surveillance data is a largely unexplored area. Clusters, termed "flags" or "alarms," arise when the number of syndromes reported on a given day exceeds a pre-set threshold. When and how to follow up on or investigate these flags is unclear. The New York City Department of Health has a team of three medical epidemiologists who review all flags appearing in emergency department triage log data or EMS response call data (Mostashari, New York City Department of Health, Personal Communication, 2001). Team members are experienced communicable disease epidemiologists, and are available to review the data seven days a week.

The team uses a number of strategies to determine whether a flag requires additional investigation. It evaluates whether the flag occurred in the same syndrome and site the day or two previously. It reviews the absolute number of persons in the flag (Is this an increase from zero to two or from one to fifteen?). On some occasions, the team accesses and reviews the actual free text of the triage log to obtain additional clinical data. The flagged emergency department may be called and asked if any increase in a given syndrome was noticed or if it can be explained. The health department may ask the emergency department to send additional clinical samples for the given syndrome on future cases to try and determine an etiological agent. Periodically, surveillance field staff have been sent to review emergency department charts, occasionally even calling patients to obtain additional information. In many instances, particularly for small numbers of cases, the team waits until the next day to see whether the flag persists or resolves. The system was designed for bioterrorism detection, and it is expected that a large-scale release would not result in a single day of increased cases. If a flag is not detected on the following day, no further evaluation is undertaken.

Other local health departments that have initiated syndromic surveillance following the events of September 11, 2001, use similar follow-up procedures. However, staff shortages, a lack of expertise in cluster detection analysis, and difficulty in sustaining intensive scrutiny of data have made ongoing efforts difficult. Health departments that do not have electronically transferred data, requiring staff to collect and enter data in addition to coordinating follow-up, are struggling to maintain syndromic systems (Blythe, Maryland Department of Health and Mental Hygiene, Personal Communication, 2002; Sockwell, Virginia Department of Health (Northern Region), Personal Communication, 2002; Cody, Santa Clara County Department of Health, Personal Communication, 2002).

Depending on the threshold of detection used in a syndromic surveillance system, the resources needed to adequately evaluate and follow up on flags could be extensive. Although "fine-tuning" of aberration-detection algorithms can reduce the number of flags, it is unclear what threshold is most appropriate for any given syndrome. The best electronic data transfer and aberration analysis programs are not likely to replace the need for trained epidemiologists and public health personnel to evaluate and respond to the flags or alarms in the data. Adequate personnel and laboratory resources will be needed to support syndromic surveillance systems, regardless of the sensitivity and specificity of aberration-detection software.

DISCUSSION OF SELECTED
SYNDROMIC SURVEILLANCE SYSTEMS

Domestic

Numerous syndrome-based surveillance systems have been implemented by state and local health departments. Many of these systems were developed in response to the bioterrorist attacks on September 11, 2001, and the subsequent anthrax outbreak. Table B-2 lists several domestic syndromic surveillance systems and selected characteristics. This is a convenience sample based on the availability of public health and academic partners to discuss their specific programs with the author, and is not intended as a comprehensive list. The programs (in Boston, Seattle, New Mexico, Hawaii, Minnesota) that have been operating the longest, beginning largely in 1999, are the sites that have received special surveillance project funding from CDC's bioterrorism cooperative agreement grants (Treadwell, CDC, Personal Communication, 2002). Florida, Chicago, and New York State have also received special surveillance project funding but were not interviewed for this report. Local health department efforts, such as the regional surveillance among the Washington, D.C., Maryland, and Virginia health departments, are operating on existing resources and have borrowed staff and expertise from other programs/areas.

Most programs listed in Table B-2 report the ability to detect increases in influenza-like illness syndromes in their surveillance data for 2001. However, formal calculations of the timeliness of the data or appropriate thresholds needed to identify influenza activity most efficiently are largely lacking. Investigators at a large multispecialty group practice in eastern Massachusetts (Harvard Vanguard Medical Associates) retrospectively reviewed electronic medical records for 1996–1999 and were able to identify three ICD-9-CM codes (cough, pneumonia unspecified, and acute bronchitis) that accounted for 91 percent of lower respiratory tract visits (n = 152,435 visits) (Lazarus et al., 2001). Increases in lower respiratory tract visits closely paralleled CDC-collected data on pneumonia and influenza deaths in 122 cities and appeared to rise "shortly before" the peak in deaths. The New York City Department of Health calculated increases in respiratory syndrome-related EMS calls that preceded sentinel physician influenza data by several weeks (see the discussion of timeliness above).

Detection of outbreaks has rarely been reported by syndromic systems. Several systems are so new that insufficient time has elapsed to detect aberrations (Paladini, Bergen County Department of Health Services, Personal Communication, 2002; Klundt, Massachusetts Department of Health, Personal Communication, 2001; Kassenborg, Minnesota Department of Health, Personal Communication, 2002). Other systems were designed as pilots to determine whether data can be efficiently transferred electronically and to address technical or security issues that might arise; outbreak detection and investigation are beyond the scope of these systems (Duchin, Public Health—Seattle and King County, Personal Communication, 2002; Stanford Report, 2001; Weiss, Stanford University, Personal Communication, 2001; Chang, Hawaii Department of Health, Personal Communication, 2002).

ESSENCE and the emergency department triage log (chief complaint) syndromic surveillance system at the New York City Department of Health have detected gastrointestinal disease outbreaks (Duchin, Public Health—Seattle and King County, Personal Communication, 2002; Pavlin, Department of Defense Global Emerging Infections System, Personal Communication, 2002). The ESSENCE syndrome counts for gastroenteritis increased above thresholds at military installations in San Diego, Maryland, New Jersey, and Kentucky during the first or second week of January 2002. An on-site outbreak investigation was conducted in San Diego, where the peak in illness occurred on January 12 and 13. Cases experienced 12–24 hours of self-limited vomiting and diarrhea. A total of 136 persons were identified in the ESSENCE database (see Figure B-2); 38 records were available for review. Records were not available for affected companies that had moved to other installations or had graduated. A potential index case was identified who worked in the chow hall while experiencing vomiting and diarrhea for 3 days; his illness onset was 2 days prior to the first outbreak cases. Efforts are under way to evaluate clinical specimens for Norwalk-like virus. Specimens are not available from the other outbreak sites. The possibility that these outbreaks could be linked is being investigated (Pavlin, Department of Defense Global Emerging Infections System, Personal Communication, 2002).

The New York City Department of Health identified the largest and most sustained alarm in the emergency department syndromic surveillance system in November 2001. On November 2, 2001, the vomiting syndrome exceeded threshold, joined by an increase in diarrhea syndrome on November 12. Increases in vomiting and diarrhea were maintained over the next 10 days. The increase was initially detected in the Bronx and subsequently involved the whole city. In November, several institutional and school outbreaks of vomiting illness were reported. Only a few specimens were obtained for testing; one sample was positive for calicivirus (Mostashari, New York City Department of Health, Personal Communication, 2001).

Investigators generally expect that syndromic surveillance will be able to detect a wide variety of diseases and conditions, not only acts of bioterrorism or emerging infections. Investigators in Boston and Northern Virginia have used a rise in emergency department volume reports to identify increased injuries from ice-related weather conditions. Both health departments note that they would not have detected this increase with currently operating traditional surveillance systems, and both sites used the data to issue public health messages regarding ice-related injury prevention strategies (Sockwell, Virginia Department of Health (Norther Region), Personal Communication, 2002; Barry, Boston Department of Health, Personal Communication, 2002).

International

Increased international travel and trade have blurred the boundaries of disease outbreaks, while improved information technology and Internet

TABLE B-2 Selected Syndromic Surveillance Systems: Domestic

Site	Date Initiated	Population Studied	Data Source(s)	Special Feature(s)	Obstacles	Future Plans
Philadelphia Republican National Convention: CDC Drop-In	7/17/00–8/11/00	Philadelphia, adjoining PA, NJ, DE counties— census data, 5 Phila. ED	First-aid stations, ED syndrome diagnoses, hospital census	Multifaceted approach, engaged surrounding counties	Provider fatigue, not sustainable, lots of coding and data entry errors	Planning regional approach, enhanced communication with all providers
Los Angeles Democratic National Convention: CDC Drop-In	8/7/00–8/22/00	11 LA County emergency departments 1 airport clinic	ED/clinic syndrome diagnoses	Manually grouped previous ED data into syndromes for baseline (36,000 visits)	Required training of hosptials, lots of data (IT) problems, not sustainable	Development of ongoing electronic data collection from ED
Maryland Department of Health	9/11/01–present	2 counties adjacent to Wash., DC— 9 hospital ED	ED triage logs— manually code and enter syndromes	Close collaboration with VA and DC health depts.	Very labor-intensive, inefficient	Developing Web-based reporting and electronic data transfer
Virginia Health Dept.-Northern Region (5 health districts)	9/11/01–present	7 hospital ED, counties adjacent to Wash., DC	ED triage logs— manually code and enter syndromes, share daily with Maryland/D.C.	Close collaboration with other states and between health districts	Very labor-intensive, data have been used for other purposes	Would like to collaborate with Maryland in web-based reporting

Santa Clara County Health Dept.	10/01/01–present	12 hospital ED in the county	Tick mark by ED triage nurse for 6 syndromes	Simple	Data entry, analysis labor-intensive; provider fatigue	Evaluating several systems, incl. Health Buddy
Baltimore City Health Department	9/11/01–present	All Baltimore ED, selected community clinics, 911 calls, dog/cat deaths, school absenteeism	ED diagnosis-based syndromes, no. dog/cat deaths, total school absentees	Comprehensive collaboration with academic centers, strong political will by the city	Not yet real-time or entirely electronic, staff needed to follow-up flags from multiple sources	Planning real-time, electronic ED syndromic system
Alleghany County, western Pennsylvania	9/11/01–present	60–70% Alleghany County	ED chief complaint, electronic	Incorporating several health systems, fully automated	HD only receives aggregate data	Expanding to 13 counties, 54 hospitals
Minnesota Department of Health	September 2000–present	St. Paul/ Minneapolis metro area	ED closures/bed capacity (web-based); electronic ICD-9 Health Partners discharge dx	Already available data source (Health Partners), flexible—can easily change codes to new syndrome	Unclear how useful, sensitive; denominator and historical data pending	Planning to add EMS data, couple Health Partner data with laboratory component
New Mexico Department of Health—U of NM, statewide medical examiner System	1999–present	Statewide	Autopsy if antecedent syndromes, specific pathological syndromes reported to NMHD	Uniform criteria for performing autopsies and reporting cases to HD; captures reportable conditions, not only BT	Broad range of timeliness, requires training of field staff	Expect to export the system to other medical examiner systems

continues

TABLE B-2 Continued

Site	Date Initiated	Population Studied	Data Source(s)	Special Feature(s)	Obstacles	Future Plans
Boston City Department of Health	1999–present	Citywide	11 ED-total volume data—electronic, Poison Control call volume, death certificate and EMS data	Jan. 2002 increase ED volume due to falls on black ice, Oct—review of volume flag noted cases seeking swabs and Cipro	83 days in 2000 exceeded threshold—real-time follow-up may be labor-intensive and frequent	Add additional sites, including adjacent county; collect additional data from some sites
Seattle-King County Health Department	1999–present	Selected sites in Seattle	3 ED and 1 large primary care clinic—electronic data transfer	Have detected influenza seasonal patterns; collaborate with academic partner	HIPAA issues with obtaining identifiers	Expand to population-based system, increase number of data sources, collect identifiers, add GIS capacity
Hawaii Department of Health	3/01–present	Statewide	Infectious disease subset of all claims from largest insurer (60–65% coverage)	ICD-9 based, electronic, insurer with excellent data processing capability	Long lagtime (18% claims available ≤ 7 days), poor coding accuracy	Continue to work toward improved timeliness, add GIS component

Massachusetts Department of Health/Harvard Vanguard Medical Associates	9/00–present	About 10% of greater Boston area (250,000 pop.)	HMO electronic medical record, electronic calls to nurse and doctors	Uses 4–5 years of historical data, good denominator data, real-time; academic partners	Special population (insured)	Developing outbreak reporting algorithms, plan to integrate with other systems
Children's Hospital Boston	not available	Children's Hospital Boston and Beth Israel Hospital	ED chief complaint, ED ICD-9 discharge diagnosis, web-based MD reporting	Reviewed 500 ED charts, chief complaint "respiratory syndrome" detected ~60%	Operating on a small pilot basis presently, no data to health dept. yet, no clusters investigated	Refine detection algorithms, add 9 hospitals for web-based reporting

SOURCES: Blythe, Maryland Department of Health and Mental Hygiene, Personal Communication, 2002; Sockwell, Virginia Department of Health (Northern Region), Personal Communication, 2002; Chernak, Philadelphia Department of Health, Personal Communication, 2001; Bancroft, County of Los Angeles, Department of Health Services, Personal Communication, 2002; Peterson, County of Los Angeles, Department of Health Services, Personal Communication, 2002; Cody, Santa Clara County Department of Health, Personal Communication, 2002; RODS; Piposzar, Alleghany County Health Department, Personal Communication, 2002; Hirshon, University of Maryland and Baltimore City Department of Health, Personal Communication, 2002; ; Kassenborg, Minnesota Department of Health, Personal Communication, 2002; Barry, Boston Department of Health, Personal Communication, 2002; Nolte, University of New Mexico, Personal Communication, 2002; Kleinman, Harvard Pilgrim Health Care and Harvard Vanguard Medical Associates, Personal Communication, 2001; Lazarus, Channing Laboratory, Brigham and Women's Hospital, Harvard medical School, Personal Communication, 2001; Chang, Hawaii Department of Health, Personal Communication, 2002; Mandl, Children's Hospital Boston, Personal Communication, 2002; Klundt, Massachusetts Department of Health, Personal Communication, 2001.

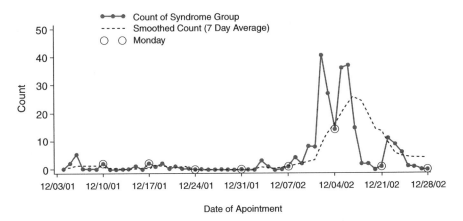

FIGURE B-2 Gastroenteritis syndrome count, ESSENCE, San Diego, 2002. Reproduced with permission. J. Pavlin, ESSENCE program, Department of Defense.

access now allow for much more rapid awareness of local disease outbreaks at distant points around the globe. Although there are few published reports of syndromic surveillance systems operating outside of the United States, efforts to enhance outbreak detection and link disease surveillance information have increased.

The World Health Organization (WHO) established a new approach to global disease surveillance in 1997 termed "outbreak verification." This system collects data from a broad range of sources, including national institutes of health, nongovernmental organizations, media, the World Wide Web, and electronic mail-based discussion groups. Follow-up is performed by outbreak verification teams in WHO regional offices. Information on outbreaks with potential international public health importance is circulated to subscribers on the Outbreak Verification List. This system is not strictly designed to detect clusters of disease syndromes, but the early nature of reports often includes disease syndromes prior to laboratory diagnosis. Between 1997 and 1999, 246 outbreaks were reported, the most common being cholera (78), acute hemorrhagic fever (24), and acute diarrheal disease (22).

Internet outbreak reporting, although not specifically designed for syndrome detection, is timely and increasingly available. As more and more countries and international organizations post information on outbreaks or syndrome clusters on publicly accessible e-mail services, such as ProMED-mail (Woodall, 1997, 2001), the use of this modality for international syndromic surveillance may increase.

A network of 22 travel/tropical medicine clinics (14 in the United States and 8 in other countries), GeoSentinel, was initiated in 1996 to collect disease- or syndrome-specific diagnoses on returning travelers, immigrants, and foreign visitors (Freedman et al., 1999). GeoSentinel was designed as a sentinel system and does not have the elements of timeliness or representativeness demonstrated by most syndromic surveillance systems, although it may serve as an early warning system.

ESSENCE collects data from DoD medical treatment facilities worldwide and is therefore international in scope. The U.S. Naval Medical Research Unit No. 2 participates in an Early Warning Outbreak Recognition System (EWORS) that collects real-time electronic syndromic data from selected hospital pediatric and internal medicine clinics and emergency departments in Indonesia (Corwin, 2000). A *V. cholerae* 0139 outbreak was identified in the 1999 pilot phase of the project.

The Israeli Ministry of Health has reported on a system of enhanced infectious disease surveillance in Israel during the six-week Gulf War, specifically looking for evidence of biological warfare (Slater and Costin, 1992). Details of the enhanced system are not available, but it apparently included analysis of daily mortality data (rather than the standard weekly procedure) and measures of pneumonia or other severe respiratory symptoms suggestive of pulmonary anthrax.

Other international reports stress early detection of outbreaks (Toubiana and Flahault, 1998; Reintjes et al., 2001; Hashimoto et al., 2000) and the importance of networks and collaborations for outbreak detection (Osaka et al., 1999; Pebody et al., 1999). However, the systems described do not collect data.

SUMMARY AND CONCLUSIONS

Syndromic surveillance is a method of obtaining information about cases exhibiting one or more disease symptoms before a definitive clinical or laboratory diagnosis is available. Outbreaks of disease due to a biological warfare agent may be difficult to diagnose. Delays in diagnosis would likely result in larger numbers of casualties and a more prolonged outbreak. Early detection, by monitoring increases in prodromal symptoms such as fever and cough, forms the basis for most current syndromic surveillance systems. More complex systems that include an advanced laboratory component, such as the CDC unexplained death and critical illness project, are being explored for the detection of emerging infections.

The implementation of syndromic surveillance is under way. Many public health officials perceive the need to provide enhanced surveillance following the attacks of September 11, and syndromic surveillance is meeting that need in some localities. Similarly, academic and industry partners are quickly embracing this surveillance technique. There is no nationally coordinated plan to guide the development of syndromic surveillance. More research is needed to guide future planning before specific recommendations can be made.

There are a number of potential benefits from syndromic surveillance:

- New opportunities for collaboration among health departments, emergency medical service providers, hospitals, information system managers, and commercial vendors
- An opportunity to reinforce the importance of identifying standards-based vocabularies, messages, and case definitions to facilitate the use and transfer of data from clinical information systems to public health surveillance
- Improved training for public health personnel in the area of information systems and disease-detection techniques
- The potential to enhance notifiable disease and noninfectious disease reporting systems.

Despite these potential benefits, however, caution is appropriate. Syndromic surveillance is a new area of public health surveillance. Studies have not yet been completed to demonstrate the value of this surveillance tool. There is scant information available regarding the best syndromes to monitor for bioterrorism or emerging infections, and among those syndromes being used, there are no generally accepted case definitions. Rather, syndrome definitions differ from site to site, and comparisons across jurisdictions may be difficult. Moreover, the best source of syndromic data is unknown. A combination of different sources may be needed to best capture an increase in early or new disease in a community. And syndromic surveillance systems, by definition, are not laboratory-based, yet supplementing syndromic data with laboratory results may greatly enhance the power and specificity of current systems.

Minimally, syndromic surveillance systems should be electronic, should not rely on provider input (be transparent), should be monitored continuously, and should have a mechanism that allows for follow-up if critical increases are detected. Methods for the detection of clusters amid background syndrome "noise" require additional evaluation to identify optimal alarm thresholds. Public health epidemiologists should be involved in the planning of detection methods and response protocols. Sustainability, personnel training needs, and cost are other major considerations. Syndromic surveillance systems should also be viewed as but one of several methods for detection of bioterrorism and emerging infections; resources should not be diverted from proven, core public health functions to syndromic surveillance programs.

Studies are needed to evaluate the incremental contribution of syndromic surveillance to other surveillance and outbreak detection programs that are in place or planned. Syndromic surveillance appears to be useful for early outbreak detection and potentially for the identification of emerging infections, but numerous questions remain.

REFERENCES

Barbera J, Macintyrre A, Gostin L, Inglesby T, O'Toole T, DeAtley C, Tonat K, Layton M. Large-scale quarantine following biological terrorism in the United States: scientific examination, logistic and legal limits, and possible consequences. JAMA 2001;286:2711–2717.

Binder S, Levitt AM, Sacks JJ, Hughes JM. Emerging infectious disease: public health issues for the 21st century. Science 1999;284:1311–1313.

Bravata D. Evidence Report/Technology Assessment. Bioterrorism: Use of Information Technologies and Decision Support Systems. Prepared for AHRQ. Draft. December 2001.

Brinsfield KH, Gunn JE, Barry MA, McKenna V, Syer KS, Sulis C. Using volume-based surveillance for an outbreak early warning system. Acad Emerg Med 2001;8:492.

Canas LC, Lohman K, Pavlin JA, Endy T, Singh DL, Pandey P, Shrestha MP, Scott RM, Russell KL, Watts D, Hajdamowicz M, Soriano I, Douce RW, Neville J, Gaydos JC. The department of defense laboratory-based global influenza surveillance system. Mil Med 2000;165(Suppl 2):52–56.

CDC. Outbreak of acute illness—southwestern United States, 1993. MMWR 1993;42:421–424.

CDC. Addressing Emerging Infectious Disease Threats: A Prevention Strategy for the United States. Atlanta, Georgia. 1994.

CDC. Outbreak of West Nile-like viral encephalitis—New York, 1999. MMWR 1999;48:845–849.

CDC. Biological and chemical terrorism: strategic plan for preparedness and response. Recommendations of the CDC strategic planning workgroup. MMWR 2000;49(RR04):1–14.

CDC. Preventing Emerging Infectious Diseases: A strategy for the 21st century. Atlanta. October, 1998. Accessed at www.cdc.gov on February 1, 2001.

CDC. Update: investigation of anthrax associated with intentional exposure and interim public health guidelines, October 2001. MMWR 2001;50:889–893.

CDC. Use of ambulance dispatch data as an early warning system for community-wide influenza-like illness, New York City. MMWR 2002 (in press).

Centers for Disease Control and Prevention. Updated guidelines for evaluating public health surveillance systems: recommendations from the guidelines working group. MMWR 2001;50(No. RR-13):1–35.

Coiera E. Use of web-based systems for clinician reporting of suspected bioterrorism events. 20 pages. A report prepared for AHRQ. June 2, 2001.

Corwin A. Developing regional outbreak response capabilities early warning outbreak recognition system (EWORS). Navy Med 2000;Sept/Oct:1–5.

Dato VM, Wagner MM, Allswede MP, Aryel R, Fapohunda A. The Nation's Current Capacity for the Early Detection of Public Health Threats Including Bioterrorism. 78 pages. Report commissioned by AHRQ. June 8, 2001.

Department of Health and Human Services. Standards for privacy of individually identifiable health information. Final rule. Fed Reg 2000;65(250):82462–82829.

Duchin JS, Karras BT, Trigg LJ, Bliss D, Vo D, Ciliberti J, Stewart L, Rietberg K, Lober WB. Syndromic surveillance for bioterrorism using computerized discharge diagnosis databases. Proc AMIA Symp 2001;897.

Espino J, Wagner M. The accuracy of ICD-9 coded chief complaints for detection of acute respiratory illness. Proc AMIA Symp 2001:164–168 (in press).

Fidler DP. The malevolent use of microbes and the rule of law: legal challenges presented by bioterrorism. Clin Infect Dis 2001;33:686–689.

Fine A, Layton M. Lessons from the West Nile viral encephalitis outbreak in New York City, 1999: implications for bioterrorism preparedness. Clin Infect Dis 2001;32:277–282.

Fraser DW, Tsai TR, Orenstein W, Parkin WE, Beecham HJ, Sharrar RG, Harris J, Mallison GF, Martin SM, McDade JE, Shepard CC, Brachman PS. Legionnaires' disease: description of an epidemic of pneumonia. N Engl J Med 1977;297:1189–1197.

Freedman DO, Kozarsky PE, Weld LH, Cetron MS. GeoSentinel: the global emerging infections sentinel network of the International Society of Travel Medicine. J Travel Med 1999;6:94–98.

Goldenberg A, Shmueli G, Caruana RA, Fienberg SE. Early statistical detection of anthrax outbreaks by tracking over-the-counter medication sales. Proc Nat Acad Sci 2002 (under consideration for publication).

Grein TW, Kamara K-BO, Rodier G, Plant AJ, Bovier P, Ryan MJ, Ohyama T, Heymann DL. Rumors of disease in the global village: outbreak verification. Emerg Infect Dis 2000:97–102.

Hajjeh RA, Relman D, Cieslak PR, Sofair AN, Passaro D, Flood J, Johnson J, Hacker JK, Shieh W-J, Hendry RM, Nikkari S, Ladd-Wilson S, Hadler J, Rainbow J, Tappero JW, Woods CW, Conn L, Reagan S, Zaki S, Perkins BA. Surveillance for unexplained deaths and critical illnesses due to possibly infectious causes, United States, 1995–1998. Emerg Infect Dis 2002;8:145–152.

Harcourt SE, Smith GE, Hollyoak V, Joseph CA, Chaloner R, Rehman Y, Warburton F, Ejidokun OO, Watson JM, Griffiths RK. Can calls to NHS Direct be used for syndromic surveillance? Commun Dis Pub Health 2001;4:178–182.

Hashimoto S, Murakami Y, Taniguchi K, Nagai M. Detection of epidemics in their early stage through infectious disease surveillance. Int J Epidemiol 2000;29:905–910.

Hoffman RE, Norton JE. Lessons learned from a full-scale bioterrorism exercise. Emerg Infect Dis 2000;6:652–653.

http://epi.health.state.nm/rsvpdesc/default.asp. Accessed December 12, 2001.

http://www.army-technology.com/contractors/nbc/idaho/. Accessed February 6, 2002.

http://www.ehealthinitiative.org/. eHealth Initiative 2001:Year in Review. Accessed February 8, 2002.

Hutwagner LC, Maloney EK, Bean NH, Slutsker L, Martin SM. Using laboratory-based surveillance data for prevention: an algorithm for detecting *Salmonella* outbreaks. Emerg Infect Dis 1997;3:395–400.

Institute of Medicine. 1987. The U.S. Capacity to Address Tropical Infectious Disease Problems. National Academy Press. Washington, D.C.

Institute of Medicine. 1988. The Future of Public Health, National Academy Press. Washington, D.C.

Institute of Medicine. 1992. Emerging Infections: Microbial Threats to Health in the United States. National Academy Press, Washington, D.C.

Jormanainen V, Jousimaa J, Kunnamo I, Ruutu P. Physician database searches as a tool for early detection of epidemics. Emerg Infect Dis 2001;7:474–476.

Jousimaa J, Kunnamo I, Makela M. Physicians' patterns of using a computerized collection of guidelines for primary health care. Int J Technol Assess Health Care 1998;14:484–493.

Kaufmann A, Meltzer M, Schmid G. The economic impact of a bioterrorist attack: are prevention and post attack intervention programs justifiable? Emerg Infect Dis 1997;3:83–94.

Kluger MD, Sofair AN, Heye CJ, Meek JI, Sodhi RK, Hadler JL. Retrospective validation of a surveillance system for unexplained illness and death: New Haven County, Connecticut. Am J Pub Health 2001;91:1214–1219.

Kortepeter MG, Pavlin JA, Gaydos JC, Rowe JR, Kelley PW, Ludwig G, McKee KT, Eitzen EM. Surveillance at US military installations for bioterrorist and emerging infectious disease threats. Mil Med 2000;165:ii–iii.

Kulldorff M. Prospective time periodic geographical disease surveillance using a scan statistic. JR Stat. Soc 2001;164, Part 1:61–72.

Lazarus R, Kleinman KP, Dashevsky I, DeMaria A, Platt R. Using automated medical records for rapid identification of illness syndromes (syndromic surveillance): the example of lower respiratory infection. BMC Public Health. 2001;1:9. Accessed at http://www.pubmedcentral.nih.gov/articlerender. fcgi?tool=pubmed&pubmedid=11722798 on December 3, 2001.

Lober WB, Karras BT, Wagner MM, Overhage JM, Fraser H, Mandl KD, Espino JU, Tsui F-C. Roundtable on bioterrorism detection: information systems-based surveillance. JAMIA. 2002 (in press).

Martin SM, Bean NH. Data management issues for emerging diseases and new tools for managing surveillance and laboratory data. Emerging Infect Dis 1995;1:124–128.

Meltzer MI, Damon I, LeDuc JW, Millar JD. Modeling potential responses to smallpox as a bioterrorist weapon. Emerg Infect Dis 2001;7:959–969.

Moser SA, Jones WT, Brossette SE. Application of data mining to intensive care unit microbiologic data. Emerg Infect Dis 1999;5:454–457.

Mostashari F, Karpati A. Towards a theoretical (and practical) framework for prodromic surveillance. Abstract. International Conference on Emerging Infectious Diseases, Atlanta. March 24–27, 2002 (accepted).

National Electronic Disease Surveillance System Working Group: National Electronic Disease Surveillance System (NEDSS): A standards based approach to connect public health and clinical medicine. J Pub Health Manage Prac 2001;7:43–50.

Osaka K, Inouye S, Okabe N, Taniguchi K, Izumiya H, Watanabe H, Matsumoto Y, Yokota T, Hashimoto S, Sagara H. Electronic network for monitoring travellers' diarrheoea and detection of an outbreak caused by *Salmonella enteritidis* among overseas travellers. Epidemiol Infect 1999;123:431–436.

Passaro DJ, Shieh W-J, Hacker JK, Fritz CL, Hogan SR, Fischer M, Hendry RM, Vugia DJ. Predominant kidney involvement in a fatal case of hantavirus pulmonary syndrome caused by Sin Nombre virus. 2001;33:263–264.

Pavlin J. Electronic surveillance system for the early notification of community-based epidemics (ESSENCE). Information Paper. Personal communication. December 17, 2001.

Pebody (RG, Furtado C, Rojas A, McCarthy N, Nylen G, Ruutu P, et al. An international outbreak of Vero cytotoxin-producing *Escherichia coli* 0157 infection amongst tourists: a challenge for the European infectious disease surveillance network. Epidemiol Infect 1999;123:217–223.

Price NO, Hacker JK, Silvers JH, Crawford-Miksza L, Hendry RM, Flood J, Hajjeh RA, Reingold AL, Passaro DJ. Adenovirus type 3 viremia in an adult with toxic shock-like syndrome. CID 2001;33:260–262.

Rainbow J, Lynfield R, Johnson JR, Danila RN. Minnesota surveillance for unexplained deaths and critical illnesses of possible infectious cause. 2000;83:61–63.

Reintjes R, Baumeister H-G, Coulombier D. Infectious disease surveillance in North Rhine-Westphalia: first steps in the development of an early warning system. Int J Hyg Environ Health 2001;203:195–199.

RODS. http://ultra.cbmi.upmc.edu/-ju/rods/.

Rotz LD, Koo D, O'Carroll PW, Kellogg RB, Sage MJ, Lillibridge SR. Bioterrorism preparedness: planning for the future. J Pub Health Manage Prac 2000;6:45–49.

Slater PE, Costin C. Infectious disease and mortality surveillance in Israel in peace and war. Pub Health Rev 1992;93:280–284.

Stern L, Lightfoot D. Automated outbreak detection: a quantitative retrospective analysis. Epidemiol Infect 1999;122:103–110.

Talan DA, Moran GJ, Mower WR, Newdow M, Ong S, Slutsker L, Jarvis WR, Conn LA, Pinner RW. EMERGEncy ID NET: an emergency department-based emerging infections sentinel network. Ann Emerg Med 1998;32:703–711.

Stanford Report. New device helps track symptoms. October 31, 2001. Accessed at www.stanford.edu/dept/news/report/news/october31/healthbuddy.html on December 21, 2001.

Toubiana L, Flahault A. A space-time criterion for early detection of epidemics of influenza-like illness. Eur J Epidemiol 1998:14:465–470.

Tsui F-C, Wagner MM, Dato V, Chang C-CH. Value of ICD-9-coded chief complaints for detection of epidemics. Proc AMIA Symp 2001:711–715 (in press).

Wagner MM, Aryel R, Dato VM, Krenzelok E, Fapohunda A, Sharma R. Availability and comparative value of data elements required for an effective bioterrorism detection system. 119 pages. Report commissioned by AHRQ. November 28, 2001a.

Wagner MM, Tsui F-C, Espino JU, Dato VM, Sittig DF, Caruana RA, McGinnis LF, Deerfield DW, Druzdzen MJ, Fridsma DB. The emerging science of very early detection of disease outbreaks. J Pub Health Manage Prac 2001b;7:50–58.

Woodall J. Official versus unofficial outbreak reporting through the Internet. Inter J Med Inform 1997;47:31–34.

Woodall JP. Global surveillance of emerging diseases: the ProMED-mail perspective. Cad Saude Publica 2001;1(Supplement):147–154.

Zelicoff A, Brillman J, Forsland DW, George JE, Zink S, Koenig S, Staab T, Simpson G, Umland E, Bersell K. The rapid syndrome validation project (RSVP). Proc AMIA Symp 2001;771–776.

Appendix C

Pathogen Discovery, Detection, and Diagnostics

David A. Relman, M.D.
Departments of Microbiology and
Immunology and of Medicine
Stanford University, Stanford, California
VA Palo Alto Health Care System,
Palo Alto, California

PATHOGEN DISCOVERY[1]

Microbial Diversity and the Limitations of Cultivation Methods

Beginning in the late 1970s and early 1980s, explorations of the natural microbial world focused on extreme environments and exploited the use of newly described molecular approaches for phylogenetic analysis and classification. Recovery of sequence-based signatures of life directly from these environments confirmed revolutionary proposals for three aboriginal lines of descent (Woese and Fox, 1977), and led to the realization that nearly all microbial life is resistant to cultivation in the laboratory. With increasing reliance on molecular methods in environmental microbiology, a picture of microbial diversity emerged that currently includes as many as 40 major divisions of bacteria; a broad and cosmopolitan domain of life known as the *Archaea*; and an intertwined early history of endosymbiotic prokaryotes, eukaryotic protists, and lateral gene transfer events (Pace, 1997; Hugenholtz et al., 1998). The inadequacies of available cultivation techniques are reflected in the fact that nearly 90 percent of all known cultivated bacterial species are contained within just 4 of the 40 divisions, even though many of the other divisions are equally or more diverse and well populated. The fact that 65 percent of all published microbiological research over a 6-year period concerned just 8 bacterial genera is a dramatic

---

[1]The discussion in this section is based on Relman (2002).

313

illustration of our strong bias toward bacteria that are amenable to cultivation (Hugenholtz, 2002).

Given these facts, it is concerning but perhaps not surprising that clinical microbiology continues to rely heavily upon cultivation-based methods. In fact, cultivation methods have improved considerably over the past several decades with advances in the scope and diversity of media components, control of environmental conditions, use of heterologous host cells, and use of growth-promoting factors (Mukamolova et al., 1998) A number of recently recognized and newly described microbial pathogens have been cultivated successfully in the laboratory, including spirochetes, rickettsia, actinomycetes, and a variety of viruses. Because the internal environmental conditions of the human body are viewed as more hospitable to life and are more easily replicated in the laboratory than are many external environmental conditions, we often assume that microbial cultivation efforts have been relatively successful. To be sure, there is no dearth of known, cultivated microbial pathogens.

On the other hand, we should not be so complacent about the completeness of our inventory of microbial pathogens, or about the sensitivity of detection methods for cultivation-amenable microorganisms. When traditional diagnostic methods are rigorously applied to syndromes of suspected infectious etiology, such as pneumonia, encephalitis, lymphocyte-predominant meningitis, pericarditis, acute diarrhea, and sepsis, only a minority of cases can be explained microbiologically. The majority of emerging infectious disease agents are zoonotic organisms, and as such are better adapted to nonhuman environmental conditions. In addition, a long list of chronic inflammatory diseases with features of infection remain poorly understood and inadequately explained from a microbiological perspective. Thus, it seems fair to speculate that the identification of pathogens in only seven bacterial divisions and the absence of any known pathogens within the domain *Archaea* may represent an imperfect understanding of the true diversity of microbes capable of causing human disease. Furthermore, it seems reasonable to conclude that current methods are lacking in sensitivity.

Molecular Approaches for Microbial Pathogen Detection and Identification: Seeking Signatures

In an effort to avoid reliance on cultivation and to establish alternative and complementary approaches, one might view the goal of microbial detection and pathogen discovery as identifying molecular signatures of infection. These signatures must be reliable in identifying a microorganism and in establishing the relationships between a previously uncharacterized organism and those that have previously been characterized. Molecular signatures can be based directly upon the features of the microbe itself or upon the features of the host response to a pathogen. And there are a variety of methods and techniques with which to acquire each of these two types of signatures (Relman, 1999).

Genomic sequence is the most frequently used "currency" in the identification of microbial signatures, and broad-range (or consensus) polymerase chain reaction (PCR) is the most practical tool for generating this currency (Relman, 1999). Furthermore, ribosomal DNA (rDNA) is among the most useful kinds of genome sequence from which organismal ancestry and interrelationships can be reliably inferred and pathogen discovery approaches designed (Relman et al., 1990, 1992). With recent improvements in the speed with which primary genome sequence can be acquired and analyzed, other detection or screening formats may become widely available and additional regions of microbial (and viral) genomes more commonly targeted. For example, high-density microarrays of oligonucleotides or amplified DNA products can be designed to screen complex pools of microbial nucleic acid for specific agents in a massively parallel and efficient manner. This technical platform obviates the need to clone and sequence large numbers of variant microbial molecules, which is particularly relevant to the analysis of clinical specimens with a significant burden of "background" microorganisms (see the further discussion below), and facilitates more sophisticated uses of pattern recognition analysis as a tool for microbial signature identification.

There are at least two alternative kinds of approaches for detecting diagnostic signatures of microbial origin that incorporate features to help discriminate between signal and noise. The first relies on differential analysis of microbial sequences in specimens from host sites that are involved and uninvolved by disease. Differential display is a screen for differences in sequence diversity and abundance between involved and uninvolved sites; representational difference analysis in essence selects for sequences of differential abundance, using PCR (Chang et al., 1994; Gao and Moore, 1996). Both approaches share the disadvantage that the sequences of differential abundance that are revealed by these methods may not be useful markers for microbial identification. A interesting study of Crohn's disease illustrates this problem (Sutton et al., 2000). The second kind of alternative approach relies upon the host immune response to identify sequences that may originate from a putative pathogen. These techniques include screening of expression or phage display peptide libraries with patient antisera or reactive T cells (Hemmer et al., 1999).

Despite a greater emphasis on efforts to discover and detect microbes by targeting them directly, the host response to infection offers attractive features for pathogen detection and classification that are unique and complementary. In theory, the host response provides microbial signatures that are, by definition, clinically relevant—that is, the host response largely defines whether infection has led to disease. It is also more intimately connected to clinical outcome and may provide signatures with prognostic value. Finally, signatures based on host response do not presuppose the presence of the putative pathogen for specimen analysis. There is further discussion of these approaches and their relative value below.

Exploring the Human Microbiome in Health and Disease

Surveys of the microbial communities associated with humans during states of health, using molecular techniques, have been initiated, albeit belatedly. These surveys are important for a number of reasons. In addition to the numerous but poorly characterized beneficial effects of the endogenous microflora on human health, a proper understanding of community membership, relative abundance, and variations therein will be critical for recognizing potential pathogens and patterns that are predictive of disease. Basic principles and paradigms in the field of ecology have not yet been applied to the study of the human microbial ecosystem. For example, we have virtually no information on the levels of microbial diversity ("richness") and abundance ("evenness") that are optimal for maintenance of local health, or of those that are associated with disease. We are only just recently learning about microbial partitioning within human micro-environments, and still understand little about interindividual variability or variability as a function of time. The validity of the "intermediate disturbance theory" (Sousa, 1984; Buckling et al., 2000) and its application to human endogenous microbial communities have not been explored. Furthermore, our capabilities to predict the effects of physical or chemical (e.g., antibiotic) perturbation on these microbial communities is extremely limited.

The subgingival crevice in the mouth is one of the more intensively studied and better understood colonized sites of the human body. Molecular surveys using broad-range rDNA PCR suggest that approximately 50–60 percent of the bacteria present at this site are distinct from all of those previously described at the taxonomic level of species—albeit a term that is loosely defined (Kroes et al., 1999; Paster et al., 2001). Some of these bacteria are not assigned to the dominant four divisions—actinobacteria, firmicutes, bacteroidetes, and proteobacteria—and belong to divisions such as TM7 and OP11 that have not previously been recognized or discussed by clinicians or clinical microbiologists, probably because they contain no known cultivated members. Molecular surveys of the endogenous flora of the human intestinal tract have only just begun. Although the clinical significance of the newly discovered community membership has not yet been established, it is clear that the human endogenous microflora play an important role in a variety of important disease states involving the skin and mucosal tissues. What is not clear, but widely speculated, is the possible role of the endogenous flora in either provoking or propagating disease at distant sites, including the central nervous system. The proposed associations between viral respiratory infections and subsequent flares of multiple sclerosis and between *Campylobacter jejuni* enterocolitis and Guillain-Barre syndrome (Ang et al., 2002) are but two examples.

Seeking Evidence of Causation

The increasing availability of molecular pathogen discovery methods and the ease with which molecular signatures are generated create a pressing problem of a different kind: How can one build a convincing body of evidence for a causative role of the putative pathogen in a disease process when the pathogen is identified with molecular signatures and has not been isolated or purified? The issues surrounding this problem are familiar to epidemiologists and have been addressed during the past half-century using distinct terminology that nonetheless is quite relevant today. One can adapt the same concepts to the kinds of data and techniques generated and used in modern approaches to pathogen detection and discovery (Fredericks, 2001). In particular, the ability to connect a signature physically to the sites of pathology where one most expects to find the putative disease agent is a helpful evidentiary component. Fluorescent in situ hybridization allows one to correlate a specific sequence with areas of pathology and tissue-based microbial structures (Fredricks and Relman, 1996; Fredricks et al., 2000). This approach also allows one to examine signature "dosage" effects. Alternatively, anatomic sites of interest can be targeted specifically for signature detection using laser capture microdissection (Emmert-Buck et al., 1996; Becich, 2000).

Recognition and Classification of Microbial Disease Based on Host Gene Expression Patterns

The limitations of methods for analysis of microbial signatures and the emergence of technology platforms for rapid, highly parallel gene expression measurements have facilitated a potentially important, independent approach for identification of microbial disease. The basic question raised is whether one can recognize and classify clinical (and preclinical) states of infection by examining host gene response patterns (Cummings and Relman, 2000; Diehn et al., 2000a). This approach offers several advantages. First, changes in gene transcript abundance occur within minutes of a new exogenous stimulus. Second, the complexity and diversity of signal transduction mechanisms that impact on human gene expression and the complexity of the output (at a genome-wide level) are extensive; therefore, discrimination between numerous diverse stimuli (e.g., different classes of pathogens) may be discernible. Third, a clinical specimen need not contain the exogenous stimulus, i.e., the infectious agent. Fourth, the intrinsic nature of the host response may be directly informative about the clinical relevance of the stimulus (host–microbe interaction) and the clinical outcome. At the present time, however, the answer to this basic question is not yet available.

The vast majority of work in this area to date has focused on the response of host cells to microbial stimuli in vitro (Boldrick et al., 2002; Nau et al., 2002). A larger body of work predates this more recent emphasis on microbial stimuli and addresses the nature of the expression patterns associated with various forms of cancer (Alizadeh et al., 2000; Ross et al., 2000; Perou et al., 1999). As many might have predicted, findings from examination of host–microbial encounters in vitro indicate the predominance of shared gene expression patterns, suggesting a stereotyped temporally controlled response to microbes in human cells (Boldrick et al., 2002). Gene expression responses exhibit microbial dose dependence, yet universal, shared dose equivalence relationships are not apparent. From these early experiments, it appears that identification of discriminatory (diagnostic) signatures may be possible. Furthermore, active, virulence-associated mechanisms may provide the basis for specific pathogen class recognition.

The transition to an analysis of humans with and without known infectious diseases ex vivo is accompanied by a number of interesting but complex questions. What is the most useful and practical type of clinical specimen from which to record genome-wide expression patterns and discern meaningful information about infection? Blood cells are attractive, given that they circulate, make contact with a wide variety of microenvironments and other cell types, and are easy to obtain. But it is unclear how well they might reflect a localized infectious process, e.g., in the brain. How much variability occurs within and between individuals during various states of health and during noninfectious stimuli? Must each individual serve as his or her own control, for proper interpretation of infection-associated responses? What kinds of host-specific genetic information and proclivities are embedded in expression data? These questions are currently being explored, but are quite wide-ranging and will require extensive sampling before they can be answered in a comprehensive fashion. One of the most intriguing questions is on what basis humans classify noxious stimuli, and, in particular, microbial causes of disease. Among the most likely uses and practical outcomes of these investigations is the identification of patterns that predict disease outcome (Alizadeh et al., 2000). Furthermore, expression analysis can be used to identify predicted membrane-associated and secreted proteins (Diehn et al., 2000b); with this approach, diagnostic and prognostic transcript abundance patterns can be converted to sets of easily measured proteins in body fluids.

MICROBIAL DETECTION AND DIAGNOSIS

Sample Collection and Processing

Current diagnostic approaches for the collection of environmental samples or clinical specimens involve primarily hands-on, ad hoc procedures using a variety of devices and instruments. In the clinical arena, these procedures result in specimens of variable quantity and quality. The process is relatively laborious and nonstandarized. A few common methods for specimen disruption are applied to each specimen type without particular regard for the possible diversity of pathogens and their various requirements, nor are special precautions used in a uniform manner to minimize degradation of pathogens or their viability. Problems with lack of standardization and nonuniformity of procedure are even more prevalent in the area of environmental microbial detection. Air and water are among the environmental specimen types that are currently collected and processed most effectively. Because of the time demands and resource constraints found in today's clinical workplace, as well as recent laboratory downsizing, recovery of fastidious microbes from clinical specimens has almost certainly suffered (Bartlett et al., 2000). For example, increasing delays from the time of sputum specimen collection to the inoculation of appropriate culture media have probably contributed to the decreasing recovery rates of *S. pneumoniae* from cases of pneumonia. Some technology developments, such as the use of microsonicators for efficient rapid microbial lysis, are likely to improve the current situation (Belgrader et al., 1999b; Taylor et al., 2001).

Detection Platforms

Traditional approaches for microbial detection and identification include microbial cultivation, immunological (e.g., antibody-based) assays, and nucleic acid detection schemes—especially amplification methods such as PCR (Tang et al., 1997; Fredricks and Relman, 1999). Cultivation is the most widely used approach in laboratories, clinics, and health care facilities throughout the world, especially in developing countries, and hence is currently the most common microbial detection platform for international surveillance. Cultivation, despite being slow, limited in sensitivity for some clinically relevant microbes, and the least technologically sophisticated, nevertheless provides the most ready assessment of complex microbial phenotypes (behaviors), such as drug resistance. Solid-phase immunological assays, such as dipsticks and optical immunoassays, have established a niche in the clinical workplace, but their utility has been demonstrated in only a limited number of infectious diseases settings (Needham et al., 1998). PCR is the most widely used method for microbial nucleic acid detection; other signal and target amplification techniques for nucleic acid detection, such as ligase chain reaction, have generated more limited commercial markets (Tang et al., 1997; Fredricks and Relman, 1999).

Although hundreds of different microbe-specific PCR assays have been described, and many of these have been applied to diverse environmental problems, a much smaller number of assays has entered routine clinical practice. Examples include assays for *N. gonorrheae*, *C. trachomatis*, herpes simplex virus, and HIV. PCR can be used to detect antibiotic resistance (Fluit et all., 2001); however, the diversity of genotypes and mechanisms associated with this phenotype and the difficulty of predicting expression from simple gene detection have hampered this approach. A modest number of recent studies have confirmed that the use of these molecular diagnostic tests can reduce patient-care costs and favorably impact patient management (Dumler et al., 1999; Ramers et al., 2000). Some of the factors that may have limited more widespread use of these theoretically appealing molecular approaches are specimen issues (see later discussion), a paucity of studies that address clinical validation, and the need for specialized expertise. Again, technology advances with PCR may in the near future shift further attention toward this platform. In particular, the development of rapid, real-time (semiquantitative) PCR with point-of-care microbial detection within 30 minutes (Belgrader et al., 1998, 1999b) may potentially alter the use of antibiotics on a widespread scale and reduce antibiotic resistance (Bergeron and Oullette, 1998). Overall, each of the three detection/diagnostic platforms provides complementary advantages and disadvantages. No one approach alone currently provides a rapid and reliable method for microbial detection in the real world.

The above comments are in general equally relevant to clinical and environmental microbial detection and identification. In the environmental detection arena, much emphasis has been placed on sensor technology. The results of these investments have led to a plethora of sensor types but relatively limited maturation of any one platform. Problems are similar to those in the clinical arena, and focus on a lack of real-world validation (see later discussion). Future efforts in environmental microbial detection will likely emphasize the integration of multiple types of environmental data, building on the principles established in the field of measurement and signature intelligence.

Performance Characteristics

A disproportionate effort in microbial detection and diagnosis has been devoted to technology platform development, rather than to standardization or validation of sample collection and processing procedures, or to test validation in a real-world setting. While analytical performance characteristics have been deliberately pursued, "clinical" performance characteristics have been relatively ignored. For example, it is important to be able to anticipate false-positive test results in a reliable and quantitative fashion. However, a proper calculation of positive predictive value requires some understanding of the pretest probability of a true positive test. In the area of environmental detection, pretest probabilities for the presence of a variety of microbial agents is probably low and difficult to determine. One is unavoidably left with a situation in which the false-positive rate is likely to be high and poorly characterized. Many of these problems also apply to the situation with clinical and preclinical diagnosis.

ISSUES AND PROBLEMS

Clinical Relevance of Laboratory Findings

The inevitable result of increasingly sensitive detection platforms is difficulty in establishing the clinical relevance of positive test results. The important distinction between infection and disease, i.e., colonization or contamination of a host with a potential biothreat agent, and pathology (disease) has challenged clinicians for a century. The same problem arises in environmental analysis. Few data are available with which to infer the level of risk to a human host of acquiring disease after detection of a potential pathogen in the environment. Sensitive and specific diagnostic tests are vitally important adjuncts to clinical diagnosis; however, screening and diagnostic tests cannot replace the crucial need for careful studies that define likelihood of exposure or examine correlations between detection and disease.

One issue of particular importance concerns the complexity and widespread distribution of microbial sequence "background" or "noise" observed in the analysis of human clinical specimens (both experimental and biological) discussed earlier. The distribution and nature of this sequence background have as yet not been well characterized. Findings of bacterial rDNA in association with blood samples from healthy humans threaten to expand the extent of this problem, and involve the analysis of anatomic compartments that have traditionally been viewed as usually sterile (Nikkari et al., 2001). A different perspective on this same apparent problem was provided in an analysis of expressed sequence tag libraries from human tissues (Weber et al., 2002; Relman, 2002). Some of the transcripts that were originally assumed to derive from the human genome appeared on closer inspection to be of microbial origin. Whether some of these molecules were intrinsic to the original specimen or introduced later remains unclear; but at least a portion can easily be attributed to agents that are common, persistent, or dormant infectious agents found within these human tissues.

Breadth of Current Assays and Approaches

There is a strong tendency in molecular diagnostics to focus disproportionate attention on a small number of pathogens that have proven to be amenable to detection. Positive findings tend to create a self-fulfilling prophecy. Few efforts are invested in improving methods for the detection of less commonly found pathogens. In addition, important lessons have been learned in recent years about the use and limitations of molecular methods for microbial pathogen discovery (see the earlier discussion). First, the assumption that sequences identified as universally conserved within a group of organisms are in fact found in all members of the group is not always justified. As previously unrecognized members of a group are revealed, small additional degrees of sequence variation are sometimes discovered. The small subunit rDNA sequences that were originally described as universal are now known to be conserved in only a subset of cellular life (Lane et al., 1985); revised sequence sites have taken their place. Second, PCR can exhibit bias and favor certain members of a mixed starting pool of molecules. The use of multiple broad-range primer pairs or reaction cosolvents may avoid a skewed perspective. Third, conserved sequences for use in broad-range PCR have not yet been identified and validated for all groups of viruses. This limitation most certainly contributed to the sizable number of cases that remained unexplained after investigation by the Unexplained Deaths and Critical Illnesses Working Group within the CDC's Emerging Infections Program (Nikkari et al., 2002). Finally, a large number of detection and diagnostic tests rely upon a small number of specific antibodies or microbial genomic sequences. This reliance creates vulnerabilities. Microbial pathogens that have variant antibody epitopes (binding sites) or sequences will fail to be detected, and may in fact be selected over time.

Specimen Problems

The problems associated with clinical and other real-world specimens are substantial, and are currently underappreciated and inadequately targeted by funding agencies. These problems became highlighted during the investigations of the Unexplained Deaths and Critical Illnesses Project under the direction of CDC and collaborating scientists (Nikkari et al., 2002; Hajjeh et al., 2002). The Unexplained Deaths Project is an enhanced passive surveillance system that identifies life-threatening cases of disease with features of infection for which routine laboratory tests fail to provide a microbiological diagnosis. It has served as a source of clinical specimens with which newer molecular diagnostic methods can be evaluated. Problems revealed in this study are common in most clinical settings. First, clinical specimens from cases of suspected but unproven infectious etiology are often obtained late in the disease course, at a time when the putative agent may no longer be present. Second, the site from which the specimen is obtained may not coincide optimally with the expected anatomic distribution of the agent. Third, the quantity of specimen may be insufficient for the expected concentration of the agent and a reasonable probability of its presence (as a single particle or genome equivalent) in the specimen. And fourth, in the real world of clinical medicine, specimen handling and storage may introduce exogenous contamination, spurious signals, or target degradation.

Standardization of Procedures

The preceding discussion has suggested that current diagnostic and detection procedures lack sufficient standardization and validation. The barriers to a successful resolution of this problem are multiple. First, additional method development and optimization for specimen collection and processing are necessary. Second, a set of uniform reagents is needed, with which multiple competing procedures and platforms can be cross-evaluated. Third, additional funds and incentives will need to be provided before an effort of the necessary breadth and rigor is undertaken by public and private organizations, as well as academic, government, and commercial ventures.

NEAR-TERM NEEDS

To address the problems and issues outlined above, a number of needs must be met. First is validation of methods in the real world. To this end, an investment in the development of procedures and in the kinds of resources described earlier must be undertaken. Second, for any given assay for a specific agent, we need additional information on the distribution and abundance of that agent and its close relatives in a wide variety of environments. As broad-range assays become more widely used in the mid- to distant future, a proportionately larger-scale effort must be undertaken to describe the microbial background of clinical and environmental sites. Third, with increasing emphasis on the use of microbial sequences for detection and diagnosis, a strong imperative is created for a broad investment in microbial genomics. In addition, the usefulness of genome sequences for microbial forensics further emphasizes the need for this investment (Cummings and Relman, 2002). Fourth, high-throughput sequencing technology and sample handling (robotics) have advanced recently in dramatic fashion. As a result, it becomes more practical and timely to consider major investments in laboratories that can handle large numbers of samples and provide surge capacity (Layne et al., 2001; Layne and Beugelsdijk, 1998). Such laboratories might facilitate standardization of methods and technology development. Finally, centralized repositories of diverse, high-affinity binding and detection reagents (e.g., antibodies, peptides, oligonucleotides, aptamers (Brody and Gold, 2000) should be established, as well as centralized repositories of genomic material and control samples. These resources would assist with standardization and validation of methods and help minimize reliance on an overly narrow set of detection reagents.

ANTICIPATING MICROBIAL THREATS

Intelligence Gathering: Human Intention

Deliberate release of a biological agent as a weapon poses a number of additional challenges in detection and diagnosis, including a much-expanded spectrum of agents and greater difficulty in calculating pretest probabilities and positive predictive values. In a timeline of events related to a bioterrorist attack, the earliest stage predates release of a bioagent and involves the evolution of a bioweapons plan or program from inception through weapon deployment. The greatest potential benefit might derive from preemptive efforts at this point in the timeline. Opportunities exist in the areas of human intelligence gathering. The science and technology communities have not been adequately tapped for their expertise in this regard. The challenge of understanding human intent in the area of biotechnology requires familiarity with science and technology culture, process, and procedure.

Intelligence Gathering: Nature

A variety of forms of evidence suggest that the diversity and number of microbial disease agents and virulence genes in nature is immense. Most of these agents and genes remain uncharacterized and unfamiliar to us, in part because they have not yet had opportunities for exposure to humans, or exposure has not been recognized. Examples of well-known reservoirs for emerging pathogens include rodents (Sin nombre virus or Lassa fever virus), birds (West Nile virus), and fruit bats (Hendra virus or Nipah virus). Within specific contexts and with appropriate epidemiological leads, one might consider a directed survey of suspected reservoirs for potential viral and microbial pathogens. Broad-range PCR would be an attractive approach for such a project (see earlier discussion). However, high-throughput sequence analysis and large-volume sample analysis will be required for recognition of meaningful patterns and establishment of significant associations with disease. These needs may ultimately require the development and use of high-density DNA microarrays designed for broad-range microbial surveys.

A Second Human Genome Project: Microbial Community Genomics

As one broad approach to the problem of poorly understood endogenous flora, one might consider a second human genome project (Relman and Falkow, 2001). Such a project would entail a comprehensive inventory of microbial genes and genomes at the four major sites of microbial colonization in the human body: mouth, gut, vagina, and skin. Community microbial genomics is a rapidly emerging experimental approach toward understanding the composition, functional capabilities, coevolution, and interactions of complex groups of microbes, many of which are resistant to cultivation or purification. This approach has already been undertaken in the study of marine and soil microbial ecology (Beja et al., 2000, 2002; DeLong, 2001; Rondon et al., 2000). A community genomics analysis of the human microbiome would provide an equally rich data set from which critical issues in human health and emerging infectious diseases could be addressed. This second human genome project could be approached with a combination of random shotgun sequencing procedures, targeted large-insert clone sequencing, and assessments of intra- and interindividual variation using high-density microarrays. From these flora arise current and future opportunistic microbial pathogens, including those that are drug-resistant. From inventories of endogenous microbial community membership, gene content, and gene expression, it may be possible to identify patterns that indicate early stages of colonization or takeover by newly acquired pathogens. With increasing degrees of population sampling in well-characterized settings and with the integration of host genome-wide expression analysis (Relman and Falkow, 2001; Hooper et al., 2001), major insights into the role of endogenous flora in health and disease will be gained.

LOOKING TO THE FUTURE

The principles that are embedded in the use of genome-wide expression patterns for classification and characterization of infectious diseases (see earlier discussion) can be viewed as an important generic feature of future

directions in microbial diagnostics and detection. Complex biological signatures and pattern recognition are relevant to the analysis of the endogenous microbial flora, protein expression profiles, secreted or exhaled volatile small molecules, and spectral properties of human cells and tissues.
Protein microarrays (Haab et al., 2001; Templin et al., 2002) are rapidly
emerging as a complementary platform for the potential generation of important biological signatures from clinical specimens. The same is true for
high-throughput mass spectroscopy methods (Petricoin et al., 2002). Patterns can be discerned that embed diagnostic and prognostic information
without the need for a clear understanding of mechanism. As mentioned
earlier, endogenous microbial flora might be the source of informative
patterns that would indicate exposure to or incipient development of infectious disease, as well as prior behavior of the host. It is already clear that
automated and miniaturized technology platforms, such as microfluidics
chips and cartridges, will speed the development of point-of-care, rapid,
hands-off diagnostic tests (Belgrader et al., 2000; Pourahamadi et al., 2000).
Technology cannot substitute for a holistic understanding of biological
systems, but exciting clinical investigation will be greatly accelerated by
new and emerging technologies.

REFERENCES

Alizadeh, A. A., Eisen, M. B., Davis, R. E., Ma, C., Lossos, I. S., Rosenwald, A., Boldrick, J.
    C., Sabet, H., Tran, T., Yu, X., Powell, J. I., Yang, L., Marti, G. E., Moore, T., Hudson,
    J., Jr., Lu, L., Lewis, D. B., Tibshirani, R., Sherlock, G., Chan, W. C., Greiner, T. C.,
    Weisenburger, D. D., Armitage, J. O., Warnke, R., Staudt, L. M., et al. Distinct types of
    diffuse large B-cell lymphoma identified by gene expression profiling. (2000) Nature
    403, 503-11.
Ang, C. W., Laman, J. D., Willison, H. J., Wagner, E. R., Endtz, H. P., De Klerk, M. A., Tio-
    Gillen, A. P., Van den Braak, N., Jacobs, B. C., and Van Doorn, P. A. Structure of
    Campylobacter jejuni lipopolysaccharides determines antiganglioside specificity and clini-
    cal features of Guillain-Barre and Miller Fisher patients. (2002) Infect Immun 70, 1202-
    8.
Bartlett, J. G., Dowell, S. F., Mandell, L. A., File Jr., T. M., Musher, D. M., and Fine, M. J.
    Practice guidelines for the management of community-acquired pneumonia in adults.
    Infectious Diseases Society of America. (2000) Clin Infect Dis 31, 347-82.
Becich, M. J. The role of the pathologist as tissue refiner and data miner. (2000) Mol Diagn 5,
    287-99.
Beja, O., Suzuki, M. T., Koonin, E. V., Aravind, L., Hadd, A., Nguyen, L. P., Villacorta, R.,
    Amjadi, M., Garrigues, C., Jovanovich, S. B., Feldman, R. A., and DeLong, E. F. Con-
    struction and analysis of bacterial artificial chromosome libraries from a marine micro-
    bial assemblage. (2000) Environ Microbiol 2, 516-29.
Beja, O., Suzuki, M. T., Heidelberg, J. F., Nelson, W. C., Preston, C. M., Hamada, T., Eisen,
    J. A., Fraser, C. M., and DeLong, E. F. Unsuspected diversity among marine aerobic
    anoxygenic phototrophs. (2002) Nature 415, 630-3.

Belgrader, P., Benett, W., Hadley, D., Long, G., Mariella, R., Jr., Milanovich, F., Nasarabadi, S., Nelson, W., Richards, J., and Stratton, P. Rapid pathogen detection using a microchip PCR array instrument. (1998) Clin Chem 44, 2191-4.

Belgrader, P., Benett, W., Hadley, D., Richards, J., Stratton, P., Mariella, R., Jr. and Milanovich, F. PCR detection of bacteria in seven minutes. (1999a) Science 284, 449-50.

Belgrader, P., Hansford, D., Kovacs, G. T., Venkateswaran, K., Mariella, R., Jr., Milanovich, F., Nasarabadi, S., Okuzumi, M., Pourahmadi, F., and Northrup, M. A. A minisonicator to rapidly disrupt bacterial spores for DNA analysis. (1999b) Anal Chem 71, 4232-6.

Belgrader, P., Okuzumi, M., Pourahmadi, F., Borkholder, D. A., and Northrup, M. A. A microfluidic cartridge to prepare spores for PCR analysis. (2000) Biosens Bioelectron 14, 849-52.

Bergeron, M. G., and Ouellette, M. Pathogenesis of pneumococcal pneumonia in cyclophosphamide-induced leukopenia in mice. (1998) Infect Control Hosp Epidemiol 19, 560-4.

Boldrick, J. C., Alizadeh, A. A., Diehn, M., Dudoit, S., Liu, C. L., Belcher, C. E., Botstein, D., Staudt, L. M., Brown, P. O., and Relman, D. A. Stereotyped and specific gene expression programs in human innate immune responses to bacteria. (2002) Proc Natl Acad Sci U S A 99, 972-7.

Brody, E. N., and Gold, L. Aptamers as therapeutic and diagnostic agents. (2000) J Biotechnol 74, 5-13.

Buckling, A., Kassen, R., Bell, G., and Rainey, P. B. Disturbance and diversity in experimental microcosms. (2000) Nature 408, 961-4.

Chang, Y., Cesarman, E., Pessin, M. S., Lee, F., Culpepper, J., Knowles, D. M., and Moore, P. S. Identification of herpesvirus-like DNA sequences in AIDS-associated Kaposi's sarcoma. (1994) Science 266, 1865-9.

Cummings, C. A., and Relman, D. A. Using DNA microarrays to study host-microbe interactions. (2000) Emerg Infect Dis 6, 513-25.

Cummings, C. A., and Relman, D. A. Genomics and microbiology. Microbial forensics—"cross-examining pathogens." (2002) Science.

DeLong, E. F. Microbial seascapes revisited. (2001) Curr Opin Microbiol 4, 290-5.

Diehn, M., Alizadeh, A. A., and Brown, P. O. Examining the living genome in health and disease with DNA microarrays. (2000a) Jama 283, 2298-9.

Diehn, M., Eisen, M. B., Botstein, D., and Brown, P. O. Large-scale identification of secreted and membrane-associated gene products using DNA microarrays. (2000b) Nat Genet 25, 58-62.

Dumler, J. S., and Valsamakis, A. Molecular diagnostics for existing and emerging infections. Complementary tools for a new era of clinical microbiology. (1999) Am J Clin Pathol 112, S33-9.

Emmert-Buck, M. R., Bonner, R. F., Smith, P. D., Chuaqui, R. F., Zhuang, Z., Goldstein, S. R., Weiss, R. A., and Liotta, L. A. Laser capture microdissection. (1996) Science 274, 998-1001.

Fluit, A. C., Visser, M. R., and Schmitz, F. J. Molecular detection of antimicrobial resistance. (2001) Clin Microbiol Rev 14, 836-71, table of contents.

Fredricks, D. N., and Relman, D. A. Sequence-based identification of microbial pathogens: a reconsideration of Koch's postulates. (1996) Clin Microbiol Rev 9, 18-33.

Fredricks, D. N., and Relman, D. A. Application of polymerase chain reaction to the diagnosis of infectious diseases. (1999) Clin Infect Dis 29, 475-86; quiz 487-8.

Fredricks, D. N., and Relman, D. A. Localization of Tropheryma whippelii rRNA in tissues from patients with Whipple's disease. (2001) J Infect Dis 183, 1229-37.

Fredricks, D. N., Jolley, J. A., Lepp, P. W., Kosek, J. C., and Relman, D. A. Rhinosporidium seeberi: a human pathogen from a novel group of aquatic protistan parasites. (2000) Emerg Infect Dis 6, 273-82.

Gao, S. J., and Moore, P. S. Molecular approaches to the identification of unculturable infectious agents. (1996) *Emerg Infect Dis* 2, 159-67.

Haab, B. B., Dunham, M. J., and Brown, P. O. Protein microarrays for highly parallel detection and quantitation of specific proteins and antibodies in complex solutions. (2001) *Genome Biol* 2, RESEARCH0004.

Hajjeh, R. A., Relman, D., Cieslak, P. R., Sofair, A. N., Passaro, D., Flood, J., Johnson, J., Hacker, J. K., Shieh, W. J., Hendry, R. M., Nikkari, S., Ladd-Wilson, S., Hadler, J., Rainbow, J., Tappero, J. W., Woods, C. W., Conn, L., Reagan, S., Zaki, S., and Perkins, B. A. Surveillance for unexplained deaths and critical illnesses due to possibly infectious causes, United States, 1995-1998. (2002) *Emerg Infect Dis* 8, 145-53.

Hemmer, B., Gran, B., Zhao, Y., Marques, A., Pascal, J., Tzou, A., Kondo, T., Cortese, I., Bielekova, B., Straus, S. E., McFarland, H. F., Houghten, R., Simon, R., Pinilla, C., and Martin, R. Identification of candidate T-cell epitopes and molecular mimics in chronic Lyme disease. (1999) *Nat Med* 5, 1375-82.

Hooper, L. V., Wong, M. H., Thelin, A., Hansson, L., Falk, P. G., and Gordon, J. I. Molecular analysis of commensal host-microbial relationships in the intestine. (2001) *Science* 291, 881-4.

Hugenholtz, P. (2002) *Genome Biol* 3, REVIEWS0003.

Hugenholtz, P., Goebel, B. M., and Pace, N. R. Impact of culture-independent studies on the emerging phylogenetic view of bacterial diversity. (1998) *J Bacteriol* 180, 4765-74.

Kroes, I., Lepp, P. W. and Relman, D. A. Bacterial diversity within the human subgingival crevice. (1999) *Proc Natl Acad Sci U S A* 96, 14547-52.

Lane, D. J., Pace, B., Olsen, G. J., Stahl, D. A., Sogin, M. L., and Pace, N. R. Rapid determination of 16S ribosomal RNA sequences for phylogenetic analyses. (1985) *Proc Natl Acad Sci U S A* 82, 6955-9.

Layne, S. P., and Beugelsdijk, T. J. Laboratory firepower for infectious disease research. (1998) *Nat Biotechnol* 16, 825-9.

Layne, S. P., Beugelsdijk, T. J., Patel, C. K., Taubenberger, J. K., Cox, N. J., Gust, I. D., Hay, A. J., Tashiro, M., and Lavanchy, D. A global lab against influenza. (2001) *Science* 293, 1729.

Mukamolova, G. V., Kaprelyants, A. S., Young, D. I., Young, M., and Kell, D. B. A bacterial cytokine (1998) *Proc Natl Acad Sci U S A* 95, 8916-21.

Nau, G. J., Richmond, J. F., Schlesinger, A., Jennings, E. G., Lander, E. S., and Young, R. A. Human macrophage activation programs induced by bacterial pathogens. (2002) *Proc Natl Acad Sci U S A* 99, 1503-8.

Needham, C. A., McPherson, K. A., and Webb, K. H. Streptococcal pharyngitis: impact of a high-sensitivity antigen test on physician outcome. (1998) *J Clin Microbiol* 36, 3468-73.

Nikkari, S., McLaughlin, I. J., Bi, W., Dodge, D. E., and Relman, D. A. Does blood of healthy subjects contain bacterial ribosomal DNA? (2001) *J Clin Microbiol* 39, 1956-9.

Nikkari, S., Lopez, F. A., Lepp, P. W., Cieslak, P. R., Ladd-Wilson, S., Passaro, D., Danila, R., and Relman, D. A. Broad-range bacterial detection and the analysis of unexplained death and critical illness. (2002) *Emerg Infect Dis* 8, 188-94.

Pace, N. R. A molecular view of microbial diversity and the biosphere. (1997) *Science* 276, 734-40.

Paster, B. J., Boches, S. K., Galvin, J. L., Ericson, R. E., Lau, C. N., Levanos, V. A., Sahasrabudhe, A., and Dewhirst, F. E. Bacterial diversity in human subgingival plaque. (2001) *J Bacteriol* 183, 3770-83.

Perou, C. M., Jeffrey, S. S., van de Rijn, M., Rees, C. A., Eisen, M. B., Ross, D. T., Pergamenschikov, A., Williams, C. F., Zhu, S. X., Lee, J. C., Lashkari, D., Shalon, D., Brown, P. O., and Botstein, D. Distinctive gene expression patterns in human mammary epithelial cells and breast cancers. (1999) *Proc Natl Acad Sci U S A* 96, 9212-7.

Petricoin, E. F., Ardekani, A. M., Hitt, B. A., Levine, P. J., Fusaro, V. A., Steinberg, S. M., Mills, G. B., Simone, C., Fishman, D. A., Kohn, E. C., and Liotta, L. A. Use of proteomic patterns in serum to identify ovarian cancer. (2002) *Lancet* 359, 572-7.

Pourahmadi, F., Taylor, M., Kovacs, G., Lloyd, K., Sakai, S., Schafer, T., Helton, B., Western, L., Zaner, S., Ching, J., McMillan, B., Belgrader, P., and Northrup, M. A. Toward a rapid, integrated, and fully automated DNA diagnostic assay for *Chlamydia trachomatis* and *Neisseria gonorrhoeae* (2000) *Clin Chem* 46, 1511-3.

Ramers, C., Billman, G., Hartin, M., Ho, S., and Sawyer, M. H. Impact of a diagnostic cerebrospinal fluid enterovirus polymerase chain reaction test on patient management. (2000) *Jama* 283, 2680-5.

Relman, D. A. The search for unrecognized pathogens. (1999) *Science* 284, 1308-10.

Relman, D. A. New technologies, human-microbe interactions, and the search for previously unrecognized pathogens. (2002) *J Infect Dis*, in press.

Relman, D. A. The human body as microbial observatory. (2002) *Nat Genet* 30, 131-3.

Relman, D. A., and Falkow, S. The meaning and impact of the human genome sequence for microbiology. (2001) *Trends Microbiol* 9, 206-8.

Relman, D. A., Loutit, J. S., Schmidt, T. M., Falkow, S., and Tompkins, L. S. The agent of bacillary angiomatosis. An approach to the identification of uncultured pathogens. (1990) *N Engl J Med* 323, 1573-80.

Relman, D. A., Schmidt, T. M., MacDermott, R. P., and Falkow, S. Identification of the uncultured bacillus of Whipple's disease. (1992) *N Engl J Med* 327, 293-301.

Rondon, M. R., August, P. R., Bettermann, A. D., Brady, S. F., Grossman, T. H., Liles, M. R., Loiacono, K. A., Lynch, B. A., MacNeil, I. A., Minor, C., Tiong, C. L., Gilman, M., Osburne, M. S., Clardy, J., Handelsman, J., and Goodman, R. M. Cloning the soil metagenome: a strategy for accessing the genetic and functional diversity of uncultured microorganisms. (2000) *Appl Environ Microbiol* 66, 2541-7.

Ross, D. T., Scherf, U., Eisen, M. B., Perou, C. M., Rees, C., Spellman, P., Iyer, V., Jeffrey, S. S., Van de Rijn, M., Waltham, M., Pergamenschikov, A., Lee, J. C., Lashkari, D., Shalon, D., Myers, T. G., Weinstein, J. N., Botstein, D., and Brown, P. O. Systematic variation in gene expression patterns in human cancer cell lines. (2000) *Nat Genet* 24, 227-35.

Sousa, W. P. Intertidal mosaics: catch size, propagule availability, and spacially variable patterns of succession. (1984) *Ecology* 65, 1918-1935.

Sutton, C. L., Kim, J., Yamane, A., Dalwadi, H., Wei, B., Landers, C., Targan, S. R., and Braun, J. Identification of a novel bacterial sequence associated with Crohn's disease. (2000) *Gastroenterology* 119, 23-31.

Tang, Y. W., Procop, G. W., and Persing, D. H. Molecular diagnostics of infectious diseases. (1997) *Clin Chem* 43, 2021-38.

Taylor, M. T., Belgrader, P., Furman, B. J., Pourahmadi, F., Kovacs, G. T., and Northrup, M. A. Lysing bacterial spores by sonication through a flexible interface in a microfluidic system. (2001) *Anal Chem* 73, 492-6.

Templin, M. F., Stoll, D., Schrenk, M., Traub, P. C., Vohringer, C. F., and Joos, T. O. Protein microarray technology. (2002) *Trends Biotechnol* 20, 160-6.

Weber, G., Shendure, J., Tanenbaum, D. M., Church, G. M., and Meyerson, M. Identification of foreign gene sequences by transcript filtering against the human genome. (2002) *Nat Genet* 30, 141-2.

Woese, C. R., and Fox, G. E. Phylogenetic structure of the prokaryotic domain: the primary kingdoms. (1977) *Proc Natl Acad Sci U S A* 74, 5088-90.

Appendix D

Forum on Emerging Infections
Membership and Publications
Board on Global Health

FORUM ON EMERGING INFECTIONS

ADEL MAHMOUD (*Chair*), President, Merck Vaccines, Whitehouse Station, New Jersey

STANLEY LEMON (*Vice-Chair*), Dean, School of Medicine, The University of Texas Medical Branch, Galveston, Texas

DAVID ACHESON, Chief Medical Officer, Center for Food Safety and Applied Nutrition, Food and Drug Administration, Rockville, Maryland

STEVEN BRICKNER, Research Advisor, Pfizer Global Research and Development, Pfizer Inc., Groton, Connecticut

GAIL CASSELL, Vice President, Scientific Affairs, Eli Lilly & Company, Indianapolis, Indiana

GORDON DEFRIESE, Professor of Social Medicine, University of North Carolina, Chapel Hill, North Carolina

CEDRIC DUMONT, Medical Director, Department of State and the Foreign Service, Washington, DC

JESSE GOODMAN, Deputy Director, Center for Biologics Evaluation and Research, Food and Drug Administration, Rockville, Maryland

EDUARDO GOTUZZO, Director, Instituto de Medicina Tropical, "Alexander von Humbolt" Universidad Peruana Cayetano Herdia, Lima, Peru

RENU GUPTA, Vice President and Head, U.S. Clinical Research and Development, and Head, Global Cardiovascular, Metabolic, Endocrine, and G.I. Disorders, Novartis Corporation, East Hanover, New Jersey

331

MARGARET HAMBURG, Vice President for Biological Programs, Nuclear Threat Initiative, Washington, DC

CAROLE HEILMAN, Director, Division of Microbiology and Infectious Diseases, National Institute of Allergy and Infectious Diseases, National Institutes of Health, Bethesda, Maryland

DAVID HEYMANN, Executive Director, Communicable Diseases, World Health Organization, Geneva, Switzerland

JAMES HUGHES, Assistant Surgeon General and Director, National Center for Infectious Diseases, Centers for Disease Control and Prevention, Atlanta, Georgia

SAMUEL KATZ, Wilburt C. Davison Professor and Chairman Emeritus, Duke University Medical Center, Durham, North Carolina

PATRICK KELLEY, Colonel, Director, Department of Defense Global Emerging Infections System, Walter Reed Army Institute of Research, Silver Spring, Maryland

MARCELLE LAYTON, Assistant Commissioner, Bureau of Communicable Diseases, New York City Department of Health, New York, New York

JOSHUA LEDERBERG, Raymond and Beverly Sackler Foundation Scholar, The Rockefeller University, New York, New York

CARLOS LOPEZ, Research Fellow, Research Acquisitions, Eli Lilly Research Laboratories, Indianapolis, Indiana

LYNN MARKS, Global Head of Infectious Diseases, GlaxoSmithKline, Collegeville, Pennsylvania

STEPHEN MORSE, Director, Center for Public Health Preparedness, Columbia University, New York, New York

MICHAEL OSTERHOLM, Director, Center for Infectious Disease Research and Policy, and Professor, School of Public Health, University of Minnesota, Minneapolis, Minnesota

GARY ROSELLE, Program Director for Infectious Diseases, VA Central Office, Veterans Health Administration, Department of Veterans Affairs, Washington, DC

DAVID SHLAES, Executive Vice President for Research and Development, Idenix, Cambridge, Massachusetts

JANET SHOEMAKER, Director, Office of Public Affairs, American Society for Microbiology, Washington, DC

P. FREDRICK SPARLING, J. Herbert Bate Professor Emeritus of Medicine, Microbiology, and Immunology, University of North Carolina, Chapel Hill, North Carolina

MICHAEL ZEILINGER, Infectious Disease Team Leader, Office of Health and Nutrition, U.S. Agency for International Development, Washington, DC

Liaisons

ENRIQUETA BOND, President, Burroughs Wellcome Fund, Research Triangle Park, North Carolina
NANCY CARTER-FOSTER, Director, Program for Emerging Infections and HIV/AIDS, U.S. Department of State, Washington, DC
EDWARD McSWEEGAN, National Institute of Allergy and Infectious Diseases, National Institutes of Health, Bethesda, Maryland
STEPHEN OSTROFF, Associate Director for Epidemiologic Science, National Center for Infectious Diseases. Centers for Disease Control and Prevention, Atlanta, Georgia

BOARD ON GLOBAL HEALTH

DEAN T. JAMISON *(Chair),* Senior Fellow, Fogarty International Center, National Institutes of Health
YVES BERGEVIN, Chief, Health Section, UNICEF
PATRICIA DANZON, Professor, Health Care Systems Department, University of Pennsylvania
RICHARD FEACHEM, Interim Secretariat, Global Fund to Fight AIDS, Tuberculosis and Malaria, Geneva
NOREEN GOLDMAN, Professor, Office of Population Research, Princeton University, Princeton, New Jersey
MARGARET HAMBURG, Vice President for Biological Programs, Nuclear Threat Initiative, Washington, DC
GERALD KEUSCH, Director, Fogarty International Center, National Institutes of Health
ARTHUR KLEINMAN, Maude and Lillian Presley Professor of Medical Anthropology/ Professor of Psychiatry and
Social Medicine, Harvard Medical School
ADEL MAHMOUD, President, Merck Vaccines
JOHN WYN OWEN, Secretary, Nuffield Trust, London
ALLAN ROSENFIELD, Dean, Mailman School of Public Health, Columbia University
SUSAN SCRIMSHAW, Dean, School of Public Health, University of Illinois at Chicago

Staff

JUDITH BALE, Director, Board on Global Health (retired December 2002)
STACEY L. KNOBLER, Director, Forum on Emerging Infections
MARK S. SMOLINSKI, Senior Program Officer
PATRICIA CUFF, Research Associate
MARJAN NAJAFI, Research Associate

KATHERINE OBERHOLTZER, Project Assistant
JASON PELLMAR, Project Assistant

PUBLICATIONS

The Infectious Etiology of Chronic Diseases
in press

The Impact of Globalization on Infectious Disease Emergence and Control
in press

The Resistance Phenomenon in Microbes and Infectious Disease Vectors
Implications for Human Health and Strategies for Containmemt
2003

The Emergence of Zoonotic Diseases
Understanding the Impact on Animal and Human Health
2002

Considerations for Viral Disease Eradication
Lessons Learned and Future Strategies
2002

Biological Threats and Terrorism
Assessing the Science and Response Capabilities
2002

Emerging Infectious Diseases from the Global to Local Perspective
2002

Managed Care Systems and Emerging Infections
Challenges and Opportunities for Strengthening Surveillance, Research, and Prevention
2000

Antimicrobial Resistance
Issues and Options
1998

Orphans and Incentives
Developing Technologies to Address Emerging Infections
1997

Appendix E
Computational Modeling and Simulation of Epidemic Infectious Diseases

Donald S. Burke, M.D.
Bloomberg School of Public Health
Johns Hopkins University

I simply wish that, in a matter which so closely concerns the well-being of mankind, no decision shall be made without all the knowledge which a little analysis and calculation can provide.

Daniel Bernoulli, on smallpox inoculation, 1766

HISTORICAL FOUNDATIONS

Mathematics and statistics have been essential to the theory and practice of infectious disease control since 1766, when Bernoulli analyzed life expectancies and death rates in his evaluation of variolation as a public health tool (Dietz, 2000). Subsequently, Philip-Charles Alexandre Louis in France and William Farr in Britain melded quantitative epidemiological measurements with philosophical concepts of social justice, a synthesis from which the statistical hygienic movement was born (Lilienfeld, 1980). The second era of epidemiology arose at the turn of the twentieth century with the proof of the germ theory and the development of mechanistic mathematical models, first by the brilliant Ronald Ross, who used his own malaria field research data to guide the construction of sophisticated mathematical models (Serfling, 1952). In the 1930s Kermack and McKendrick formulated the now familiar "S-E-I-R" (susceptible, exposed, infected, and removed) deterministic differential equations models for the transmission of infectious diseases (Serfling, 1952). Stochasticity—the role of chance—was subsequently added to the models.

In its third era (the past few decades), epidemiology has moved away from its classical foundations in infectious diseases to focus on chronic diseases, and, of necessity, reverted to an emphasis on statistical identification of risk factors rather than elucidation of mechanisms and dynamics. Some leaders in the field rue this development. Dr. Mervin Susser, a highly respected statesman–epidemiologist, recently admonished his fellow epidemiologists to adopt a multilevel, systems analysis, "eco-epidemiology" approach (Susser and Susser, 1996a, 1996b). Others have argued that modern epidemiology must fully embrace new powerful computational technologies to analyze, model, and simulate the dynamics of disease generation and propagation (Koopman, 1996).

TOWARD A NEW SCIENCE OF EXPERIMENTAL EPIDEMIOLOGY

Epidemiology is not commonly considered to be an experimental science. The discipline concerns itself with large populations of ill (or potentially ill) humans, and rigorously controlled experimental designs are rarely practical or ethical. When prospective epidemiological studies are undertaken, as in Phase III efficacy trials of vaccines, study population size limitations are such that usually only one new intervention can be evaluated. Mathematical and statistical modeling is invaluable in the design and interpretation of epidemiological studies, but is not well suited to simulation of interventions and outcomes. Extraordinary increases in the speed and memory of inexpensive computer processors now make it possible to create and run computations that were impossible only a few years ago, giving rise to computational simulations of unimagined speed, granularity, and stochasticity. Such simulations could serve as dry "laboratories" for a new science of experimental epidemiology in which new population-level interventions could be designed, evaluated, and iteratively refined on simulated epidemics, with tangible benefits for real-world epidemic prevention and control efforts. Successful development of this new science will require interdisciplinary collaborations between epidemiologists and other computationally oriented academic disciplines (Levin et al., 1997). Indeed, some exciting developments have already appeared at these epidemiological/computational interfaces and are briefly reviewed here. They include harmonic decomposition, agent-based modeling, network modeling, and creation of digital organisms.

Harmonic Decomposition Analysis

The tempo, mode, and spatial distribution of an epidemic infectious disease are well understood to reflect external forcing events (e.g., weather or climate), host immune factors (e.g., herd immunity), microbial evolu-

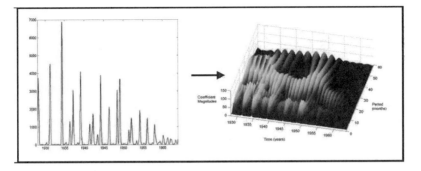

FIGURE E-1 Continuous wavelet transform decomposition of 1928–1964 Baltimore measles time series data showing that the incidence curve is decomposable into a shorter component with a periodicity of 12 months, and a longer component with a variable periodicity of 24–36 months. The longer component correlates closely with changes in birth rates.

tion, and population-level control efforts, as well as the complex dynamic interplay among these factors. Recently, new analytic techniques borrowed from physics, such as Fourier analysis and wavelet analysis, have permitted the decomposition of temporo-spatial epidemic harmonics (the aggregate signal) into modes, each of which may reflect only one of the underlying factors. For example, Fourier analysis has been used to decompose dengue and malaria data sets to reveal the weather-independence of interepidemic variability (Rogers et al., 2002; Hay et al., 2000). Of special interest is demonstration of the power of wavelet analysis to decompose measles epidemic harmonics to reveal recurrent spatial spreading patterns not evident in the undecomposed epidemic data. Such preliminary successes with decompositional techniques suggest they will make it possible to analyze and explain the dynamics of many infectious diseases (Grenfell et al., 2001; Strebel and Cochi, 2001).

Agent-Based Models

Agent-based computational models are computer programs in which a population of individual entities is created, and each individual is endowed with simple rules for interactions with the environment and with other individuals (Holland, 1995). Agents are typically programmed as two-dimensional entities that are distributed across a two-dimensional surface in proximity to other similar agents (but there is no inherent limit on this dimensionality). As the model runs, agents move over the surface and interact with each other. As has been generally observed in the field of complexity studies, remarkably complex behaviors can emerge at a group level from very simple rules governing interagent behaviors. Indeed, Wolfram (2002) suggested that one simple variety of agent-based computational models, termed cellular automata (immobile, identical, grid-based agents), can be used to model all manner of complex scientific phenomena. To date, agent-based models have been used primarily in social and economic modeling. Epstein and Axtell (1996) made an early seminal contribution, and, more recently, a full supplement of the *Proceedings of the National Academy of Sciences* was devoted to agent-based modeling in the social sciences (Bankes, 2002). A few promising studies have appeared in which agent-based modeling is used to examine infectious diseases (e.g., influenza) and the immune response (Hofmeyr and Forrest, 2000). The rapid rise in freely available computational power should permit the development of a wide variety of infectious disease agent-based simulations (Swarm Development Group website).

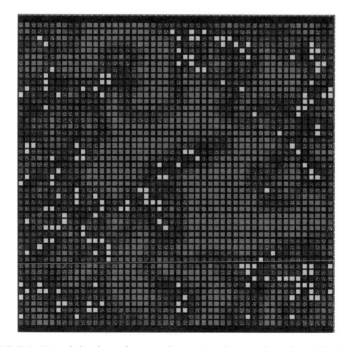

FIGURE E-2 Visual display of a two-dimensional agent-based model. Each square represents an individually programmable, mobile agent. Color-coding allows easy visual tracking of agents with different properties.

Network Models

Social networks have long been known to play a major role in determining the rate and pattern of epidemic spread of microbial diseases in human societies. Attention has focused in particular on the role of population heterogeneities and subnetworks in the spread of sexually transmitted diseases, especially HIV/AIDS; however, little work has been done on the role of network topology in the spread of other infectious diseases. More recently, physicists and computer scientists have become concerned about the spread of infectious agents (e.g., computer viruses, worms, etc.) through the Internet and the World Wide Web.

This welcome new interest in network topology has spawned a minor revolution in network modeling. It is now clear that many natural and human-made networks, from actors (the Kevin Bacon game) to the U.S. electrical power grid to the Internet, all follow a "scale-free" distribution (Barabasi, 2002). The observation that a wide variety of unplanned network topologies may follow a stereotyped pattern has led to research on how networks add nodes and grow (the "emergence" of networks); the factors involved are just beginning to be understood. Furthermore, the crucial role of occasional long-distance internodal connections in shortening global mean path lengths (the "small world" phenomenon) and accelerating epidemic spread has come to be appreciated (Watts, 1999). Recent

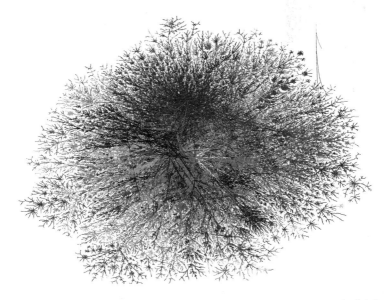

FIGURE E-3 Internet routing map (80,000 nodes). See http://www.cs.bell-labs.com/~ches/map/.

work on the tolerance of various abstract network topologies to errors or attacks has been convincingly modeled, and general strategies for improving network stability have been proposed. It appears clear that network models inspired by the Internet will productively inform the modeling of microbial pathogen networks (Albert et al., 2000; Pastor-Satorras and Vesignani, 2001; Lloyd and May, 2001).

Digital Microbes

Evolutionary principles have been widely incorporated into machine learning, artificial intelligence, and computer programming for decades. Indeed, in genetic algorithms—the first and now a standard evolutionary computation technique—code strings are iteratively mutated, recombined, and selected for fitness, just as if they were nucleic acid strings evolving in nature (Burke et al., 1998). Genetic algorithms are now widely employed by computer programmers to solve practical computationally intensive problems, such as protein folding, but only a few studies have appeared in which evolving code strings are used to simulate microbial evolution and adaptation. Preliminary studies suggest that the rules governing code string evolution may be independent of the stuff from which the evolving code strings are made, and that experiments on digital microbes—with code string evolution and epidemiology "in silicon"—may be a productive way to understand and solve problems that are difficult to study in nature (Ray, 1995; Wilke et al., Adami et al., 2000; Radman et al., 1999).

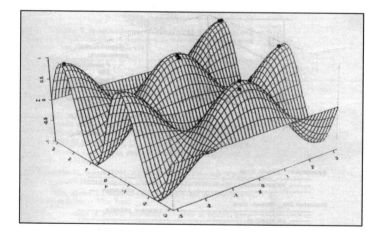

FIGURE E-4 Representation of evolving bit strings in a fitness landscape. In this example populations of strings are shown as dots colonizing local fitness optima in sequence space.

BIOTERRORISM MODELS

An immediate problem facing the United States is whether to reinstitute routine smallpox vaccination of the entire population. Rational alternatives would be to withhold routine vaccination, and use smallpox vaccine only in "ring immunization" of contacts once cases had appeared, or immediately preimmunize some subset of the population and be prepared to implement ring immunization. Critics of modeling argue that models cannot provide clear evidence for or against any option; advocates counter that the purpose of modeling and simulation is not to provide an answer, but to furnish a tool for improving the decision-making process. Indeed, all decisions are based on models (mental or otherwise), but the use of computational models forces all assumptions to be made explicit, and permits a search for nonlinear intervention effects that may not be discovered using intuitive mental models. Particularly in dealing with a hypothetical threat such as smallpox, models and simulations can allow the testing of intervention strategies in silicon that simply cannot be tested in advance, and could never be tested in a real-world bioterrorism emergency.

NEW NATIONAL INITIATIVE IN COMPUTATIONAL EPIDEMIOLOGY

The Center for Discrete Mathematics and Theoretic Computer Science, created by the National Science Foundation, recently established a five-year special focus on computational and mathematical epidemiology (Center for Discrete Mathematics and Theoretic Computer Science webpage, 2001). The objectives are to develop and strengthen collaborations and partnerships between mathematical scientists (mathematicians, computer scientists, operations researchers, statisticians) and biological scientists (biologists, epidemiologists, clinicians), and to identify and explore methods in mathematical science—especially discrete mathematics and algorithms, models, and concepts developed in the field of theoretic computer science—not yet widely used in studying epidemiological problems.

REFERENCES

Adami C, Ofria C, Collier TC. Evolution of biological complexity. Proc Natl Acad Sci 97: 4463–4468 (2000).

Albert R, Jeong H, Barabasi A-L. Error and attack tolerance of complex networks. Nature 406: 378–382 (2000).

Bankes SC. Agent-based modeling: A revolution? Proc Natl Acad Sci 99 (Suppl 3): 7199–7200 (2002).

Barabasi A-L. *Linked: The new science of networks.* (2002).

Burke DS, De Jong KA, Grefenstette JJ, Ramsey CL, Wu AS. Putting more genetics into genetic algorithms. Evol Comput 6: 387–410 (1998).

Center for Discrete Mathematics and Theoretical Computer Science. http://www.isd.atr.co.jp/~ray.pubs/tierra.

Dietz K, Heesterbeek JAP. Bernoulli was ahead of modern epidemiology. Nature 408: 513–514 (2000).

Epstein JM, Axtell RL. *Growing artificial societies. Social science from the bottom up.* MIT Press, Cambridge, MA (1996).

Grenfell BT, Bjornstad ON, Kappey J. Travelling waves and spatial hierarchies in measles epidemics. Nature 414: 716–723 (2001).

Hay SI Myers MF, Burke DS, et al. Etiology of interepidemic periods of mosquito-borne disease. Proc Natl Acad Sci 97: 9335–9339 (2000).

Hofmeyr SA, Forrest S. Architecture for an artificial immune system. Evol Comput 8: 443–473 (2000).

Holland JH. *Hidden order: How adaptation builds complexity.* Addison Wesley (1995).

Koopman JS. Emerging objectives and methods in epidemiology. Am J Public Health 86: 630–632 (1996).

Levin SA, Grenfell B, Hastings A, Perelson AS. Mathematical and computational challenges in population biology and ecosystems science. Science 275: 334–343 (1997).

Lilienfeld AM (Ed). *Aspects of the history of epidemiology: times, places, and persons.* Johns Hopkins University Press, Baltimore (1980).

Lloyd AL, May RM. Epidemiology: How viruses spread among computers and people. Science 292: 1316–1317 (2001).

Pastor-Satorras R, Vespignani A. Epidemic spreading in scale-free networks. Phys Rev Let 86: 3200–3203 (2001).

Radman R, Matic I, Taddei F. Evolution of evolvability. Ann N Y Acad Sci. 870: 146–155 (1999).

Ray TS. Evolution, ecology, and optimization of digital organisms. http://www.isd.atr.co.jp/ray/pubs/tierra. 1995.

Rogers D, Randoph S, Snow RW, Hay SI. Satellite imagery in the study and forecast of malaria. Nature 415: 710–715 (2002).

Serfling RE. Historical review of epidemic theory. Human Biology 24: 145–166 (1952).

Strebel PM, Cochi SL. Waving goodbye to measles. Nature 414: 695–696 (2001).

Susser M, Susser E. Choosing a future for epidemiology: I. Eras and paradigms. Am J Pub Health 86: 668–673 (1996a).

Susser M, Susser E. Choosing a future for epidemiology: II. From black box to Chinese boxes and eco-epidemiology. Am J Pub Health 86: 674–677 (1996b).

Swarm Development Group. http://www. swarm.org.

Watts D. *Small worlds. The dynamics of networks between order and randomness* (1999).

Wilke CO, Wang JL, Ofria C, Lenski RE, Adami C. Evolution of digital organisms at high mutation rates leads to survival of the flattest.

Wolfram S. *A new kind of science.* Wolfram Media (2002).

Appendix F

Committee and Staff Biographies

MARGARET A. HAMBURG, M.D. *(co-chair)*, is Vice President for Biological Programs, Nuclear Threat Initiative, Washington, D.C. Before taking on her current position, Dr. Hamburg was the Assistant Secretary for Planning and Evaluation, U.S. Department of Health and Human Services, serving as principal policy advisor to the Secretary of Health and Human Services. Prior to this, she served for almost six years as the Commissioner of Health for the City of New York. As chief health officer in the nation's largest city, Dr. Hamburg's many accomplishments included the design and implementation of an internationally recognized tuberculosis control program that produced dramatic declines in tuberculosis cases; the development of initiatives that raised childhood immunization rates to record levels; and the creation of the first public health bioterrorism preparedness program in the nation. She is a graduate of Harvard College and Harvard Medical School and completed her residency in Internal Medicine at the New York Hospital/Cornell University Medical Center. She currently serves on the Harvard College Board of Overseers. She has been elected to membership in the Institute of Medicine (IOM), the New York Academy of Medicine, the Council on Foreign Relations, and is a Fellow of the American Association of the Advancement of Science and the American College of Physicians.

JOSHUA LEDERBERG, PH.D. *(co-chair)*, is Professor emeritus of molecular genetics and informatics and Sackler Foundation Scholar at the Rockefeller University, New York. His lifelong research, for which he re-

343

ceived the Nobel Prize in 1958, has been in genetic structure and function in micro-organisms. He has a keen interest in international health and was co-chair of the previous Institute of Medicine study (1990–1992) on Emerging Infections. He has been a member of the National Academy of Sciences since 1957 and is a charter member of the Institute of Medicine.

BARRY J. BEATY, PH.D., is Professor of Microbiology, Immunology, and Pathology at Colorado State University. He is a University Distinguished Professor and founder and former Director of the Arthropod-borne and Infectious Diseases Laboratory, a center of excellence in training and research in vector-borne and zoonotic diseases. Dr. Beaty's research interests include arbovirology, vector biology, and the epidemiology and control of zoonotic diseases. He has published more than 200 scientific papers, with emphases on the genetic and molecular bases of vector-pathogen and rodent-pathogen interactions, molecular manipulation of mosquitoes, development of clinically relevant diagnostics, and investigations of novel approaches to predict and prevent zoonotic disease emergence. Dr. Beaty is a member of the National Academy of Sciences and the WHO Steering Committee on the Biology and Control of Vectors (Molecular Entomology), and is one of the Program Leaders of the MacArthur Foundation Network on the Biology of Parasite Vectors. He has numerous research and training activities ongoing in vector-borne disease endemic countries.

RUTH L. BERKELMAN, M.D., is the Rollins Professor and Director, Center for Public Health Preparedness and Research at the Rollins School of Public Health at Emory University. She came to Emory University in 2000 following 20 years with the Centers for Disease Control and Prevention, where she had served as an Assistant Surgeon General both in the position as Sr. Adviser to the Director, CDC, and as Deputy Director, National Center for Infectious Diseases. In the mid-1990s, she led CDC's efforts to address the threat of emerging infectious diseases. Her career began as an Epidemic Intelligence Service (EIS) Officer, and her expertise is primarily in infectious diseases and disease surveillance. Dr. Berkelman is board certified in pediatrics and internal medicine, and is a graduate of Harvard Medical School. She is active in the Infectious Diseases Society of America and the American Epidemiologic Society, and she currently serves on the Policy and Scientific Affairs Board of the American Society of Microbiology. She also consults with the Nuclear Threat Initiative on reduction of the threat of biologic weapons.

DONALD S. BURKE, M.D., is Professor of International Health and Epidemiology and Director of the Center for Immunization Research at the Johns Hopkins Bloomberg School of Public Health. Previously he served 23 years at the Walter Reed Army Institute of Research, including 6 years at the Armed Forces Research Institute of Medical Sciences in Bangkok, Thailand. His research focuses on the epidemiology and prevention of human epidemic virus diseases including HIV/AIDS, dengue, flavivirus encephalitis, and hepatitis. He is past President of the American Society of Tropical Medicine. He has served on the NRC Roundtable for the Development of Drugs and Vaccines Against AIDS, the NRC Committee on Climate, Ecology, Infectious Diseases, and Human Health (as Chairman), the IOM Committee to Review the Department of Defense Global Emerging Infections Surveillance and Response System, and currently serves on Board of the IOM Medical Follow-up Agency.

GAIL H. CASSELL, PH.D., is Vice President of Scientific Affairs and Distinguished Research Scholar in Infectious Diseases, Eli Lilly and Company, former Vice President, Infectious Diseases Research, Drug Discovery Research, and Clinical Investigation, at Eli Lilly & Company. Previously, she was the Charles H. McCauley Professor and (since 1987) Chair, Department of Microbiology, University of Alabama Schools of Medicine and Dentistry at Birmingham, a department that, under her leadership, has ranked first in research funding from the National Institutes of Health since 1989. She is a member of the Director's Advisory Committee of the National Centers for Disease Control and Prevention. Dr. Cassell is past President of the American Society for Microbiology, a former member of the National Institutes of Health Director's Advisory Committee, and a former member of the Advisory Council of the National Institute of Allergy and Infectious Diseases. She has also served as an advisor on infectious diseases and indirect costs of research to the White House Office on Science and Technology and was previously Chair of the Board of Scientific Counselors of the National Center for Infectious Diseases, Centers for Disease Control and Prevention. Dr. Cassell served 8 years on the Bacteriology-Mycology-II Study Section and served as its chair for 3 years. She serves on the editorial boards of several prestigious scientific journals and has authored more than 250 articles and book chapters. She has been intimately involved in the establishment of science policy and legislation related to biomedical research and public health. Dr. Cassell has received several national and international awards and an honorary degree for her research on infectious diseases.

JIM YONG KIM, M.D., PH.D., a physician–anthropologist, is a Founding Trustee of Partners in Health (PIH), a Harvard-affiliated non-profit organization that supports health projects in poor communities in Peru, Mexico, Guatemala, Haiti, Russia, and the United States. His main areas of expertise are infectious diseases and access to pharmaceuticals in poor populations and he chairs a WHO Working Group on multidrug-resistant tuberculosis. Dr. Kim also serves as Director of the Program in Infectious Disease and Social Change at Harvard Medical School and is Chief of the Division of Social Medicine and Health Inequalities at Brigham and Women's Hospital, Boston. He was lead editor of *Dying for Growth: Global Inequality and the Health of the Poor*, a volume that examines the socioeconomic forces that impact health outcomes of the poor throughout the world. He has recently edited, along with the WHO, *The Global Plan to Stop TB*, the first consensus business plan for the global TB control community.

KEITH P. KLUGMAN, MBBCH, PH.D., is Professor of International Health, the Rollins School of Public Health, and Professor of Medicine, Division of Infectious Diseases, at Emory University, Atlanta, Georgia. He is a Visiting Researcher at the Respiratory Diseases Branch of the Centers for Disease Control and Prevention. He is currently Director of the Respiratory and Meningeal Pathogens Research Unit of the Medical Research Council and the National Health Laboratory Service at the University of Witwatersrand in Johannesburg. Dr. Klugman has a Ph.D. in physiology and specialist qualifications from South Africa and the United Kingdom in pathology and microbiology. He is a Fellow of the Royal Society of South Africa, a member of the Wellcome Trust Tropical Diseases Interest Group, the Executive Committee of the International Society of Chemotherapy, the U.S. National Committee of the International Union of Microbiological Societies, and has authored more than 250 publications in peer-reviewed journals. He is internationally known for his research on antibiotic-resistant bacteria, opportunistic respiratory infections associated with HIV, and bacterial vaccines.

ADEL A.F. MAHMOUD. M.D., PH.D., is President of Merck Vaccines at Merck & Co., Inc. He formerly served Case Western Reserve University and University Hospitals of Cleveland as Chairman of Medicine and Physician-in-Chief from 1987 to 1998. Born in Cairo, Egypt, Dr. Mahmoud received his M.D. degree from the University of Cairo. He was selected a WHO fellow to study for the Ph.D. degree at the University of London, School of Hygiene and Tropical Medicine, which he was awarded in 1971. Dr. Mahmoud prepared the first specific anti-eosinophil serum, which was used to define the role of these cells in host resistance to helminthic infections. Dr. Mahmoud's work to examine the determinants of infection and disease in schistosomiasis and other infectious agents led to the development of innovative strategies to control those infections, which have been adopted by the World Health Organization as selective population chemotherapy. Dr. Mahmoud was elected to membership of the American Society for Clinical Investigation in 1978, the Association of American Physicians in 1980 and the Institute of Medicine of the National Academy of Sciences in 1987. Dr. Mahmoud is a fellow of the American College of Physicians, and a member of the Expert Advisory Panel on Parasitic Diseases of the World Health Organization. He is a past-President of the Central Society for Clinical Research and the International Society for Infectious Diseases. Dr. Mahmoud currently serves as Chair of the Forum on Emerging Infections and is a member of the Board on Global Health, both of the Institute of Medicine. He also chairs the U.S. delegation to the U.S.-Japan Cooperative Medical Sciences Program.

LINDA O. MEARNS, PH.D., is a Senior Scientist at the National Center for Atmospheric Research, Boulder, Colorado and Deputy Director of the Environmental and Societal Impacts Group (ESIG). She holds a Ph.D. in Geography/Climatology from UCLA. She has performed research and published in the areas of crop–climate interactions, climate change scenario formation, climate change impacts on agro-ecosystems, and analysis of climate variability and extreme climate events in both observations and climate models. She is a member of the IPCC Task Group on Scenarios for Climate Impact Assessment, and was co-convening Lead Author for the chapter on Climate Scenario Development in IPCC Working Group I for the IPCC Third Assessment Report (2001), and a Lead Author on two other chapters in Working Groups I and II: one on Regional Projections of Climatic Change and the other in WGII on Scenarios. She has just completed an integrated assessment project on the effects of changes in climate variability on crop production in the southeastern United States. Her current projects include an Integrated Assessment of Environmental Problems on the North Slope of Alaska, Climate Change Effects on Crops in the Yangtze River Area of China (funded by NASA), and Uncertainty in Datasets used for Agricultural Assessments (NSF-MMIA). She also served on the National Academy Panel on Climate, Ecosystems, Infectious Diseases, and Human Health, March 1999–June 2001. She also leads the NCAR Climate Impacts Assessment Science Initiative, which includes plans to form a climate/health research and educational program.

FREDERICK MURPHY, D.V.M., PH.D., is Dean-Emeritus and Professor in the School of Veterinary Medicine at the University of California Davis. Formerly, he was the director of the National Center for Infectious Diseases at CDC. He is recipient of the Presidential Rank Award and is a member of the German Academy of Natural Sciences. He has been a leader in viral pathogenesis, viral characterization, and taxonomy; his interests include public health policy, vaccine development, and new, emerging, and re-emerging diseases. Dr. Murphy is a member of the Institute of Medicine. He is co-chair on the Institute of Medicine Committee on Occupational Health and Safety in the Care and Use of Nonhuman Primates and is a member of the National Academy of Sciences Committee on International Security and Arms Control/Institute of Medicine Board on International Health, Committee for Russian/U. S. Collaborative Program for Research and Monitoring of Pathogens of Global Importance, and the Institute of Medicine Committee on Prion Diseases.

MICHAEL T. OSTERHOLM, Ph.D., M.P.H., is the Director of the Center for Infectious Disease Research and Policy (CIDRAP) at the University of Minnesota where he is also Professor, School of Public Health. Previously, Dr. Osterholm was the state epidemiologist and Chief of the Acute Disease Epidemiology Section for the Minnesota Department of Health. Following the September 11 terrorist attacks, Dr. Osterholm has served as an advisor to the U.S. Secretary of the Department of Health and Human Services (HHS) on issues related to bioterrorism and public health preparedness. He has received numerous research awards from the National Institute of Allergy and Infectious Diseases and the Centers for Disease Control and Prevention (CDC). He served as principal investigator for the CDC-sponsored Emerging Infections Program in Minnesota. He has published more that 240 articles and abstracts on various emerging infectious disease problems and is the author of the best selling book *Living Terrors: What America Needs to Know to Survive the Coming Bioterrorist Catastrophe*. He is past president of the Council of State and Territorial Epidemiologists. He serves on the National Academy of Sciences, Institute of Medicine Forum on Emerging Infections. He has also served on the IOM Committee on Food Safety, Production to Consumption, and as a reviewer for the IOM report on chemical and biological terrorism.

CLARENCE J. PETERS, M.D., is the John Sealy Distinguished University Chair in Tropical and Emerging Virology at the University of Texas Medical Branch in Galveston and is Director for Biodefense in the Center for Biodefense and Emerging Infectious Diseases at that institution. Before moving to Galveston in 2001, he worked in the field of infectious diseases for three decades with NIH, CDC, and the U.S. Army. He has been Chief of Special Pathogens Branch at the Centers for Disease Control in Atlanta, Georgia and previous to that, Chief of the Disease Assessment Division and Deputy Commander at USAMRIID. He was the head of the group that contained the outbreak of Ebola at Reston, Virginia and led the scientists who identified hantavirus pulmonary syndrome in the southwestern United States in 1993. He has worked on global epidemics of emerging zoonotic virus diseases including Bolivian hemorrhagic fever, Rift Valley fever, and Nipah virus. He received his M.D. from Johns Hopkins University and has more than 275 publications in the area of virology and viral immunology.

Dr. Peters is currently also a member of the National Academy of Sciences Committee on Research Standards and Practices to Prevent the Destructive Application of Biotechnology.

PATRICIA QUINLISK, M.D., M.P.H., is a medical epidemiologist practicing at the Iowa Department of Public Health where she functions as the Medical Director and the State Epidemiologist. Her background includes training as an clinical microbiologist (MT(ASCP)), training microbiologists while a Peace Corps Volunteer in Nepal, a Master's of Public Health from Johns Hopkins with a emphasis in infectious disease epidemiology, medical school at the University of Wisconsin, and training as an field epidemiologist in the Centers for Disease Control and Prevention's (CDC) Epidemic Intelligence Service. For the last ten years, she has conducted annual epidemiologic training courses in Europe, and teaches regularly at the University of Iowa, Des Moines University (Medicine and Health Sciences), Iowa State University, and other educational institutes around Iowa. She serves, or has served, on several national advisory committees including the National Vaccine Advisory Committee, the Sub-Committee for Vaccine Safety and Communication, the Advisory Committee of the U.S. Marine Corps Chemical/Biological Incident Response Force, the Department of Defense's Panel to Assess the Capabilities for Domestic Response to Terrorist Acts Involving Weapons of Mass Destruction (the Gilmore Commission), and as President of the Council of State and Territorial Epidemiologists (CSTE). In addition to the present committee, she is a member of the IOM Committee on the Psychological Consequences of Terrorism.

P. FREDERICK SPARLING, M.D., is the J. Herbert Bate Professor of Medicine, Microbiology and Immunology Emeritus at the University of North Carolina (UNC) at Chapel Hill and is Director of the North Carolina Sexually Transmitted Infections Research Center. Previously he served as Chair of the Department of Medicine and Chair of the Department of Microbiology and Immunology at UNC. He was President of the Infectious Disease Society of America in 1996–1997. He was also a member of the Institute of Medicine's Committee on Microbial Threats to Health (1991–1992). Dr. Sparling's laboratory research is in the molecular biology of bacterial outer membrane proteins involved in pathogenesis, with a major emphasis on gonococci and meningococci. He is pursuing the goal of a vaccine for gonorrhea. Dr. Sparling is an active committee member for the Forum on Emerging Infections.

ROBERT G. WEBSTER, PH.D., holds the Rose Marie Thomas Chair of Virology in the Department of Infectious Diseases at St. Jude Children's Research Hospital. He was admitted to the Royal Society of London in

1989, in recognition for his contribution to influenza virus research. In 1998 he was appointed to the National Academy of Sciences. In addition to his position at St. Jude, Dr. Webster is Director of the U.S. Collaborating Center of the World Health Organization dealing with the ecology of animal influenza viruses. Dr. Webster's interests include the structure and function of influenza virus proteins and the development of new vaccines and antivirals. His work extends from characterization of the natural history of influenza in wild birds to the emergence of influenza pandemics in humans and domestic animals.

MARK L. WILSON, SC.D., is currently Director of the Global Health Program and Associate Professor of Epidemiology at the University of Michigan, where his research and teaching cover the broad area of ecology and epidemiology of infectious diseases. After earning his doctoral degree from Harvard University in 1985, he worked at the Pasteur Institute in Dakar Senegal (1986–1990), was on the faculty at the Yale University School of Medicine (1991–1996), and then joined the University of Michigan. Dr. Wilson's research addresses the environmental determinants of zoonotic and arthropod-borne diseases, the evolution of vector–host–parasite systems, and the analysis of transmission dynamics. He is an author of more than 100 journal articles, book chapters and research reports, and has served on numerous governmental advisory groups concerned with environmental change and infectious disease epidemiology. He recently served as a member of the NRC Panel on Climate, Ecosystems, Infectious Diseases and Human Health.

MARY E. WILSON, M.D., is Associate Professor of Medicine at the Harvard Medical School and Associate Professor in the Department of Population and International Health at Harvard School of Public Health. She received an M.D. from the University of Wisconsin in 1971, and was chief of infectious diseases at Mount Auburn Hospital in Cambridge for more than 20 years. She co-edited the book *Disease in Evolution: Global Changes and Emergence of Infectious Diseases.* Dr. Wilson has long been interested in infections in travelers and immigrants, and has studied the role of migration and movement of materials in the appearance and expression of infectious diseases. Other interests include tuberculosis and use of vaccines, especially in travelers. She was recently a member of the Institute of Medicine Committee on Strategy for Minimizing the Impact of Naturally Occurring Infectious Diseases of Military Importance: Vaccine Issues in the U.S. Military.

STAFF BIOGRAPHIES

MARK S. SMOLINSKI, M.D., M.P.H., is Senior Program Officer at the Institute of Medicine and Study Director for *Microbial Threats to Health.* Mark received his medical degree from the University of Michigan, training in Internal Medicine at Oakwood Hospital in Dearborn, Michigan, and training in Preventive Medicine at the University of Arizona where he received his Master's in Public Health. He was a member of the investigation team during the hantavirus discovery in Southwestern United States. Mark was stationed as a CDC Epidemic Intelligence Officer in San Diego, and the principal public health investigator on an outbreak of pertussis among adults in a correctional facility, tetrodotoxin poisoning from puffer fish in California, and sexual behavior surveillance in the San Diego core STD prevalence areas. His experience includes epidemiologic field work in the Republic of Georgia. Most recently, Mark was the Luther Terry Fellow at the U.S. Department of Health and Human Services in the Office of Public Health and Science where he was a member of the Healthy People 2010 development team and had primary responsibility for *Healthy People 2010: Understanding and Improving Health,* which focuses on the Leading Health Indicators and a community health framework. Mark joined the Institute of Medicine in May 2001.

PATRICIA A. CUFF, M.S.,R.D., M.P.H., is Research Associate for the Institute of Medicine study on *Microbial Threats to Health.* She received an M.S. in Nutrition and an M.P.H. in Population and Family Health from Columbia University in 1995. Patricia has worked extensively in the field of HIV nutrition as a counselor, researcher, and lecturer on the topics of adult and pediatric HIV for 13 years. She has also participated in research projects of HIV-infected youths in Romania. Patricia joined the staff at the Institute of Medicine in April 2001.

KATHERINE A. OBERHOLTZER, is Project Assistant for the Institute of Medicine study on *Microbial Threats to Health.* Katherine received her B.S. in Integrated Science and Technology with a concentration in Biotechnology from James Madison University in 2000. She is currently pursuing her Professional Editing Certificate at the George Washington University. Katherine has worked as the Meeting Coordinator for the Maryland AIDS Education and Training Center of the Institute of Human Virology at the University of Maryland, Baltimore. Katherine joined the staff at the Institute of Medicine in December 2000.

Index

Z